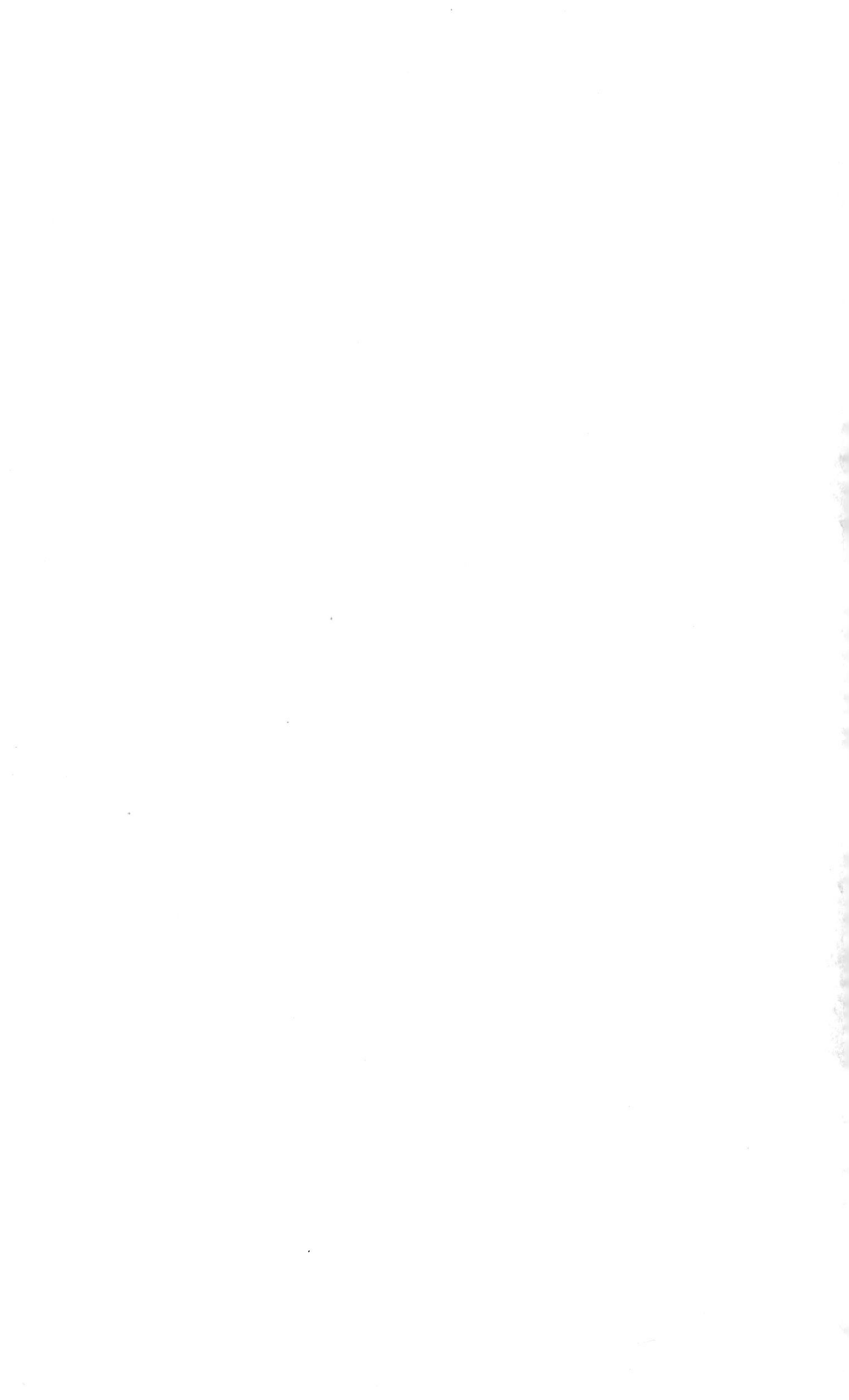

New Directions
in
HEALTH PSYCHOLOGY

New Directions *in* HEALTH PSYCHOLOGY

Edited by
**Ajit K. Dalal
Girishwar Misra**

$SAGE www.sagepublications.com
Los Angeles • London • New Delhi • Singapore • Washington DC

Copyright © Ajit K. Dalal and Girishwar Misra, 2012

All rights reserved. No part of this book may be reproduced or utilised in any form or by any means, electronic or mechanical, including photocopying, recording or by any information storage or retrieval system, without permission in writing from the publisher.

First published in 2012 by

SAGE Publications India Pvt Ltd
B1/I-1 Mohan Cooperative Industrial Area
Mathura Road, New Delhi 110 044, India
www.sagepub.in

SAGE Publications Inc
2455 Teller Road
Thousand Oaks, California 91320, USA

SAGE Publications Ltd
1 Oliver's Yard, 55 City Road
London EC1Y 1SP, United Kingdom

SAGE Publications Asia-Pacific Pte Ltd
33 Pekin Street
#02-01 Far East Square
Singapore 048763

Published by Vivek Mehra for SAGE Publications India Pvt Ltd, typeset in 10/12 Goudy Old Style by Star Compugraphics Private Limited, Delhi and printed at Chaman Enterprises, New Delhi.

Library of Congress Cataloging-in-Publication Data Available

ISBN: 978-81-321-0755-2 (HB)

The SAGE Team: Sharel Simon, Pranab Jyoti Sarma

Dedicated to

Anand C. Paranjpe, K. Ramakrishna Rao and
Rama C. Tripathi

Thank you for choosing a SAGE product! If you have any comment, observation or feedback, I would like to personally hear from you. Please write to me at contactceo@sagepub.in

—Vivek Mehra, Managing Director and CEO,
SAGE Publications India Pvt Ltd, New Delhi

Bulk Sales

SAGE India offers special discounts for purchase of books in bulk. We also make available special imprints and excerpts from our books on demand.

For orders and enquiries, write to us at

Marketing Department
SAGE Publications India Pvt Ltd
B1/I-1, Mohan Cooperative Industrial Area
Mathura Road, Post Bag 7
New Delhi 110044, India
E-mail us at marketing@sagepub.in

Get to know more about SAGE, be invited to SAGE events, get on our mailing list. Write today to marketing@sagepub.in

This book is also available as an e-book.

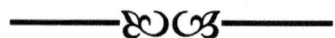

Contents

List of Tables and Figures ix
Preface xiii
Acknowledgements xvii

1. Psychology of Health and Well-being:
   Emergence and Development 1
   Ajit K. Dalal and Girishwar Misra

Part I
Conceptual Foundations

Introduction 49

2. Evolution of the Concept of Mental Health: From Mental
   Illness to Mental Health 57
   R. Srinivasa Murthy
3. Stress and Coping from Traditional Indian
   and Chinese Perspectives 77
   M.N. Palsane and David J. Lam
4. Concept of Psycho-social Well-being: Western and
   Indian Perspectives 95
   Durganand Sinha
5. Cultural Perspectives on Nature and Experience of Happiness 109
   Ashok K. Srivastava and Girishwar Misra

Part II
Social and Developmental Context of Health

Introduction 135

6. Puberty, Sexuality and Coping: An Analysis of the
   Experiences of Urban Adolescent Girls 141
   Namita Ranganathan

7 Mental Disorders in Women: Evidence from a
   Hospital-based Study   155
   U. Vindhya, A. Kiranmayi and V. Vijayalakshmi
8 Research on Families with Disabled Individuals:
   Review and Implications   179
   Lina Kashyap

Part III
Perspectives on Healing

Introduction   205

9 The Guru as Healer   211
   Sudhir Kakar
10 Working through Emotional Pain: A Narrative Study
   of Healing Process   232
   Jyoti Anand
11 Yoga and the State of Mind   249
   R.L. Kapur
12 Psychotherapy and Indian Thought   259
   Alok Pandey

Part IV
Overcoming Distress

Introduction   285

13 Anasakti and Health: An Empirical Study of *Anasakti*
   (Non-attachment)   289
   Namita Pande and Radha Krishna Naidu
14 Living with a Chronic Disease: Healing and Psychological
   Adjustment in Indian Society   304
   Ajit K. Dalal
15 Near-death Experience in South India: A Systematic
   Survey in Channapatna   318
   Satwant Pasricha
16 Resilience for Well-being: The Role of Experiential Learning   329
   Sweta Srivastava and Arvind Sinha

Part V
Challenges Ahead

	Introduction	353
17	Health Modernity: Concept and Correlates *Amar Kumar Singh*	357
18	Life Events Stress, Emotional Vital Signs and Hypertension *Sagar Sharma*	389
19	Perception of AIDS in Mumbai: A Study of Low Income Communities *Shalini Bharat*	409
20	Disaster and Trauma: Who Suffers and Who Recovers from Trauma, and How? *Damodar Suar*	429

About the Editors and Contributors	469
Index	476

List of Tables and Figures

TABLES

7.1	Diagnostic Categories of Mental Illness	162
7.2	Socio-demographic Profile of Women Patients	165
7.3	Distribution of Male and Female Patients	168
7.4	Prevalence of Common Mental Disorders in Male and Female Patients	171
13.1	Coefficients of Correlation between SSS, WSS, ADR, *Anasakti* and Strain	296
13.2	Means of SSS, WSS, ADR and Strain Scores of the Criterion Groups	297
13.3	Multiple Regression Analysis for Total Sample: *Anasakti*, WSS and ADR as Independent Variables, Strain as Dependent Variable	298
14.1	Rank Order of Causal and Recovery Beliefs as Reported by the Patients	310
14.2	Correlations of Causal Dimensions with Delay in Seeking Treatment and Perception of Hospital Environment	311
14.3	Affective Reactions of Hospital Patients	311
14.4	Correlation of Health Beliefs with Psychological Recovery/Adjustment Measures	312
14.5	Correlation of Psychological Recovery/Adjustment with Medical Recovery	313
15.1	Prevalence of Revival and NDE Cases in the Survey Villages	322
15.2	Main Features of NDE Cases	324
16A.1	Basic Statistics Pertaining to Time Point One	346
17.1	Dimensions and Themes of Modernity	369
17.2	Health Modernity Scale (HMS): Dimensions and Illustrative Items	370

17.3	Health Status and Its Correlates in India	376
17.4	Infant Mortality Differentials in India (1979)	381
18.1	Life Events Stress (Negative and Positive Impacts), Trait Anger, Modes of Anger Expression and Trait Anxiety in Hypertensives and Normotensives	395
18.2	Stepwise Discriminant Analysis with Respect to Patients with Hypertension vs. Normotensive Controls (N = 80 in each group)	396
20.1	Disasters from 1997–2006	432
20.2	Normal Traumatic Reactions to Disaster	439
20.3	Risk and Protective Factors of Trauma	451
20.4	Psychosocial Interventions at Various Phases of a Disaster	462

FIGURES

1.1	Domains of Health: Restoration, Maintenance and Growth	20
5.1	All Economic Growth Contributes to Well-being	116
5.2	Some Economic Growth is Neutral with Respect to Well-being	117
5.3	Some Economic Growth May Detract from Well-being	117
16.1	Initial Conceptual Schemes	336
16.2	Showing the Revised Model of Relationship among Variables Based on Obtained Results	345
17.1	Extent of Health Modernity	374
17.2	Extent of Health Modernity	375
20.1	Disaster Management Cycle	456

Preface

Dharmarth kama mokshanam arogyam mulamuttaman.
(Health is the key resource for the pursuit of duty, pursuit of wealth, fulfilment of desires and liberation.)

We are living in an age of unprecedented technological developments that are changing the contours of time and space; developments that configure our life-world beyond imagination. The developments have created comforts and helped amplify our capabilities to transform our notions of who we are and how our experiences are organized. The reigning ideology of modernity with its assumptions of individualism and materialism has nurtured a view of human being which establishes the physical self as the ultimate reality and consumerism as the pathway. The resulting lifestyle is sedentary, and increasingly more and more of physical and mental activities are being assigned to machines. This is leading to various lifestyle diseases like diabetes, coronary heart disease (CHD), obesity, stress and anxiety, hypertension, depression, and so on.

In the prevailing discourse, health is embedded within a reductionist framework in which the human body or physique is treated as the ultimate reality. This perspective fits well within the medical model which is the primary basis of health care and policy planning around the globe. It is, therefore, not surprising that health is held as the absence of bodily dysfunction or disease. It took years to recognize the positive side of health and build on the psycho-social knowledge to improve one's state of subjective well-being. Health is now seen in a broader sense encompassing prevention of disease, treatment, growth and rehabilitation and, above all, a wholesome existence.

Refreshingly, the Indian tradition lays considerable emphasis on positive health and has provisions not only for the cure and prevention of diseases but also to enhance health. The indigenous systems of Yoga, Ayurveda and various folk traditions have delineated a number of practices and interventions to augment health and well-being. Most of them are rooted in a broad-based ontological conceptualization in which a person is a composite entity consisting of body, mind and spirit. In this scheme, the state of health and well-being is dynamically located at the intersection of person and environment. That is why, Ayurveda and Yoga emphasize on *samatva* or balance between the inner and the outer (person and environment) which share common properties (i.e., *vata, pitta* and *kaf*). This is based on the view that life depends on the continuous interchange between the body and the environment.

In the Indian view, the entire world is supposed to be constituted by the same basic elements (*mahabhutas*). However, the specific constitutions of different individuals are quite diverse. Every human being has his or her own nature (*prakriti*) and temperament or inclination (*svabhava*). Thus, while everyone is constituted of the three primordial or basic attributes called the *Tri-Gunas*, i.e., *sattva, rajas* and *tamas*, they do differ in terms of the pattern of their relative salience. The unique pattern of behaviour exhibited by a person depends on the combination of these attributes. The lifestyle and (ill)healt-related behaviours and practices also function in relation to these attributes. The difficulties arise when there is a deviation from the balanced state, and therefore restoration of health and well-being requires steps to compensate for the imbalance. The remedies prescribed include (re)organization of diet, thought and action (*ahar, vichar* and *vyavahara*).

It is widely recognized that the modernist view is lopsided and the existential conditions necessarily demand attention to individuality as well as relatedness. The pursuit of well-being, however, is currently marred by the preoccupation with material pursuits and consumption. This perpetuates the chain of suffering and pain. The consumerist culture gives prominence to the accumulation of money and unmindful consumption of social and environmental resources in the service of the egoistic self. The feeling of agency and control over the environment becomes central and communion remains secondary and subservient to the egoistic self. This seems rewarding from a short-term perspective. However, the same becomes dangerous and painful when viewed from a long-term perspective. Environmental challenges like global warming and greenhouse effect clearly demonstrate the dreadful consequences of the short-term perspective of the limited self. Self-aggrandizement is becoming a curse, although we are blind to it. A relational and inclusive view of self recognizes the legitimacy of others and treats them as constitutive. The boundary of the self then becomes a bridge for communion and facilitates the welfare of everyone. In fact, the shift towards an inclusive self becomes a transcendental and spiritual journey.

The hallmark of the Indian perspective is inner-directedness and spirituality, which, however, has been wrongly and unfortunately labelled as other-worldly and, therefore, not considered veritable for growth and development at the physical–social plane. A holistic analysis suggests that it is otherwise. Self-transcendence extends the vision in a comprehensive and encompassing manner, in which there is space for everyone in a relational matrix. Complementarity and interdependence among all the elements become the organizing principles. It opposes greed and the tendency to accumulate, which is on the rise (as encouraged by the consumerist culture) and is rapidly destroying the social fabric and ecology in many parts of the world.

In psychology, the subfield of health and well-being is rapidly growing and has become one of the most popular areas of research and teaching. There is a burgeoning body of literature now to view health and well-being from a culturally informed perspective. In India there are a number of universities and institutions where health is being researched from the psychological perspective. Interest has also grown to explore the indigenous healing systems. The resources in the area of health and well-being, though mostly in journals and books, have largely remained inaccessible to Indian readers. There is an urgent need to make this resource material available to teachers, researchers, students and practitioners. This volume was planned to not only fill this gap but to enlarge the scope of academic deliberations by drawing attention to the diverse theoretical, methodological and applied engagements with health and well-being.

This volume is an outgrowth of personal experiences, as teachers and researchers, that the editors had in this field over the last two decades. The genesis of this volume also lies in the numerous interactions we had in formal and informal settings in seminars, discussions and classroom teaching. We had occasions to reflect on the issues as reviewers in the Indian Council for Social Science Research (ICSSR) surveys and journal articles. In the process of selecting articles for this volume, we have consulted a wide range of colleagues, and scanned published Indian work of the past two to three decades. Also, some articles were specially commissioned for this volume.

The chapters included in this volume are organized into five parts, dealing with the following themes: Conceptual Foundations, Social and Developmental Context of Health, Perspectives on Healing, Overcoming Distress and Challenges Ahead. The first chapter offers a general review of the field by the two editors of this volume. Each part has a general introduction which presents an overview of the field along with a brief exposition of the theme included in that section. The first part, 'Conceptual Foundations', comprises four chapters which introduce the field of health psychology to the reader. They relate to the conceptual, cultural and traditional perspectives on health and well-being. The second part, 'Social and Developmental Context of Health', includes chapters which deal with health issues pertaining to adolescence, women and disabled persons. These chapters are based on empirical work, considering the developmental and social aspects of health in different contexts. The chapters in the third part, 'Perspectives on Healing', take a holistic view of health from the indigenous and contemporary perspectives. Healing, in these chapters, has been discussed from the traditional psycho-spiritual perspective and its relevance for recovery from the diseased state as well as for realizing one's growth potential. In the fourth part, 'Overcoming Distress', the concern is to relate health and well-being with concepts like non-attachment and resilience, and also with illness conditions. This part presents Indian studies that have researched different psychological attributes which shape our responses to stressful situations and make us less or more vulnerable, leading to differential experiences of well-being. The last part, 'Challenges Ahead', includes chapters that bring up health and health-related issues in different life domains. These chapters deal with some of the emerging health-related concerns in recent times. The chapters included in this part pertain to the areas like attitude towards health, life events and stress symptoms, dealing with AIDS and natural disasters. Overall, these 20 chapters constitute a sample of important contributions which students, teachers and professionals may like to consult while engaging in courses in the area of health and well-being.

The preparation of the volume has been facilitated by the support of our colleagues, friends and students. The support of our immediate families was very crucial in the completion of this project, which went through several roadblocks and uncertainties at different stages. We are also grateful to all the authors and publishers who gave their consent to include their chapters in this volume. We hope that the volume will help understanding the issues of health and well-being in the Indian context and invite its readers for a critical engagement with the challenges faced by the society.

Ajit K. Dalal
Girishwar Misra

Acknowledgements

1. R. Srinivasa Murthi (1989). Evolution of the concept of mental health: From mental illness to mental health. In Mane (Ed.), *Mental health in India* (pp. 17-41). Mumbai: TISS Publications.
2. M.N. Palsane and David J. Lam (1996). Stress and coping from traditional Indian and Chinese perspectives. *Psychology and Developing Societies*, 8(1), 29-53.
3. Durganand Sinha (1990). Concept of psycho-social well-being: Western and Indian perspectives. *NIMHANS Journal*, 8(1), 1-11.
4. Namita Ranganathan (2003). Puberty, sexuality and coping: An analysis of the experiences of urban adolescent girls. *Psychological Studies*, 48(1), 56-63.
5. Jyoti Anand (2004). Working through emotional pain: A narrative study of healing process. *Psychological Studies*, 49(2-3), 185-102.
6. Lina Kashyap (1991). Research on families with disabled individuals: Review and implications. In TISS Unit for Family Studies (Ed.), *Research on families with problems in India: Issues and implications, Vol. 2* (pp. 269-98). Mumbai: Tata Institute of Social Sciences.
7. Sudhir Kakar (1991). The Guru as a healer. In Kakar, S. *The analysts and the mystic*. New Delhi: Penguin India.
8. R.L. Kapur (1994). Yoga and the state of mind. *Seminar*, 415, 30-34.
9. Ajit K Dalal (1999). Health beliefs and coping with chronic illness. In G. Misra (Ed.), *Psychological perspectives on stress and health* (pp. 100-125). New Delhi: Concept.
10. Satwant Pasricha (1992). Near-death experience in south Iindia: A systematic survey in Channapatna. *NIMHANS Journal*, 10(2), 111-18.
11. Sweta Srivastava and Arvind Sinha (2005). Resilience for well-being: The role of experiential learning. *Psychological Studies*, 50(1), 40-49.
12. Amar Kumar Singh (1984). Health modernity: Concept and correlates. *Social Change*, 14(3), 3-16.
13. Sagar Sharma (2003). Life events stress, emotional vital signs and hypertension. *Psychological Studies*, 48(3), 52-65.
16. Shalini Bharat (2000). Perception of AIDS in Mumbai: A study of low income communities. *Psychology and Developing Societies*, 12(1), 43-66.

NEW PAPERS

1. Psychology of Health and Well-being: Emergence and Development
   Ajit K. Dalal and Girishwar Misra
2. Cultural Perspectives on Nature and Experience of Happiness
   Ashok K. Srivastava and Girishwar Misra
3. Mental Disorders in Women: Evidence from a Hospital-based Study
   U. Vindhya, A. Kiranmayi and Vijayalakshmi
4. Psychotherapy and Indian Thought
   Alok Pandey
5. *Anasakti* and Health: An Empirical Study of *Anasakti* (Non-attachment)
   Namita Pande and Radha Krishna Naidu
6. Disaster and Trauma: Who Suffers and Who Recovers from Trauma, and How?
   Damodar Suar

1

Psychology of Health and Well-being: Emergence and Development

AJIT K. DALAL AND GIRISHWAR MISRA

> *The body and mind constitute the substrata of diseases and happiness (i.e., positive health). Balanced utilization (of time, mental faculties and objects of sense organs) is the cause of happiness.*
>
> —Charaka Samhita, 1: 1.55

INTRODUCTION

Health and well-being constitute one of the most relevant areas of contemporary psychological research and practice. With the increase in variety and complexity of health hazards in life, there is growing concern about the psychological factors that improve and impair the health status of a person. Health happens to be one of those few domains which illustrate the inherent unity of mind–body as the basis of academic discourse. Indeed, the concepts of health and well-being are so broad in scope that they cannot be confined to the narrow disciplinary boundaries. Its analysis, therefore, draws from many social as well as natural science disciplines, such as medicine, medical sociology and public health.

This chapter presents an overview of the historical development of health psychology as a psychological specialty and shares the substantive, conceptual, methodological and applied developments in this field, in general, and in the Indian context, in particular. It also offers an outline of the indigenous perspective from the stand point of Ayurveda and orients towards some of the contemporary and future concerns in the discipline.

THE BEGINNINGS OF HEALTH PSYCHOLOGY

Emergence of the field of health psychology has taken place in the context of realization that an understanding of biological mechanisms alone is insufficient to maintain or promote health. Interestingly enough, psychological stress has only recently been recognized in the modern medical circles as an important etiological factor underlying a wide range of diseases and disorders. The causal linkages between people's emotional state and illness, although known for ages, have just started receiving serious attention from the health researchers. For example, on the basis of available research, we now know that to understand and alleviate the physical pain, one has to examine the attitudes, expectations, beliefs and emotional support which the patient has, not just his or her response to the drug treatment. As Capra (1983) mentioned, it is quite ironic that physicians themselves are the ones who suffer most from the mechanistic view of health, ignoring the role of stressful life experiences. Their life expectancy is 10–15 years less than that of general population, with high rate of physical illness, drug abuse, suicide and other kinds of social pathology (see Nandy, 1988). In contrast, the psychosocial models of health posit that instead of viewing patients as mere passive recipients of certain treatment regimen, they should be considered as equal partners acting jointly in achieving the common goal of (better) health. Dalal and Ray (2005) have discussed at length the psycho-medical model of patient care as a more effective and viable alternative to the biomedical model.

The contention that psychological state influences the health of a human being has a long history in the traditions of Indian thought systems. The ancient Vedic texts have dealt with the issues of physical and mental health. They subscribed to an essential unity of the mind and the body, and proposed theories and practices to deal with a large number of health-related problems. For instance, the Atharvaveda and the Yajurveda provide ample descriptions of a variety of mental disorders, such as *vibheeti* (fear from nature, water, death, etc.), *Gandharva* and *Apsara* syndrome (referring to sex disorders, associated with a particular group), *moha* (attachment, eroticism), *unmad* (insanity), *grahi* (hysteria) and *vishada* (distress). The Atharvaveda has mentioned in detail the symptoms of these disorders and also about their remedial measures. These texts show the mental, physical and moral aberrations were closely linked to certain societal conditions (see Mondal, 1996). In the traditional medicinal system of India—Ayurveda (the science of life)—this has been a common practice to make psychological treatment integral to the entire treatment process.

In modern times, too, India had taken an early initiative to promote social science research in the field of health. The Bhore Committee Report (1946) that formed the basis of India's health policies clearly recognized the role of social and economic factors in the development of health services, particularly in promoting traditional practices and community participation to ensure primary health care. It is an irony that, in spite of rich heritage, India's health care system is primarily based on Western medicine. As will be discussed later, the Western system of medicine treats a person just as a body, ignoring his or her feelings, beliefs and cultural background.

In its short history, modern scientific psychology, until recently, has not shown much interest in physical health, which was considered a specialty of medical science. Psychological research was primarily concerned with mental health problems. Clinical psychologists restricted themselves to investigate the classification of mental illnesses and determining its etiology, and to diagnose and treat the afflicted patients. Another emphasis has been on examining the stressful life experiences and their psychological consequences. Clinical psychologists provided psychotherapeutic treatment to patients with all kinds of mental health problems. However, their role remained subsidiary to those of the psychiatrists. This clear demarcation between mental and physical health was consistent with the notion of mind–body dualism. Traditionally, clinical psychology did not deal with somatic problems. Its concepts, theories and methods are ill-equipped to understand the psychological aspects of physical health problems. This is how health psychology began to emerge as a field distinct from clinical psychology. The emerging discipline of health psychology got recognition at international level only in 1970s, and the first journal in the area of health psychology was started in 1982. Since then, health psychology has been one of the most rapidly growing fields of psychology.

In the last two decades, psychological factors have come to be identified as the major cause of a wide range of physical diseases and disabilities. For example, Type A Personality (a person showing the characteristics of being impatient, ambitious, impersonal, etc.) is considered to be a major risk factor in the coronary heart disease (CHD). Prolonged psychological stress is found to be responsible for hypertension, peptic ulcer and many other diseases. Again, psychological factors have been found important in the recovery from the physical ailments. The role of psychologists is now well-recognized in the treatment of organic diseases. Patient compliance, doctor-patient communication, attitude change, self-care, etc., are some of the potential areas to which health psychologists are making important contributions. The scope of health psychology is now encompassing the strategies for health promotion and making preventive health measures more effective. Psychological rehabilitation of patients with chronic diseases and disabilities is another field that is gaining popularity.

Prior to the emergence of the specialty of health psychology, the academic and professional concerns of this kind were dealt with in specialties like abnormal psychology, community psychology and clinical psychology. Out of these, the closest was clinical psychology. Health psychology's identity as a distinct discipline is a recent accomplishment. Whereas clinical psychology primarily deals with mental health problems: detection, prevention and psychotherapeutic treatment of mental diseases, including appraisal of mental health, health psychology outgrew from its parent discipline to deal with physical health and illnesses also. While clinical psychology dealt with the pathology of mind as their specialty, health psychology became chiefly concerned with the role of mind in shaping the health status of a person.

The field of health psychology grew with the realization and research evidence that psychological knowledge can make important contribution in the wide range of health-related domains, such as coping with stress, pain management, sleep disorders, healing of hospital patients, doctor-patient communication, patient compliance, self-care, etc. Again, the scope of health psychology is much broader than medical psychology that restricts itself to psychological factors in physical illnesses and does not cover the whole spectrum of health issues. The other similar development is that of behavioural medicine. Traditionally, this subspecialty evolved to apply learning theories to the field of health. It employed behaviour modification techniques for evaluation, prevention and treatment of diseases and disabilities. Today, the field of behavioural medicine has transcended its behaviourist origin and the term is interchangeably used with health psychology. Historically, health psychology has its roots in social psychological traditions and has applied this knowledge base in dealing with health-related issues. Consequently, the field is still dominated by social and cognitive psychologists. Nevertheless, it is presently one of the fastest growing branches of psychology.

THE CHANGING SCENARIO

The emerging discipline of health psychology is going through a metamorphosis in the recent years (Carpenter, 2001). In the past, the point of contact between psychology and health has often been seen in economic terms, i.e., how to save the cost of medical treatment (see Cummings, 1999). What kind of psychological treatment will cut down the cost of medical treatment? In this sense, psychology was seen as an ancillary discipline. As health psychology is growing a close, symbiotic interaction between the mind and the body is taking the centre stage. The contemporary view of healthy behaviour has outgrown the expressions we habitually use—outdated words, concepts and beliefs within the Descartean mould. Health is no longer considered a static condition; rather, it is seen in terms of challenges and opportunities. We must open ourselves to a dynamic view of health that acknowledges the implications of a new holistic paradigm of thinking emerging from body-mind research leading to a comprehensive understanding of healthy behavioural response.

Even 20 years back, the reference of spirituality was avoided in psychological research on health. Today the scenario is changing, and spirituality and religion are now considered important factors in causing the disease as well as in healing. In the Western behavioural science, spirituality is now ready to take the centre stage (Sloan and Bagiella, 2001). A special issue of the *American Psychologist* on 'Spirituality, Religion and Health', published in January 2003, is a clear evidence of the increased interest and research activities in this area. It is a genuine frontier of research, one in which psychologists have both much to offer and much to learn (Miller and Thoresen, 2003). This is a radical departure from the secular and non-spiritual orientation of mainstream Western psychology, having wider implications for the growth of health psychology.

As an emerging discipline in India, health psychology is still in its infancy. Though there are many exciting possibilities of research and application, there is lack of appropriate teaching programmes and research agenda in this field. In recent times, research in three fields has significantly contributed to the growth of health psychology in India. First is the research in the area of Yoga that has established close linkages between the mind and the body. A body of research (for example, Swami Rama, Ballentine and Swami Ajay, 1976) refers to relaxation and other mind-control techniques to alleviate physical suffering. Second is the stress research. The deleterious effects of stress on health have been systematically examined in a number of studies and its etiology in the occurrence of a large number of diseases has been uncovered. The research in this field has grown beyond the traditional stress models and the role of cultural and personality factors in moderating the adverse health-related effects of stress have been a major research preoccupation (see Misra, 1999; Pestonjee, 2002; Sharma, 1988). Third is the systematic exploration into the healing traditions of India. The traditional healers have developed many psychological techniques to alleviate suffering of the patients afflicted by various diseases (Kakar, 1982). Renewed interest in Ayurveda, the Indian system of medicine, which intricately interweaves both medicinal and healing aspects of the treatment, has brought forth the potential role of psychological factors.

There is a greater interest now in exploring the possible role that psychologists can play in improving the health status and recovery from illness or injury. As in other branches of psychology, most of the theories and concepts are borrowed from the Western research, and the conceptual richness of Indian tradition has not been explored. There are, however, a few sporadic attempts which bear many promises of emerging as new research trends. Some important research in the area of health psychology has been reviewed by Dalal (2001) in the Fourth Indian Council of Social Science Research (ICSSR) Survey of Research in Psychology. The most recent review of Indian research is by Sharma and Misra (2010). There are other attempts to review the growth of health psychology in India (Chandaram and Pellizzari, 2003; Misra and Varma, 1999; Singh, Yadav and Sharma, 2005). This review endeavours to present a panoramic perspective on the emergence of the field of health psychology in India.

As a hybrid psychological science of health, this new discipline is multi-disciplinary, multi-method and applied in nature. It concerns all, common men as well as the researchers and practitioners, whose primary concern is to improve the quality of health and well-being. This new discipline draws not only from the Western scientific tradition, but also from diverse sources from scriptures, literary work, folklores, life stories and ethnographic work. It practically touches almost all aspects of human life. In this background, any attempt to present a holistic view of health becomes a daunting task. The scope of this review chapter is limited to locating Indian works in the overall field of health psychology and exploring new research possibilities.

A WHO Definition of Health

The most acceptable definition of health is given by the World Health Organization: 'Health is the state of complete physical, mental and social well-being, and not merely an absence of disease or infirmity' (WHO, 1978).

The concept of health, as defined by WHO, is a significant departure from the medical model of health. It is a definition of positive health. It goes beyond the mere absence of a disease: the focus being on maintaining good health rather than on the treatment of different diseases. This definition views health as a multi-dimensional concept—the four dimensions and components of health being physical, mental, social and spiritual. The spiritual dimension of health was added much later in the WHO definition. The emphasis is on proper balance among the four components of health. This revised view recognized the various levels of existence in human life. A human being is not merely a physical body. We are also located in the social and moral space and consider spiritual living, too, as a genuine part of our existence. This view of health is more inclusive and non-body-centred. It goes well with the notion of human existence in terms of five sheaths (*koshas*). A related aspect is the emphasis on balance (*sama*) or equilibrium. Health is like a dynamic field in which different elements operate in communion and harmony.

Health thus refers to proper functioning of the body and the mind as well as the capacity to participate in social activities, performing the roles and abiding by the moral principles. It takes into consideration the nutritional status, immunity from diseases and better quality of social and family life. In fact, the concept of good health is considered as synonymous to the general well-being of a person. The concern is not with cure, i.e., treating and preventing organic malfunctioning, but with healing the person, i.e., regenerating a sense of well-being and fitness to deal with one's life conditions. Clearly, the emphasis in WHO definition is on the positive rather than on the negative side of health.

The WHO definition not only considers health as mere absence of disease but also emphasizes absence of infirmity, or physical and mental disability. It thus implies rehabilitation as an integral part of any health care programme. Being very comprehensive, it brings into the fold of health care not only the medical practitioners but also family members, community leaders and herbal and spiritual experts.

Health and Well-being

In the backdrop of the expanded definition of health, as discussed in the preceding section, oftentimes the terms health and well-being are used together, if not as synonyms. Health and well-being comprises people's evaluations, both affective and cognitive of their lives (Diener and Suh, 1997). It is an outcome of a complex interplay of biological, socio-cultural, psychological, economic and spiritual factors. Analyzing the discourse on health, Nandy (2000) calls for attending to the plurality of the notion of health and emphasizes on the need to bring to our psychological inquiry 'something of the sagacity, insights and cumulative wisdom of the people with whom we live' (p. 111). The conceptualization of the state of well-being is closer to the concept of mental health and happiness, life satisfaction and actualization of one's full potential. Verma and Verma (1989) have defined *general well-being* as the subjective feeling of contentment, happiness, satisfaction with life's experiences and of one's role in the world of work, sense of achievement, utility, belongingness and no distress, dissatisfaction or worry.

The *Taittiriya Upnishad* has elaborated that happiness, joy and well-being are the moments when there is an unobstructed manifestation of *ananda* (bliss), which is our original or true nature. It is the opaqueness of our mental faculties that obstruct the manifestation and experience of *ananda*. The principle that is responsible for opaqueness, inertia, dullness, darkness, depression, etc., is called *tamas*. The principle that is responsible for brightness, illumination, transparency, etc., is called *sattva*. Greater is the transparency of the mental faculties, i.e., *sattva*, greater is the experience of *ananda* (see Kiran Kumar, 2002). The Indian traditional perspective offers an ideal state of human functioning and constitutes health and well-being as a state of mind (somewhat equivalent to the concept of subjective well-being [SWB]) which is peaceful, quiet, serene and free from the conflicts and desires. The Indian notion of a healthy person is of an auto locus person (*swastha*) who flourishes on the recognition of life force derived from the material reality (*mahabhutas*) and, therefore, offers remedies for being healthy by opening a dialogue with its environment and recognition of order (*dharma*) in the entire life world (*sristi*). The nutrition (*ahar*), world of leisure (*vihar*) and thoughts (*vichar*) need to be synchronized in proper order. Health and well-being are both personal as well as social. The desire for the well-being of everyone (*kamaye duhkhtaptanam praninamartinshanam*) has been a core Indian concern that has pan-human relevance. Undoubtedly, such a conceptualization of health and well-being is significant in its own right (Sharma and Misra, 2010).

The Biomedical Model of Health Care

The biomedical model has governed the thinking of most of the health practitioners for the last one and half centuries in the West. It has now managed to attain worldwide acceptance and has been adopted as an official health care programme by almost all countries. India too is no exception where official health policies and programmes have primarily relied on the biomedical model. The vast network of hospitals, dispensaries, down to primary health centres (PHC) are manned by the professionals trained in the biomedical tradition.

The biomedical model considers disease as a form of biological malfunctioning, some kind of biochemical imbalance or neurophysiological disturbance. In this, the body is held as a machine that can be analysed in terms of parts, i.e., a system of synchronized organs. A disease is seen as impaired functioning of a biological mechanism and the doctor's role is to intervene, either physically or chemically, the malfunctioning of the specific body part (Capra, 1983). The model is based on the assumption of mind–body dualism in which psychological and social processes are considered independent of the disease process. Though the emotional state of the patient is considered important, it is kept outside the purview of medical treatment.

Historically, the biomedical model is a logical outgrowth of the philosophical and scientific developments in Europe in the age of enlightenment. It is consistent with the individualistic and capitalistic worldview of the post-industrial societies. The biomedical theory of disease grew around the conviction that most diseases are caused by invaders from the outside 'micro-organisms or germs'. The discovery of antibiotics in the 1930s and 1940s gave impetus to the modern medicine; the 'miracle drugs' seized public imagination. There were great hopes that medical science would eventually discover an effective drug therapy to eradicate every known disease; that there will be 'a pill for every ill'. This belief was so strong that even emotional and mental disorders were treated with various drugs, ignoring their psychogenic antecedents. The biomedical model of health care has not fulfilled the expectations it aroused. Adherence to this model has helped in reducing mortality by controlling prevalence of contagious diseases. The human lifespan is increasing all over the world, though the actual contribution of biomedicine towards this success is debated. Improved economic status, social hygiene and health consciousness have also made significant difference in this scenario. Moreover, though mortality is going down, an increasingly large population continues to suffer from various chronic and degenerative diseases.

Apart from the growing disillusionment, the biomedical model has serious limitations in terms of its adequacy for health practices. The model treats a patient as an organism, a biological entity. The proponents of this model were more interested in the disease than the patient. Thus, when the curative aspect is taken up, the emphasis is on the nature of diseases, its various symptoms and on the ways to remove them. In this process, the patient is only a recipient of certain medication and no cognizance is taken of the psychological state of the patient. Biomedical practices envisage no role for the patient and his or her support group in the process of diagnosis and in deciding about the course of treatment. The interest in the patient as a person is only incidental. As Siegel (1986) has rightly observed, '(Medical) practitioners still act as though disease catches people, rather than understanding that people catch disease by becoming susceptible to the germs of the illness to which we are constantly exposed' (p. 2).

Thus, most of the health schemes focus on providing better medical facilities rather than involving the patient towards a common goal of attending sickness. Quite often, medical practitioners learn from their personal experiences that diagnosis would be more accurate and treatment more effective if the patient's socio-economic and cultural background, beliefs, needs and anxieties are also taken into consideration. Nevertheless, it is presumed that the patient would be receptive, willing to supply all necessary information and would conform to the treatment regimen. This may be so, at the most, in case of hospitalized patients. In cases of chronic diseases, patients and their families do not always accept the passive role and frequently engage in their own, at times, 'in some secret forms of curing', depending on their appraisal of the disease and its future course (Engel, 1977). The biomedical model views the practices of faith and spiritual healing with scepticism, and with that, all the cultural traditions of managing health problems are shelved.

The biomedical model breaks down when it comes to the preventive health care, where there are no cooperative-captive patients, where people are under no compulsion to comply with the prescribed health procedures. People may even pay no heed when they are told about the adverse health consequences of some of their habits, like smoking. There may be differences in phenomenological meanings of illness and health. In brief, unless people are willing to cooperate, no preventive health care is possible or can be sustained.

STRESS AND HEALTH PARADIGM

In today's world where stress has become a very common experience, it is one of the most used and abused terms in the public discourse. In common usage, 'stress is pressure or the tension created by the pressure; it is unpleasant and undesirable'. A large number of symptoms in medical diagnoses are attributed to stress. Today, stress management has become a booming enterprise. The focus in this endeavour is both on environmental factors, called stressors, and on internal factors, the mental state of strain. In psychological research, the emphasis is more on the complex process by which people respond to the stressors that is perceived as challenge or threat.

Lazarus and Folkman (1984) have emphasized on appraisal of the stressors as a critical factor in stress experience. His three-stage model of appraisal: primary appraisal, secondary appraisal and reappraisal, suggests that coping efforts are primarily contingent on the mode of appraisals. To respond to any situation, first, it is to be interpreted as a potential threat, danger, challenge or impertinent. Second, one needs to evaluate the response choices. Of course, such evaluation will depend on the perception of the event itself. On the basis of this, a person makes coping choices and reappraises the stressors. This is a dynamic process and continues till the stressors cease to exist.

When people fail to handle their stress experiences, the mental and physical health problems start surfacing. People utilize different types of coping strategies. The two broad categories are: *problem-focused* and *emotion-focused*. While the former attends to the nature of the problem and its solution, the latter deals with engaging the self. Coping often depends on the availability of resources and perception of control. Researchers distinguish between primary and secondary control (Misra, 1994; Rothbaum, Weisz and Snyder, 1982). While primary control refers to person's control over the environmental factors, secondary control aims to bring changes in one's own self and involves the degree to which the person adapts to the environmental stresses. When the environmental stresses persist, people experience burn out. It may, however, be remembered that there are certain stresses that are positive in terms of their consequences. These are called U stresses.

Stress and Body's Immune System

There is increasing evidence that grief, depression and other negative feelings are linked with the increased risk of organic (like cancer) and infectious (like cold) diseases. For example, recent bereavement has been linked with the increased risk of a number of diseases, such as CHD, tuberculosis, allergies and peptic ulcers (Taylor, 2006). Stress-related negative emotions tend to suppress body's immune system over an extended time, rendering the person vulnerable to a host of diseases.

The immune system protects the body from the invading micro-organisms—bacteria, virus, fungi and parasites. These are called antigens. The immune system of the body, rather than being a centralized system, operates through a blood circulatory process throughout the body and gets activated wherever antigens are encountered. Called lymphocytes, there are special types of white blood cells, medically called as T-cells, B-cells and natural killer–cells (NK cells). These blood cells multiply, differentiate and mature in bone marrow, thymus, lymph nodes and spleen and in other body parts. The lymphocytes produce their own antigens to mobilize a direct attack to kill the invading foreign micro-organisms in the blood stream. Glasser (1976) pointed out that the immune system must be extraordinarily efficient in destroying the invading bacteria and viruses on an ongoing basis to keep us healthy. Even when they temporarily give in, they always keep the fight going on. It is only when the body's immune system is destroyed by a virus called Human Immunodeficiency Virus (HIV) that people become highly vulnerable to all kinds of infections.

In recent years, a new field of psychoneuroimmunology has emerged to examine the mediating role of psychological factors in immune deficiency. The body's immune system is presumed to be interacting with the central nervous system and endocrine system on one hand, and with psychological and social aspects of life on the other. Vaillant and Mukamal (2001) have discussed involuntary mental mechanisms that adaptively alter the inner and/or outer reality to minimize the level of stress. Many studies have demonstrated the linkages between stress and poor immunity. More chronic the stress, more severe is the damage caused to the immune system. Kiecolt-Glaser and others (1984) found that examination stress results in poorer immunocompetence, more so for the lonely students. Kiecolt-Glaser and others (1987) found that women who were recently separated had lower immunity than married women.

The effect of stress on the body's immune functioning is, however, mediated by a number of factors, including nature and severity of stressors. For example, the stressors which are uncontrollable produce more adverse effects than those which are controllable. Again, people who were more depressed were found to be more susceptible to infectious diseases and slower recovery rate. Schleifer and associates (1989; 1993) discovered on the basis of empirical work and meta-analysis that depression was associated with immunodepression, primarily among older and hospitalized patients. Also, a mild physical stress experienced in the recent past was sufficient enough to enhance immunity against the adverse effects of the present stress experience.

However, not much is still known about the possible physical mechanism through which psychosocial factors operate and play an important role. Several lines of work suggest that psychosocial stress alters the composition of brain chemicals, triggering chain reactions in the central nervous system and the hypothalamus which regulates the secretions of the endocrine system and increase the level of corticoid in the blood. The corticoid in the blood is presumed to damage lymphocytes and lower the efficiency of the immune system. Chronic stresses, negative emotions and lack of social support often silently block the breeding of NK-cells in the blood stream. These findings are, however, suggestive of the possible linkages and could be mediated by a large number of concomitant factors.

Stressful Life Events

Be it a failure in an examination or an interview, or the death of someone near and dear, all of us experience such tragic events in our lives and usually cope with them successfully. Of course, this is not true with everyone, every time. It is now well-established that the mortality rate is much higher among widows and widowers than among married persons of the same age. Studies have shown a sharp rise in mortality rate during the first six months of widowhood. The experience of death of a close relative or friend has been noted to be related to fatal heart attack (Taylor, 2006).

The pioneering work of Selye (1976) has suggested that stressful events lead to health impairing physiological changes and illness. People fall ill because of some kind of pressure their lives go through. Following Selye's work, stress was defined in medical science as a specific physiological condition, the *general adaptation syndrome*. This syndrome or physiological change is caused by a person's own adaptive response to the stresses experienced. This means that although the syndrome itself is specific (specific changes in bodily systems), the condition of stress it results in a generalized state of the person (Radley, 1994).

Stress works through the central nervous system. This means that the relationship of a stressor to the internal state is contingent on the meaning of that event for the person. Also, stress engenders changes to which a person must adapt. As change happens to be an essential aspect of life, it is hard to conceive of a state of stress which is qualitatively different from any other state of being alive. The experienced stress thus affects general health status by lowering immunity, rather than causing a specific disease. Despite intense research activity in this area, a clear relationship between stress and disease is yet to be established. Many factors mediate the responses to stressful conditions. As a result, there are important individual differences in responses to stress.

Though Selye did not test his model empirically, his work aroused much interest in this field. Holmes and Rahe (1967) developed a measure of overall stress due to life events. They tried to establish linkages between the level of stress and strain (physical, psychosomatic and mental illness). The Schedule of Recent Experiences developed by them is a self-administered questionnaire containing 43 life events to which subjects responded by checking those events that they have experienced in the recent past (six months to one year). The schedule was based on the rationale that life changes per se are stressful, regardless of their desirability. More than 300 such scales were developed since the publication of Holmes and Rahe's scale, but no clear-cut pattern of any relationship between life events and strain has emerged. Many scales developed later separately examined positive and negative events. A measure of negative events was found to be a better predictor of strain than just a change measure (Agarwal and Naidu, 1988).

One of the reasons for the lack of a linear relationship between life stressors and illness could be person's own appraisal orientation. Lazarus (1966) posits that a stressful life event can be appraised as potentially *harmful* (as with illness and injury) or *threatening* (to self-esteem) or *challenging* (offering opportunity for gain and growth). Such differential appraisal of the same stressor gives rise to different emotions and coping responses. When the appraisal of threat persists in the face of failure to cope with the stress, it leads to greater incidence of disease.

In view of a clear relationship between stressful life events and illness, many researchers have shifted their attention to the study of daily hassles (irritants) which seem to have cumulative effect on the occurrence of chronic diseases. Daily hassles are stable, repetitive and low intensity problems encountered in daily life. The impact of these low intensity stresses persists. Their affect on body systems is gradual, but in the long run it may be more damaging than the cataclysmic events. Noise, environmental pollution, job dissatisfaction and crowded neighbourhood are few examples of such daily hassles. As Baum and Valins (1977) argued, such stressors are more health-impairing when these cannot be avoided. People scoring high on life events and daily hassles were more prone to falling ill in the near future. A relative excess of daily irritants (hassles) over pleasant experiences is associated with an increased risk of hospitalization. High level of daily hassles was found to be a significant predictor of increased utilization of outpatient services. In the Indian context, Thakar and Misra (1999) have reported negative relationship between daily hassles and well-being among working women.

AYURVEDA: AN INDIGENOUS MODEL OF HEALTH AND WELL-BEING

> *An individual is an epitome of the universe, as all the material and spiritual phenomena of the universe are present in the individual, and all those present in the individual are also contained in the universe ... As soon as he realizes his identity with the entire universe, he is in possession of true knowledge which stands him in good stead in getting salvation.*
>
> —Charaka Samhita (4: 5.3,7)

Ayurveda, the ancient medical system of India, offers a different perspective on life and health in which wholeness, integration, freedom, connectivity, creativity and enjoyment figure as central concerns. The etymology of the word 'Ayurveda' summarizes its primary objective—A Science of Life and Longevity (*ayus* meaning 'life, vitality, health, longevity', and *veda* meaning 'science or knowledge'). Its main concern is to support and prolong healthful human life. The authorship of the most basic text of Ayurveda is attributed to Charaka, who essentially compiled the proceedings of a conference, known as the *Charaka Samhita*. Ayurvedic medicine was already well-developed by the time of Buddha. The famous Indian universities of that period, Nalanda and Taxshila, produced many great physicians.

Ayurvedic psychosomatics have taken a different, relatively untravelled road. Consistent with its thesis of the identity of mind and body, Ayurveda posits that any disturbance, physical or mental, manifests itself both in the somatic and in the psychic spheres, through the intermediary process of the vitiation of the 'humors'. Ayurvedic therapy aims at correcting the *doshas* or the imbalances and derangements of the bodily humours (namely, *vata* or bodily air, *pitta* or bile and *kapha* or phlegm) and restoring equilibrium. As Fields (2001: 52) has articulated:

Healing involves restoration of balanced states of being within the organism—that is, at the level of the doshas or constituent principles of the mind/body complex, and between organism and environment. Broadly conceived, equilibrium in Ayurveda means the stable and harmonious functioning of our organs and systems, psyche and spirit, but also, a balanced and creative relationship with our fellow creatures and nature as a whole.

It does so by coordinating all of the material, mental and spiritual resources of the whole person, recognizing that the essence of these potencies is the manifestation of cosmic forces. In principle, Ayurvedic therapy for all diseases cannot be other than a blend of the psychological and the physiological. In practice, the psychological part of the treatment rarely goes beyond suggestion, exhortation, consolation and a recommendation of meditative procedures. Even for diseases of primarily mental origins and with predominantly mental symptoms, it is overwhelmingly a psychological therapy for the psyche. There are three therapies with regard to their location of action: 'scientific' therapy, which uses proper diet, activities and remedies according to season and climate, at the level of the physical body; 'conquest of the mind', involving restraint of the mind from the desire for unwholesome objects; and 'divine' therapy, including all sorts of spiritual rituals and penance. Medical intervention at the physical level is of four types: diet, activity, purification and palliation (Svoboda, 1992).

Ayurveda is a principal architect of the Indian concepts of person and the body (Kakar, 1982). As a paradigm, it shows how body, mind and spirit interactions can be predicted, balanced and improved upon to enable people to live gracefully and harmoniously. For Ayurveda, spirit and matter, soul and body, although different, are not alien, insofar as they can be brought together in a healthy relationship with consequences that are mutually beneficial. Its prime concern is not with 'healing' in the narrow sense of curing illness, but in the broader sense of promoting health and well-being and prolonging life. The goal of this enhanced vitality is the achievement of all the values that life has to offer, both secular and religious. Healing therefore is no less than liberation. In Ayurveda, balance or equilibrium (*sama*) is synonymous with health. Also, the maintenance of equilibrium is health and, conversely, the disturbance of the equilibrium of tissue elements characterizes the state of disease. The person in Ayurveda is conceived of as simultaneously living in and partaking of different orders of being—physical, social and spiritual. Inclusion of spirituality as a fourth dimension, in addition to the three dimensions of physical, mental and social vitalizes the other three aspects. It may be noted that the boundaries between these levels are fluid as they are interconnected and complement each other. The recognition of similar composition of man and creation is a fundamental postulate of Ayurveda. How healthy a person is depends upon one's level of consciousness. Every thought changes one's physiology; one becomes precisely what one believes oneself to be. Healthy thoughts create health; dark, hopeless thoughts make one's body lose hope and surrender to disease. Medicine and religion differ only in their fields of activity; if the mind and spirit are at peace, the body too will be in the same state, but if one's field of consciousness is populated by conflict, frustration and distress, one's physiology will descend into disease. The principal word for health in Sanskrit, *svastha*, means 'established in oneself' or 'self abiding'. It is nothing but establishment in one's own essential nature. Incidentally, Patanjali also considers this state as the goal of Yoga. This seems to be appropriate for the holistic view of the human being as a unity incorporating psychophysical as well as spiritual dimensions. Material or bodily and spiritual, both kinds of concerns deserve our attention.

Ayurveda, as a pragmatic science, proscribes the ways to establish people in themselves. Ayurveda is steadfast in insisting that medicine should always be centred on the whole person (*rashi purusha*) rather than on the disease. The Ayurvedic approach may thus be understood as being 'holistic' in nature. This paradigm approaches disease from 'inside out'. The fundamental principle of holistic philosophy is that illness results when emotional, psychological or spiritual stresses become overwhelming and thus cause a weakening of the body. The body reflects or manifests the deeper struggles of the person's inner life. The holistic paradigm suggests that the 'energy' level of a human being, meaning the inner emotional and spiritual world, precedes, and in fact determines, all that is experienced at the physical level.

While delineating health, Ayurveda emphasizes on one's relationship with the environment, seasons and events within which one is situated. Depending on the incongruence/congruence between the person and the environment, anything can become health/disease-promoting. Thus, this view is decentred and non-dispositional in an important way. Ritu Satmya, for example, is the principle of adaptation that states that food should be according to the season (rainy, winter and hot). As Zimmerman (1987) has noted, the ideal is to accustom oneself to hit on the right choice of regimen, so that the nature of what is eaten is rendered appropriate to the nature of the one who eats it. Thus, it is a health-promoting adaptation. In addition to adaptation, Ayurveda also includes non-susceptibility as an important determinant of health. It is resistance to diseases, or immunity from diseases. It is reflected as vitality at the level of body that makes resistance to both biological illness and physical injury. At the psychological level, non-susceptibility is reflected in mental clarity and equilibrium from which one can respond from other person's behaviours and communications, and from within one's own psyche, without extreme reactions of suffering or behaviour damaging to self or others. It may be noted that *tamas* and *rajas gunas* are pathogenic factors affecting the mind. One, therefore, as *Bhagavadgita* recommends, must pursue towards the goal of being in the state of *sthitapragya*.

The normal functioning of a person, according to Charaka, includes the following criteria: alleviation of pain, normal voice, normal complexion, increased strength, appetite, proper digestion and nourishment of body, proper elimination of waste, proper sexual functioning, sufficient sleep at the proper time, absence of dreams indicating morbidity, happy awakening and unimpaired mind, intellect and sense organs (*Charaka Samhita*, 3: 8.89). Achieving these goals is the objective of therapy but it is pursued according to the type of constitution of a particular person. Thus, the particular combination of the three *doshas* is looked into. In fact, health and disease are relative to the state of *doshas*. As a result, the presence or absence of disease is coterminus with the state of equilibrium of *doshas*.

Also, body is considered to be an instrument in achieving higher goals and a person must look after it properly for the sake of these goals. The terms *sharira* and *deha* used for body indicate that it breaks and is a container or envelope, respectively. It has many connotations in various traditions. Ayurveda views body as the ground of well-being at material as well as spiritual levels. Zimmerman (1987) considers Ayurveda as an ecological theory and considers body as a place, and its condition depends on the factors like climate, season, diet and custom. The therapeutic intervention is therefore two fold, i.e., rendering the environment appropriate to the needs of the person and rendering patient's diet and regimen appropriate to the ecological conditions. Ayurvedic health care concentrates on all the three, i.e., body, mind and self (*sharira, manas, atman*) (see Misra, 2005).

Ayurveda views therapy as a sort of spiritual advancement through co-operation of physical and spiritual. Charaka calls human body as a vehicle of congruous junctions (*samyogavahi*). The physician has to orchestrate proper conjunctions, foods and medicinal substances, with the person's given constitution and the circumstances. A patient's visit to a healer is a pilgrimage, at the culmination of which comes the healing ritual performed by the doctor (guru), which helps remove one's 'sins', dietary and otherwise, from where one has stored them deep within oneself, so that the body's fire element cleanses oneself of them. Ayurveda favours gradual over sudden cure to protect one's vitality, which controls the immune system. The gradual elimination of addictions gives the system necessary time to acclimatize itself to living without a crutch.

The basic principles of Ayurvedic treatment are immutable; how they are applied differs from case to case. Treatment is supposed to be totally individualized, and so, different diseases may sometimes share a single therapy and a single disease may be treated differently in different patients according to the 'measure' of the factors involved. 'Treatment is rooted in measure': the effect any particular therapy has on any particular patient depends on its dosage, which depends upon the patient's constitutional type, the climate, the *doshas* involved, the strength of the patient versus the strength of the disease, the patient's age and constitution, the specific syndrome, the patient's social environment, the goal of treatment, the physician's preferred methods of treatment, etc. Time cycles, including 'disease time' and the 'joints' of the seasons, are especially important because the *doshas* are controlled differently at different times (Svoboda, 1992).

Ayurveda remains a living tradition, a way of living. For centuries Ayurveda has guided the lifestyle of people and has helped in organizing the practices of daily leaving, including food preferences, leisure activities and preventive and promotive health measures in India. The knowledge of Ayurvedic medicines has flown from guru to disciple. Though in reality, as many studies have shown, professionalized Ayurvedic doctors have become wholly body-oriented, unlike the traditional *vaidyas* who are still holistic in their orientation. But as Svoboda (1992) remarked, as long as Ayurveda remains a way of life, as a universal art of healing, it will always exist and pervade individual consciousness. By promoting the value of freedom from limitations and sufferings, it continues to show a solid and secure way of curing the psychophysical limitations including the limitations of human understanding. In the contemporary period, there is revival of interest in the Ayurvedic system of healing (see Chopra, 1990).

HEALTH AND WELL-BEING: A SCHEMATIC MODEL

In view of the preceding discussion, it is now possible to present a comprehensive model to incorporate the various facets of health and well-being and to schematically present the whole gamut of psychological conditions which are linked with health, as causes, concomitants and consequences.

In this schematic model presented in Figure 1.1, the field of health is presented as comprising of the three main domains, conceived as: *restoration, maintenance* and *growth* of life processes. The first domain is essentially the illness domain where the primary focus is on bringing the person back from the state of illness (incongruity/disjunction) to the state of health or re-establishing the congruence and conjunction. Here, health practically implies the process of recovery from the disease. Thus, it involves curative and healing interventions that can free the patient from the bodily suffering and pain. Patients, health practitioners, caregivers and hospitals are immediately concerned with this domain. Disability rehabilitation also falls within it.

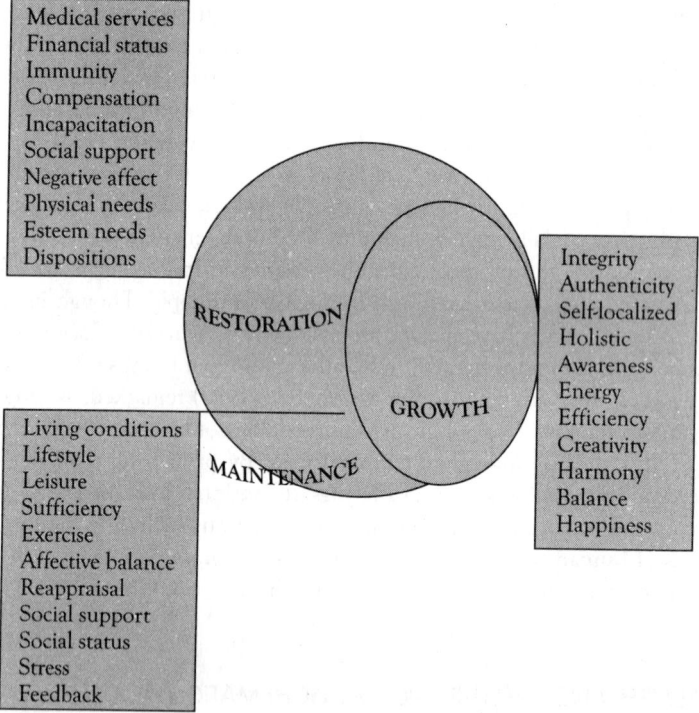

Figure 1.1: Domains of Health: Restoration, Maintenance and Growth

The second domain of health is that of maintenance, which until recently has been unattended by the masses. The major concern of this domain is to engage in the activities to maintain good health and protect oneself from diseases and disabilities. Health is not static or fixed. It is a dynamic process and one's present health status never guarantees that it will remain the same in future. People who primarily belong to this domain are agents of their health. They have to be motivated to act proactively to enhance their immunity or power of resistance to diseases, resilience, physical and mental vitality and active participation in family and communal lives. In other words, this domain involves the personal as well as social or relational space. On the one hand the person has to perform exercise, Yoga, work and take proper diet, on the other he or she has to be active in continuing and nourishing the social relations with family, co-workers and environment.

The third domain of health is growth-centred. It can be referred to as psycho-spiritual health. The person evolves and goes beyond the isolated and limited self. In this domain, health is seen from a much wider perspective in which it encompasses the total existence (physical, social and spiritual) of a person. The awareness or consciousness of a person is to be established in both the physical as well as moral or ethical spaces. The person strives to achieve a level of functioning that ensures effective personal functioning to further harmony with others. The blossoming of inherent potential takes place and with energy, creativity and efficiency the person maintains equilibrium. The journey with restoration from disease (*vyadhi*) moves towards the state of self-realization, equanimity and calmness leading to bliss often conceptualized in terms of *samadhi*.

It should be clear by now that there is a great deal of overlap and permeability in the three domains of health, though these are hierarchically organized. The salience of these domains in one's life space keeps on shifting (shrinking or expanding). The relative space occupied by the growth domain would determine the quality of health one has. Second, the antecedents and consequents are linearly arrayed in the case of restorative health, where the main interest is in identifying the factors which cause the disease and lead to recovery.

In the case of maintenance domain, the causality is bi-directional. In that, emotions, beliefs, expectations play a balancing role, and are both— the causes and the consequences. In the growth domain, an individual can create and control these psychological factors, so as to deploy them for performing efficiently. Third, the interaction of mind, body and self is a crucial condition in all the three domains. However, whereas in the restoration domain the emphasis is more on the mental states affecting the body condition, in the maintenance domain it is the harmonious relation between the two which is of prime importance; in the growth domain, the focus is on psychological factors and a harmonious relation among mind–body–soul (self).

PSYCHOLOGICAL FACTORS SHAPING HEALTH AND WELL-BEING

Psychological research in the area of health has gradually accumulated to provide overwhelming evidence to argue that the mental states do affect the physical health in substantial degree. A variety of psychological factors including personal dispositions, moods states, attitudes, beliefs, expectations and affective states are documented as both causes and concomitants of one's health and well-being.

Individual Dispositions and Temperament

Health psychologists have identified several personality dispositions having significant bearing on the health status of people. These dispositions predispose a person to a negative emotional state, such as depression, anxiety and nervousness, or lead to maladaptive coping behaviours. The experience of control and positive attitude has been found important in the success of surgery. Also, recovery of the surgical patients has been reported to be contingent on patient's emotional state prior to the surgery (see Cohen and Lazarus, 1979). Janis (1958) found a curvilinear relationship between anticipatory fear and post operative recovery.

The personality variable of Type A behaviour pattern is found to significantly contribute to the occurrence of CHD (Glass, 1976). A predominantly Type A person shows extreme competitiveness, a sense of urgency (always feels rushed or is impatient when delayed), excessive involvement in work, aggressiveness and hostility. People displaying this behaviour pattern seem to be engaged in chronic, ceaseless and unnecessary struggle with themselves, with others and with circumstances. In contrast, Type B behaviour pattern is characterized by a low level of competitiveness, time urgency and hostility. They are easygoing and philosophical.

In a study of eight-and-half-year follow-up of more than 5,000 people, Rosenman and others (1976) confirmed that Type A behaviour is strongly related to CHD incidence. The mortality from this disease was twice as high in Type A patients than in Type B patients. Their study revealed that those who exhibited competitive lifestyle were more likely to develop CHD even when biological risk factors (like smoking) were controlled. Their later work (Jenkins, 1976) indicated that different aspects of Type A behaviour were associated with myocardial infarction, angina pectoris and silent heart attack.

A similar search for a cancer-prone personality has not been as successful. There is some evidence that those who develop cancer are unable to express positive feelings, make an extensive use of repression and use ego defence less frequently (Bahnson, 1981). Longer survival rate among cancer patients was associated with more frequent expression of hostility and other negative feelings (Derogatis, Abeloff and Melisaratos, 1979; Pennebaker, 1990). Different personality patterns, known as Type C personality, are identified to be cancer-prone. Type C people are basically nice guys who never show anger and other negative reactions in public (Temoshok, 1987). They are helping, cooperative, smiling type, never hurting others, but at the same time never expressing their true feelings. These are lonely people, even shy of seeking help when need be. Derogatis et al. (1979) discovered that Type C people have four times higher risk of cancer than the others.

Along similar lines, Suzanne Kobasa proposed a new personality factor called hardiness to differentiate people who do and who do not get sick under prolonged stress (Kobasa, 1979). Hardiness includes three characteristics: (a) *personal control* – people's belief that they can influence events in their lives; (b) *commitment* – people's sense or purpose of involvement in events, activities and people in their lives; and (c) *challenge* – tendency to view changes as opportunities to growth rather than as threat to security. Hardy people are better able to deal with stressors and are less likely to fall sick. Kobasa (1979), in a study of highly stressful executives, found that those who fall sick scored low on hardiness scale. However, because of the correlational nature of most of these studies, it is not yet ruled out that it is illness which could be shaping hardiness.

Cognitive and Attitudinal Factors in Recovery

As stated by Lazarus and Folkman (1984), people construe a stressful life event in their own idiosyncratic ways. Many studies have focused on the manner in which people appraise the severity of life events, their causal explanations and ramifications. Some people are more negative in their subjective construction of an event, view the situation as uncontrollable and feel helpless and hopeless. Abramson, Seligman and Teasdale (1978) postulated a pessimistic explanatory style, characterized by internal (self), stable and global explanations of the negative events. The pessimistic explanatory style and depression have been found to be positively related. In a 35-year longitudinal study, Peterson, Seligman and Vaillant (1988) found that pessimistic explanatory style was not linked with poor health at the age of 25, but significantly predicted poor health above the age of 45 years. One explanation was that at a young age people have physical resources to absorb negativity, but these get depleted as their age advances. A prospective study of CHD and optimism found that 'a more optimistic explanatory style, or viewing the glass as half full, lowers the risk of CHD in older men' (Kubzansky, Sparrow, Vokonas and Kawachi, 2001) and discussed other research showing a link 'between pessimism, hopelessness and risk of heart disease' (Kubzansky et al., 2001). Agarwal and Dalal (1993) found that beliefs in the doctrine of *karma* and God, which give rise to hope, facilitated recovery from myocardial infarction.

Positive orientation or thinking about the crisis is another important cognition that has wide implications for recovery from any disease. Studies (Scheier and Carver, 1985; Scheier, Weintraub and Carver, 1986) have shown that optimism (generalized expectancy of good outcomes) is associated with problem-focused coping, seeking social support, seeing the positive side of the illness and acceptance of uncontrollable outcomes. Taylor (1983) observed that positive comparison was often used by cancer patients for self-enhancement in the event of an accident or illness. The patients who compared themselves with those who were in worse conditions recovered earlier. In a study by Agarwal, Dalal, Agrawal and Agrawal (1994), positive life orientation emerged as an important predictor of medical, as well as of psychological, recovery of myocardial patients.

Health Beliefs and Affective Reactions

A wide variety of reactions are observed when people are told about the diagnosis of a chronic illness. Quite often the initial reaction is that of denial or disbelief, which averts the onset of any emotional crisis. Denial also gives some time to adjust to the impinging reality. Other typical reactions are of high anxiety and emotional disturbance and clouded thinking. On the other hand, there are people who accept the diagnosis rather stoically. Chronic illness is something people have to live with and have to make long-term alterations in their lifestyle. There could be wide fluctuations in the mood of patients with changes in their physical condition and nature of disability. Pain and discomfort are other factors influencing the affective state. Many of these affective reactions may be transitory or of diffused kind, whereas other reactions are specific to the appraisal of the symptoms. Broadly speaking, affective reactions could be of two types: (a) general responses to the situation, like fear, sadness, unpleasantness, anxiety, etc.; and (b) belief dependent affective reactions. The affective reactions are often very specific reactions and are based on causal beliefs, perceived control and appraisal of the situation. They include anger, depression, disappointment, pity, etc.

Studies have been done to establish the linkages between affective reactions to an undesirable life condition and causal and control related beliefs. Causal appraisal gives rise to a qualitative distinction among the feelings. Weiner (1985) found that in the case of giving help, lack of effort on the part of the help-seeker aroused anger, whereas physical disability led to aroused feeling of pity. Dalal and Tripathi (1987) in a study of help-seeking behaviour found the linkages between control beliefs (situation controllable or uncontrollable) and affective reactions, stable and reversible. Some attribution-affect linkages found in their two experimental studies were uncontrollable sympathy, controllable anger and dislike.

The onset of a chronic illness and subsequent hospitalization result in more frequent arousal of the feelings of anxiety, depression, suppressed anger and helplessness (Westbrook and Viney, 1982). In an Indian study by Agarwal and Dalal (1993), the dominant affective reactions found in the hospitalized patients were helplessness, depression and metaphysical rationalization. There were some gender differences, the female patients showed greater degree of anger and anxiety, whereas male patients more often showed disengagement and rationalization. It was also noted that anger was the least frequent reaction. In a study by Kohli and Dalal (1998) on cancer patients, evidence of anger response was very low. They showed greater degree of acceptance and rationalization in terms of the theory of *karma*, where people look for justification in their own wrong-doings in the previous births. Higher attribution to metaphysical factors probably explains why Indian patients display low anger reaction.

It seems that the feeling which is more often expressed as a result of loss of control is that of helplessness. People show acute helplessness when they feel loss of control in a tragic situation. When all previously acquired skills fail to yield any desirable results and the patients start doubting their own ability to exercise any control, then the feeling of helplessness overtakes. Abramson, Seligman and Teasdale (1978) posited that the affective reaction depends on the causal attributions they make. If the cause is perceived as being permanent rather than temporary, then the feeling of helplessness will be long-lasting. If the cause is perceived as influencing many situations rather than just one, then the feeling of helplessness is likely to generalize to other situations. Finally, if the cause is perceived as being internal rather than external, the person is likely to suffer a loss of self esteem. As Wortman and Brehm (1975) argued, whether a person would experience anger or helplessness depends on his or her causal attributions.

The feeling which is reported most frequently in the people suffering from chronic illness is that of depression. Depression is characterized by a dejected mood, loss of desire to do things, general tiredness and inability to concentrate. The depressed person thinks that nothing can be done to change the undesirable life conditions. Like anger and helplessness, the feeling of depression sets in at a later stage of the chronic illness. During the initial phase of the illness, the patients may be too preoccupied with the diagnosis and the hospital procedure to feel depressed. The depressive responses surface at a later stage when the patient has tried much treatment unsuccessfully and now has to cope with a host of new problems related to adjustment in his day-to-day living. Many studies suggest that the emotional reaction of depression is beneficial in a sense that it is preparatory to later adjustments that must be made as a consequence of illness. However, acute or prolonged depression is certainly pathological.

Health Impairing Behaviours and Lifestyle Changes

In general, behavioural factors exert influence on health and illness of people in four ways: health enhancing, health impairing, health protective and illness management. Diet, exercise and meditation are health enhancing behaviours; tobacco chewing, alcoholism will come under health impairing behaviours. The examples of health protective behaviours are immunization, maintaining hygiene and pollution-free environment, whereas illness management refers to taking initiatives to recover from an impending illness. Here, we may focus more on the behaviours which have adverse consequences for health; directly or indirectly, they become causative factors in the onset of a disease.

Much of the Western literature in dealing with health-impairing behaviours has focused on smoking, obesity and to a lesser extent on alcoholism. What people eat and how much they weigh are considered behavioural processes which in concert with genetic and metabolic characteristics shape the health of a person (Baum and Posluszny, 1999). An unhealthy diet appears to directly enhance the risk of a disease, as low level of nutrition may contribute to pathophysiology of a disease, as tobacco chewing, smoking, drug use and alcohol consumption may have direct effects on bodily systems and impair their efficiency. In low income countries like India, under-nutrition and malnutrition become a major risk factor.

Consumption of tobacco in different forms is pervasive all over the world. Once tobacco use becomes a habit, it is highly resistant to change. The primary active ingredient in tobacco is nicotine, which has stimulant properties that increases Sympathetic Nervous System (SNS) arousal, alertness and reduces appetite. Smoking and other forms of tobacco use are major contributors to heart diseases, hypertension, stroke, cancer and other diseases. Passive exposure to tobacco smoke is also problematic and has similar effects as that of smoking. Consumption of tobacco in different forms is very common in India and has been found to be significantly associated with cancer.

Alcoholism, drugs and other narcotics are no lesser evil and are much more rampant than smoking. However, media and research exhibit more concern with smoking. In the case of alcoholism, it is suggested in many studies that it is not alcohol consumption per se which affects health but the pattern of drinking, rather, its abuse. Moderate level of drinking is considered to be good for health in many Western studies. Alcohol consumption becomes a health hazard when it is used as a mechanism for stress alleviation. Its association with social and moral aspects of behaviour often poses serious health problem at individual and family levels.

Stress is supposed to affect diet and weight in many ways. People who are under stress or in negative mood are often seen eating more. They seek, what is called 'comfort foods' or foods that make them feel better. Most of these foods are relatively high in fat and salt or sugar, meaning that stress may increase consumption of less healthy food. Such people gain weight and loose stamina to fight stress. In some cases, increased metabolic demand during stress may increase consumption of food without necessarily affecting weight. The growing craze for fast and junk food and synthetic drinks is becoming a serious health problem for the teenagers.

Whereas obesity and weight gain is a problem for a section of the society, a much larger section of the society which is below poverty line suffers from malnutrition. While good nutrition enables one to lead a socially and economically active life, malnutrition has an adverse impact on health and life expectancy, and increases mortality rate. It retards physical growth, leads to functional impairment, disability and diminished productivity and reduces resistance to disease. People who are most vulnerable to malnutrition are those below poverty line and the socially disadvantaged, infants, preschool children and pregnant women. The problem of malnutrition is a resultant of unavailability of food, low purchasing power of the people and population growth.

In poverty conditions, these are the women who are often more malnourished. Studies have shown that in India, diets of girl children and women are inadequate due to discriminatory practices. Women are discriminated in terms of both quantity and quality of the food available to them. The low dietary intake and maternal malnutrition is a major cause of low birth weight children. Malnutrition of the mothers again causes child mortality and mental retardation. Low status of women in the society and social practices are greatly responsible for this sorry state of affairs.

Exercise, on the contrary, is related to promoting positive health. Physical exercises play important role in managing weight, stress, as well as in keeping oneself physically and mentally fit. Although heavy exercises adversely affect health, moderate and regular exercises keep a person physically and mentally fit.

Two kinds of physical exercises essential for good health are stretching exercises, such as Yogic *asanas* and aerobic exercises, such as jogging, swimming and bicycling. These exercises produce different effects and are equally essential for a healthy living. Whereas stretching exercises have a calming effect, aerobic exercises increase arousal level of the body. Yogic *asanas* provide systematic stretching to all the muscles and joints of the body and massage the glands and other body organs. They relax muscles and decrease their activity level. Aerobic exercises have activating and stimulating functions—to energize heart, lungs and muscles. These exercises increase heart rate and breathing and reduce the cholesterol level.

COPING WITH CHRONIC DISEASES

The question of interest here is 'What do people go through while facing a disease which is of a chronic nature?' Research shows that the kind of psychological responses people make and the stages they go through depend on many factors. One is the nature of the disease itself. The onset of the disease could be sudden, as in the case of a heart attack, or gradual, in which case the patients get sufficient time to deal with the disease. The disease could be life threatening, as cancer, or may go through in acute-chronic cycle, as in asthma. It could be a physically disabling disease, requiring a lot of changes in one's life routine, like arthritis, or just demanding more care, like diabetes. Some diseases take a heavy toll on one's financial, social and psychological resources, some others are just a nuisance for the person. Again, the severity of the disease, their social background, support system and individual dispositions play a crucial role in determining the stages the patients go through in the process of coping with a chronic disease (Dalal, 2001).

In a large number of cases, the initial reaction to the diagnosis of chronic disease is that of shock and disbelief. People try to actively seek disconfirming evidence. It takes time to reconcile with the idea that they are suffering from a disease with which they have to live with for a long period of time, may be for the rest of their lives. They swing between hope and despair. The realization that their disease is of chronic nature may result in extreme mood swings, from depression to hostility. At a later stage, with psychological acceptance of chronic disease, people tend to seek more information about the disease, about the remedial and palliative aspects and its possible implications for their lives. They explore about their own role in containing and preventing the after-effects and integrating the disease within their own lives. People in their endeavour to live with the disease go through the cycles of stability, improvement, remission, relapse and renewed efforts.

How people live with chronic diseases is one of the most fascinating and challenging issue of research. The research evidence shows very little consistency in the findings. There are many reasons for this inconsistency. One, a bulk of research is from the medical perspective, where the emphasis is on the disease and not on the person. The effort is to understand the nature of the disease, to arrive at an accurate diagnosis and to plan out the treatment procedure. Patients' own perspective and their own perception and feelings are of little interest. Second, patients' own role in managing the disease is still the least explored. Like the attending doctor, the patient is also actively involved in understanding the disease and trying out various remedial measures.

Patients' own beliefs about illness play an important role in this venture. It is suggested in many studies that patients' own beliefs about their health and treatment regulate their health behaviour to a far greater extent than the doctors' beliefs or what the objective medical data suggest (Williams and Calnan, 1996). However, there are few longitudinal studies examining these aspects. Third, the role of cultural factors is relatively ignored in psychological research. Though there is substantial anthropological and sociological work to highlight cultural differences in health practices and treatment modalities, psychologists have yet to provide a comprehensive understanding of how these beliefs get translated into concrete action. Psychological research may fall into some pattern if cultural beliefs and their psychological imports are more systematically understood. To put it briefly, the research focusing on health beliefs shares some common understanding about the human nature. They are summarized as follows:

1. People are generally actively involved in understanding the meaning of their illness. This understanding is essential to prepare and appropriately respond to any health crisis.
2. People differ widely in the way they subjectively construct the experience of illness. Their beliefs about the illness and life in general provide the basic inputs for these subjective constructions.
3. The subjective constructions and representations of illness in terms of their meaning, causes and control influence their recovery (or adjustment) significantly, at times more significantly than the real nature of the disease.
4. People are motivated to make efforts to recover from the crisis situation. In fact, it is assumed that the efforts to recover begin with the onset of the chronic disease itself.
5. People are not only motivated but also possess a self curing mechanism. In the crisis situation, this mechanism gets activated and people on very rare occasions need institutional support to deal with the psychological crisis. People not only recover or successfully adjust but also learn to be more resourceful in facing a similar crisis in future.
6. People can be helped and trained to cope with the adversities by bringing appropriate changes in their own beliefs and attitudes.

Social Support System

The notion of social support in health psychology is conceptualized as including both social embeddedness and emotional support that informs the people suffering from diseases that they are valued and cared about (Cobb, 1976). Social support, either elicited or provided spontaneously, goes a long way in determining how people deal with the life challenges and threats. Supportive interactions and the presence of supportive relationships in people's lives have been shown to play a major role in emotional well-being and physical health. Mother Teresa said it best: 'Being unwanted is the worst disease that any human being can ever experience' (as quoted in Muggeridge, 1997, p. 17). Although supportive ties may create dilemmas for both the providers as well as the recipients of social support, belongingness to a reliable support system of kin and friends often reduces the risk of disease and enhances the recovery from mental and physical illness (Uchino, Uno and Holt-Lunstad, 1999).

Family as a support system has been specifically analyzed by S. Sharma (1999). There are two major mechanisms that explain how social support reduces the negative impact of stress on health and well being, i.e., *direct-effects hypothesis* and *buffering-effect hypothesis*. Moreover, the efficacy of social support is likely to be dependent on: (a) who is providing the support; (b) what kind of support is provided; (c) to whom is the support provided; (d) for what problem is the support provided; and (e) when and for how long is the support provided (see Sharma, 1999). Such issues are partly reflected in a recent study by Miltiades (2002) where the effect on the psychological well-being of India-based parents was examined whose adult children had migrated to the United States of America. It was seen that the availability of alternative support systems (the extended family support, the hired help) did not alleviate the feelings of 'loss', depression and loneliness in such parents. Thus, the appropriateness of a special kind of support seems to be dependent on the match between the type of support and the nature of problem encountered at a point in the life course, and also who is the provider of that support.

PROMOTING HEALTH AND WELL-BEING

Asian traditions focus on advanced stages of development and states of well-being, the Western systems provide details of psychopathology and early development (see Leslie, 1998). Integrating these two perspectives may enable us with a 'full spectrum' model of health which traces etiology, causes and treatment of illness (recovery) to maintenance of good health through various stages of growth and enlightenment.

The growth model focuses on realization of human potential for transcendent experiences and cultivation of wisdom that touches the higher levels of consciousness. In some way, the person works at the transpersonal level by recognizing continuity and interconnectedness of the living beings. The emphasis here is on higher order needs of the extended or inclusive self, which are more encompassing. The pain and suffering of such a person has no bounds as they are not personal. Such kind of enlightenment seeks the common ground and gazes at the issues for all beings (*prani*) and for everyone (*sarva*). Sharing and expanding the sense of self demands not only creativity but also a discipline of a very high order. The journey from fragmentation to integration or from self to self is very challenging but certainly capable of bringing unparallel joy and bliss. The vision celebrates the idea that 'I am everywhere and everyone is in me'. The differentiation is crossed in favour of integration. The person becomes more inward-looking, keen about transcending the vagaries of physical environment and bodily (physical) concerns and focusing more and more on self-growth. Wellness then becomes a virtue (Conrad, 1994). In fact, this aspect of health is a major contribution of Indian positive psychology.

Normally people are engaged in diverse social interactions and respond according to the specific demands. Their self-experience is often fragmented. The same person when engages in growth processes organizes his or her self and tries to rediscover the hidden potential. The person is empowered by recognizing his abilities to think act and feel in an integrated fashion. This often occurs while one encounters a guru or gets guidance from some elder or reading books or engaging with relevant discourses. The company of noble people (*satsangati*) who are enlightened or knowledgeable ones or experiential exposure to relevant events often plays a critical role in it, which works like a paradigm shift for the person. The life, the world and the modes of experience are positively transformed.

It may be noted that the self-transformation mentioned here is not merely an inward journey in which the person tries to escape from the reality. That does not characterize growth and evolution. Developing a reality orientation too is an integral part of that transformation. Such a person will have a more comprehensive appreciation of reality. He or she will be able to have a broader picture of reality. Such an informed view may help avoiding the trivialities that engage common people who limit their efforts and confine to short-term gains. A focus on growth inherently involves future orientation and going beyond the given. Such people display great resilience in the face of loss and trauma. Resilient people often display ability to maintain a stable equilibrium. They are found to respond to bereavement with lesser degree of grief (Bonanno, 2004).

Growth also involves vitality, thriving and a positive attitude. The recent developments in positive psychology clearly indicate that positive moods and feelings are not merely indicators of health rather than they contribute to it. They build and broaden the base for health. In other words, a person's happy or good mood not only exhibits his present health status but also leads to more happiness and positive health (Fredrickson, 2001). Increasingly many studies show the effects of optimism and hope towards a person's well-being and health. Unfortunately the focus of research has largely been preoccupied with the negative aspect (illness and pathology) and absence of disease has been treated as health. The studies on health, therefore, frequently use the measures that include the list of disorders and problems rather than positive aspects of health. It is in the case of quality of life and SWB that attention is paid to positive health.

Finally, the developments in positive psychology indicate that a growth orientation requires change in the lifestyle with a space for activities like meditation, Yoga and looking within. In today's stressful and tension ridden life, these efforts contribute to peace, happiness and well-being of the people. The self of contemporary man is saturated (Gergen, 1988; 1994), i.e., stuffed with too much information and opportunities. It is populated by myriad of things of all kinds—good, bad, trivial and meaningful. The market and media complicate the situation by drawing attention to the apparent achievements and attractions that disturb the equilibrium. It is, therefore, important to bring self-regulation and self-control in a relational world to the centre stage.

HEALTH SCENARIO IN INDIA

Health policies, programmes and practices mirror the culture, society and political scenario, and India is a good case in this regard. As mentioned earlier, Ayurveda remained the basis of daily living and treatment of diseases for ages. In addition, Siddha and Unani-Tibb have also been practiced. The Western notion of health and illness has not been the only way towards medical care (Khare, 1996). After the arrival of the British, Western medicine started dominating the scene and became the official health care programme of the country. After the political independence, there was a rapid expansion of health care infrastructure and medical institutions. India has the largest rural health care network in the world with 24,000 PHCs and 3,000 community health centres. In 1998, there were about 670,000 hospital beds for a 900,000,000 population. These investments have brought down the infant mortality rate to 85 and enhanced the life expectancy from 32 years in 1947 to 63 years in 2001.

In 1982 when the Government of India reformulated National Health Policy and adopted officially WHO declaration of 'Health for All by 2000', many significant changes were introduced at the policy level (Chatterjee, 1993). It brought forth the role of community and social sciences in promoting public health care. An apex committee of ICSSR and Indian Council of Medical Research (ICMR) was formed to bring changes in the curriculum of medical education and to bring in more input from social science research. Many of the changes in 1982 Health Policy and that in Alma Ata Declaration were already enunciated in the Bhore Committee Report way back in 1946. In-between years, the policy diverted towards high technology medicine, urban hospitals and colleges and disease-based planning. The New Health Policy was supposed to be a corrective devise to mould it in the direction of community-based services. Non-governmental Organizations (NGOs) were expected to play a major role in this endeavour.

In the context of these developments, creation of rural health infrastructure facilities became a major activity in the 1980s and a massive expansion of Sub-health Centres took place with emphasis on maternal and child care, family welfare and hygiene education. Each PHC was targeted to have one doctor and one community health officer (medical doctor, of course). This expansion was so rapid that the targets of developing infrastructure by 2000 were met in 1991 itself. In terms of manpower planning, a remarkable achievement was the training of 40 million Community Health Workers (CHWs) within five years (1977-1982), almost one CHW for each village in the country, constituting the largest health care cadre in the world (Chatterjee, 1993). These CHWs were trained by the medical doctors to take care of the common diseases and to function as links between the community and medical staff. This rapid expansion did compromise in quality in many ways. Nobody knew what kind of training these CHWs should be imparted and very soon these workers began to perceive themselves as village medical practitioners. Later on, Indian Medical Association opposed this scheme and termed these CHWs as quacks, who were indeed more popular than the medical doctors in many places. In 1981 when the Government of India transferred this scheme to the states, many states who did not commit to this scheme initially started backing out. Lack of availability of state fund made this scheme almost defunct, with CHWs demanding stipend for their work and often resorting to mass protest. These workers were rechristened as Multi-purpose Health Workers, and later as health guides. This most ambitious scheme of the government lost its direction and relevance in the present time.

In 1990s, a major shift in the policy took place in which the management of health was turned over to local self-government, namely, panchayati raj. Initially there was a lot of enthusiasm and hope that it will make health services more accountable to the local communities. But, like many other schemes, it also got mired in many controversies and rarely showed the desired results. Unfortunately, panchayats are not true representatives of the people but are dominated by the power elite and power brokers who cater only to their wasted interest. In the feudal system, which still prevails in rural India, decentralization and bottom up approach rarely succeeds. It is anachronistic to the present ethos and functioning of the government.

Another major development was privatization of the medical education and treatment. The government opened up the health sector for the private enterprises in a hope that while they will cater to the better-off section of the society, the government will be able to concentrate on the health of the poor strata of the society. The pressure of international agencies, like WHO and World Bank, paved the way for this shift in policy. With the complete breakdown of government health care programme, health is now turning into a most lucrative industry. The brunt of this fallout is mostly experienced by the poor who have nowhere to go for treatment. On one hand, where Kerala has shown the way to successfully provide universal health care, the Bihar, Madhya Pradesh, Rajasthan and Uttar Pradesh (BIMARU) states have witnessed a total collapse (Baru, 2003). It is important to note that modern public health interventions are merely the manifestation of colonial gene which our health planners have inherited (Bagchi and Soman, 2005). The apathy of the colonial rulers is matched only by the shocking indifference of the Indian political leaders who paid scant attention to the quality of health care. Now in the present era, profits and markets are shaping the health services. Health is being considered as individual responsibility rather than a systemic service expected of the state.

SOME EMERGING ISSUES FOR RESEARCH

Health and well-being is still an emerging area in psychology and in spite of all promises and possibilities, the discipline has yet to mature as an independent enterprise in India. We have not been able to build on rich healing traditions and holistic curative practices. With the failure of Western medicine in managing morbidity, there are intense efforts worldwide for the search of alternative health care systems and India has much to offer in this respect. In this context, some of the important themes of research in which potential of research, theory-building and applied work exists are briefly indicated.

Stress Research

Stress is still one of the most popular research topics in India. An overview of the body of existing literature suggests that research in this area had primarily followed the stress–strain (mental health) models and have tried to find efficient coping strategies in different demographic groups. The emphasis was on the measurement of life stresses, coping strategies and well-being and to establish linkages among them. The focus is now gradually shifting to the perception and experience of stress, long-term consequences of stress, personal control, coping strategies and their consequences for health. The Indian techniques of meditation and relaxation have much to contribute to stress alleviation programmes. Indian psychologists have yet to outgrow the narrow disciplinary boundaries and the limitations of their professional training to focus on the 'real' issues.

The research in this domain needs to focus on the positive consequences of experiencing stress and its potential for personal growth, resilience and enrichment. Also, the role of worldview is rarely taken into account. Seeking pleasure and avoiding pain is important but the possible image of a world totally free of pain and misery is something that has been rejected in the Indian thought. The image of world has been more realistic by recognizing its limitations and the goals of pleasure have been moderated accordingly. To be happy in a world which is in flux, one needs to bring changes within also when caught in stress and illness. Perhaps the happiness and well-being despite the adversity is possible only with a different kind of reality perspective that has space for pain and misery too. This does not mean to view life pessimistically. Instead, it creates a realistic vision that has positive contribution to the quality of life.

Healing Practices

The traditional healing systems in India still constitute an uncharted area of research. The pioneering work of Neki (1973), Kakar (1982), Joshi (1988; 2000), etc., have laid a good foundation for this stream of work to build on. We still need to know how traditional healing works, how culture, mind and body transact as a complex system, not only to heal the person but also to facilitate personal and social well-being and happiness. Indian texts have rich source material to understand suffering and healing as psychological states. Many of them are in practice. However, the Indian researchers have been less innovative and somewhat reluctant to address substantive issues. For instance, spirituality is one such issue which has not been attended to. The rich array of concepts, theories and practices available in the Indian tradition has remained unexplored. Yoga uses body to transcend it. Yoga as a therapy involves physical practice as well as a way of cultivation of consciousness. It treats liberation as healing. *Tantra, mantra* and music are also used for therapeutic practices. The Indian perspective does not dichotomize the material and spiritual. As Crawford (1989) maintains, 'for ayurveda, spirit and matter, soul and body, although different, are not alien, insofar as they can be brought in a healing relationship with consequences that are mutually beneficial'. The researchers, however, have not attended to the issues that emanate from this kind of indigenous view. The Tibbia, Siddha and other traditions of medicine too have also not been examined adequately to examine their contributions to health and well-being. Interestingly, these traditions seek remedies within the self and immediate environment and therefore are more accessible. However, owing to negligence and aversion, they are becoming obscure. In recent years, some impetus has been given to them but systematic efforts are very few (see Kapur and Mukundan, 2002 for children's health). As yet, there are not many studies to understand the underlying mechanisms and integrating them within the contemporary scientific research.

Efficacy of Psychological Interventions

Studying the efficacy of psychological interventions is another promising area of research in which there are many possibilities. Health psychologists need to work in unison with health practitioners of both traditional and medical variety. Such intervention studies are the need of the hour. A call for the 'Health For All by 2000' and its aftermath have brought many shifts in the research agenda in the field of social sciences, in general, and health psychology, in particular. One, the impressive achievements in the health sector has brought down the mortality significantly but at the same time increased the instances of morbidity. Though we know a good deal about the causes and cases of mortality, psychosocial and cultural dimensions of morbidity conditions are not much researched into. This area needs much attention by the social scientists.

Enhancing the Health Status

There is a realization among the researchers, practitioners and policy-makers in the health sector that health status has complex linkages with poverty, deprivation, population growth and education. No direct relationship between poverty and health was found in several studies. This calls for a more interdisciplinary approach in research to find ways to improve health status of the people. Health research needs to come out of the narrow disciplinary groves and has to accept the more challenging task of helping people improve their physical and mental health. Research in this area has to be futuristic, i.e., to assess the health requirements of the burgeoning population and the role of technology in providing health care. Community-oriented health services are going to be a major research area for the social scientists in the years to come. The health policies and planning has to involve people, voluntary organizations, activists and social scientists, not just medical professionals. Encouraging community participation and linking health with the wider developmental issues has to get reflected in the research agenda. To this end, health communication is going to play a key role. We need research in this area.

Mapping the Meaning of Health and Illness

In this context it may be mentioned here that the meaning of health and illness are culturally derived. How do people understand that they are sick? What do they do to recover ad stay healthy? What happens when people have to live with a long-term illness? How do the prevailing cultural beliefs about how to stay well affect people in their everyday activities? These questions are of prime importance when we want to understand health behaviour of people. Patient-centred care is emerging as a key concept in modern medicine also. This makes a stronger case for employing social constructivist approach (Gergen, 2001) in health research. From this position, illness is a process of an ongoing interaction between culture and people. From this perspective, medical view is just one among many constructions. There are other promises of developing people-centred health care programmes. Accordingly, a health practitioner or a healer has to be something more than an expert in the field but has to be sensitive to the way people construe health and illness. Research in this area is sadly lacking. Finally, as Nandy (2000: 111) has succinctly put it:

> The concept of health does not emerge only from textbooks, it is also scattered all around us in various disguises and is waiting to be discovered by us.

We must have the intellectual modesty and alertness to pick up these concepts to enrich and pluralize our idea of health.

We need to attend to the cultural and sub-cultural variations in the notions of health, illness and well-being.

Rethinking Well-being

Well-being is one of the cherished goals of humanity. It refers to the state of optimal psychological functioning and experience and defines the idea of 'good life'. As has been mentioned earlier, well-being or SWB is people's chief concern in life. SWB is defined in many ways. While liberation (*moksha*) from suffering was considered the summum bonum of life by the ancient Indians, Amartya Sen (1999) notes that freedom is a more rational goal for development than gross national product. He found that in cultures where relative freedom has expanded, both quality of life and economic growth have taken place. In large part, the past research in psychology concerned itself with psychopathology. It is under the positive psychology movement that attention is now being paid to well-being and the issues of empathy, love, wisdom, gratitude, resilience and authenticity (see Snyder and Lopez, 2002). It is found that material security and luxury alone are not sufficient for experiencing well-being as many poor countries score high on the measure of happiness. In fact, viewing well-being in terms of pleasure or happiness is one perspective only. There is another perspective that emphasizes on actualization of human potential or one's true nature. The former presents the *hedonic* view while the latter reflects *eudaimonic* view (Ryan and Deci, 2001). The relationship of personal wellness and collective well-being also needs to be investigated. The social well-being as a positive state associated with optimal functioning within one's social network and community (Keyes, 1988) incorporates social integration, social contribution, social coherence, social actualization and social acceptance. The relationship of well-being with a host of variables such as self-esteem, emotion, physical health, social class, wealth, attachment and relatedness are being investigated. In Indian thought, two kinds of pleasures are described: one is mere pleasure (*preyas*); the other is those pleasures which are good or desirable (*shreyas*). Recently, attention is being paid to happiness. Seligman's (2002) *Authentic Happiness* and the idea of signature strengths—the personal traits associated with various virtues—are interesting proposals (see Peterson and Seligman, 2001). On the whole, the domain of well-being requires serious research attention.

Culture and Health

Health psychology also needs to attend the cultural complexity of the contemporary world. The Western perspective as universal is problematic. As Lewis-Fernandez and Kleineman (1994) have pointed out, understanding of health and pathology in the West has been bound to three culture-bound ideologies, namely, self is egocentric, mind–body dualism and culture as epiphenomenon. The cross-cultural, cultural psychological work and anthropological work have shown convincingly that these assumptions do not hold true in many Asian, Latin and African cultures. People do hold interdependent, relational and encompassing notions of self (Mascolo, Misra and Rapisardi, 2004), which go beyond the self-contained and autonomous conceptualization of self. The body–mind continuity and inter-relationship is also widely accepted and people consider and experience human suffering in an integrated somatopsychological mode: as simultaneous mind and body distress. They do not classify psychopathology as organic disorders which are experienced as psychological distress and psychological problems which are somatized (Lewis-Fernandez and Klineman, 1994). Also, the meanings and practices are often culturally specific and they play important role in shaping the experiences of distress and well-being. In this context, it is important to note that culture is not a static category or phenomenon. It is dynamic in nature and operates as a process. In a world where several cultures are clashing and synthesizing at the same time, health practices and beliefs are also subject to change and reconfiguration. Processes of globalization, migration and communication revolution are restructuring the world of experience. This scenario is posing new challenges and giving opportunities for health psychologists. It is through innovative research, teaching and training that the emerging issues in the area of health psychology can be scientifically dealt with.

References

Abramson, L. Y., Seligman, M. E. P. and Teasdale, J. (1978). Learned helplessness in humans: Critique and reformulation. *Journal of Abnormal Psychology*, 87, 49–74.

Agarwal, M. and Dalal, A. K. (1993). Beliefs about the world and recovery from myocardial infarction. *Journal of Social Psychology*, 133, 385–94.

Agarwal, M. and Naidu, R. K. (1988). Impact of desirable and undesirable life events on health. *Journal of Personality and Clinical Studies*, 4, 53–62.

Agrawal, M. Dalal, A. K., Agrawal, R. K. and Agrawal, D. K. (1994). Positive life orientation and psychological recovery of myocardial infraction patients. *Social Science and Medicine*, 38, 25-130.
Bagchi, A. K. and Soman, Krishna. (2005). *Maladies, preventives and curatives-debates in public health in India.* New Delhi: Tulika Books.
Bahnson, C. B. (1981). Stress and cancer: The state of the art. *Psychometrics*, 22, 207-20.
Baru, R. (2003). Privatization of health services. *Economic and Political Weekly*, 38(42), 4433-37.
Baum, A. and Valins, S. (1977). *Architecture and social behavior: Psychological studies of social density.* Hillsdale, NJ: Earlbaum.
Baum, A. and Posluszny, D. M. (1999). Health psychology: Mapping bio-behavioral contributions to health and illness. *Annual Review of Psychology*, 50, 137-63.
Bhore Committee Report. (1946). *Health survey and development committee.* New Delhi: Government of India.
Bonanno, G. A. (2004). Loss, trauma, and human resilience: Have we underestimated the human capacity to thrive after extremely aversive events?. *American Psychologist*, 59, 20-28.
Capra, F. (1983). *The turning point.* Glasgow: Flamingo.
Carpenter, S. (2001, November). Curriculum overhaul gives behavioral medicine a higher profile. *Monitor on Psychology*, 32, 78-79.
Chandaram, P. and Pellizzari, J. R. (2003). Health psychology: South Asian perspectives. In Shahe Kazarian and David R. Evans (Eds), *Handbook of cultural health psychology* (pp. 411-44). San Diego: Academic Press.
Charaka. (1962). *Charaksamhita* (K. N. Pandey and G. N. Chaturevedi Hindi translation). Varanasi: Chowkhambha Vidya Bhavan.
Chatterjee, M. (1993). Health for too many: India's experiments with truth. In J. Rohde, M. Chatterjee and D. Morley (Eds), *Reaching health for all* (pp. 342-77). New Delhi: Oxford University Press.
Chopra, Deepak. (1990). *Quantum healing: Exploring the frontiers of mind-body medicine.* New York: Bantam Books.
Cohen F. and Lazarus, R. S. (1979). Coping with the stresses of illness. In G. C. Stone, F. Cohen and N. E. Adler (Eds), *Health psychology: A handbook.* San Francisco: Jossey-Bass.
Cobb, S. (1976). Social support as a moderator of life stress. *Psychosomatic Medicine*, 38, 300-14.
Conrad, P. (1994). Wellness as virtue: Morality and the pursuit of health. *Culture, Medicine and Psychiatry*, 18, 385-401.
Crawford, S. Cromwell. (1989). Ayurveda: The science of long life in contemporary perspective. In Anees A. Sheikh and Katherina S. Sheikh (Eds), *Eastern and Western approaches to healing: Ancient wisdom and modern knowledge* (pp. 3-32). New York: John Wiley.
Cummings, N. A. (1999). Medical cost offset, meta-analysis, and implications for future research and practice. *Clinical Psychology: Science and Practice*, 6, 221-24.

Dalal, A. K. (2001). Health psychology. In J. Pandey (Ed.), *Psychology in India revisited, Vol. 1* (pp. 356-411). New Delhi: Sage.

Dalal, A. K. and Ray, Shubh (Eds). (2005). *Social dimensions of health*. Jaipur: Rawat.

Dalal, A. K. and Tripathi, M. (1987). When the help is denied: A study of attribution linked affective reactions. *International Journal of Psychology, 22*, 1-15.

Derogatis, L. R., Abeloff, M. and Melisaratos, N. (1979). Psychological coping mechanisms and survival time in metastatic breast cancer. *Journal of American Medical Association, 242*, 1504-08.

Derogatis, L. R., Abeloff, M. and Melisaratos, N. (1979). Psychological coping mechanisms and survival time in mentalistic breast cancer. *Journal of the American Medical Association, 242*, 1504-08.

Diener, E. and Suh, E. M. (1997). Measuring quality of life: Economic, social and subjective indicators. *Social Indicators Research, 40*, 189-216.

Engel, G. L. (1977). The need for a new medical model: A challenge for biomedicine. *Science, 196*, 129-36.

Fields, G. P. (2001). *Religious therapeutics: body and health in yoga, Ayurveda and tantra*. New York: State University of New York.

Fredrickson, B. L. (2001). The role of positive emotions in positive psychology: The broaden-and-build theory of positive emotions. *American Psychologist, 56*, 218-26.

Gergen, K. J. (1988). *The saturated self*. New York: Basic Books.

———. (1994). *Realities and relationships*. Cambridge Mass: Harvard University Press.

———. (2001). Psychological science in a post modern context. *American Psychologist*, 56(10), 803-13.

Glass, D. C. (1976). *Behavior patterns, stress and coronary disease*. Hillsdale, NJ: Earlbaum.

Glasser, W. (1976). *Positive addiction*. New York: Harper & Row.

Holmes, T. H. and Rahe, R. H. (1967). The social readjustment scale. *Journal of Psychosomatic Research, 11*, 213-18.

Janis, I. L. (1958). *Psychological stress*. New York: Wiley.

Jenkins, C. (1976). Recent evidence supporting psychologic and social risk factors for coronary disease. *New England Journal of Medicine, 294*, 987-94.

Joshi, P. C. (1988). Traditional medical system in the central Himalayas. *The Eastern Anthropologist, 41*, 77-86.

———. (2000). Relevance and utility of traditional medical systems (TMS) in the context of a Himalayan tribe. *Psychology and Developing Societies, 12*, 5-29.

Kakar, S. (1982). *Shamans, mystics and doctors*. New Delhi: Oxford University Press.

Kapur, Malvika and Mukundan, Healata. (2002). *Child care in ancient India from the perspectives of developmental psychology and pediatrics*. New Delhi: Sri Sad Guru Publications.

Keyes, C. L. (1988). Social well-being. *Social Psychology* Quarterly, 62, 121-40.

Khare, R. S. (1996). Dava, daktar and dua: Anthropology of practiced medicine in India. *Social Science and Medicine, 43*, 837-48.

Kiecolt-Glaser, J. K., Fisher, L. D., Ogrock, P., Stout, J. C., Speicher, C. E. and Glaser, R. (1987). Marital quality, marital disruption and immune function. *Psychosomatic Medicine*, 9, 13-34.

Kiecolt-Glaser, J. K., Garner, W., Speicher, C. E., Penn, G. M., Holliday, J. and Glaser, R. (1984). Psychosocial modifiers of immunocompetence in medical students. *Psychosomatic Medicine*, 46, 7-14.

Kobasa, S. C. (1979). Stressful life events, personality, and health: An inquiry into hardiness. *Journal of Personality and Social Psychology*, 37, 1-11.

Kohli, N. and Dalal, A. K. (1998). Culture as factor in causal understanding of illness: A study of cancer patients. *Psychology and Developing Societies*, 10, 115-29.

Kubzansky, L. D., Sparrow, D., Vokonas, P. and Kawachi, I. (2001). Is the glass half empty or half full? A prospective study of optimism and coronary heart disease in the normative aging study. *Psychosomatic Medicine*, 63, 910-16.

Kumar, K. (2002). An India conception of well-being. In J. Henry (Ed.), *European positive psychology proceedings* (pp. 124-35). Leicester, U.K.: British Psychological Society.

Lazarus, R. S. (1966). *Psychological stress and the coping process*. New York: McGraw Hill.

Lazarus, R. S. and Folkman, S. (1984). *Stress, appraisal and coping*. New York: Springer.

Leslie, Charles (1998). *Asian medical systems: A comparative study*. Varanasi Motilal Banarasidas.

Lewis-Fernandez, Roberto and Kleinman, Arthur. (1994). Culture, personality and psychopathology. *Journal of Abnormal Psychology*, 102, 67-71.

Mascolo, M. F., Misra, G. and Rapisardi, C. (2004). Individual and relational conceptions of self in India and the United States. In M. F. Mascolo and Jin Li (Eds), *Culture and developing selves: Beyond dichotomization* (pp. 9-26). *New Directions for child and adolescent development No. 104*. San Francisco: Jossey-Bass.

Miller, W. R. and Thoresen, C. E. (2003). Spirituality, religion, and health. *American Psychologist*, 58, 24-74. (Special section.)

Miltiades, H. B. (2002). The social and psychological effect of an adult child's emigration on nonimmigrant Asian Indian elderly parents. *Journal of Cross Cultural Gerontology*, 17, 33-55.

Misra, G. (1994). Psychology of control: Cross-cultural considerations. *Journal of Indian Psychology*, 17, 22-39.

—— (Ed.). (1999). *Psychological perspectives on stress and health*. New Delhi: Concept.

——. (2005). From disease to well-being: Perspectives from an indigenous tradition. In R. Singh, A. Yadava and N. R. Sharma (Eds). *Health Psychology* (pp. 281-94). New Delhi: Global Vision.

Misra, G. and Varma, S. (1999). Introduction: Concerns in the study of stress and health. In G. Misra (Ed.), *Psychological perspectives on stress and health* (pp. 25-38). New Delhi: Concept.

Mondal, P. (1996). Psychiatry in ancient India: Toward an alternative standpoint. *NIMHANS Journal*, 14(3), 166-99.

Muggeridge, M. (1997, September 9). In a 1968 BBC interview: 'Being unwanted is the worst disease'. *Daily Telegraph*, p. 17.

Nandy, A. (1988). *Science, hegemony and violence: A requiem for modernity*. New Delhi: Oxford University Press.

———. (2000). Towards a new vision of health psychology. *Psychological Studies*, 45, 110-13.

Neki, J. S. (1973). Guru-chela relationship: The possibility of a therapeutic paradigm. *American Journal of Orthopsychiatry*, 43, 755-66.

Pennebaker, J. W. (1990). *Opening up: Healing powers of confiding in others*. New York: Morrow.

Pestonjee, D. M. (2002). *Stress and coping*. New Delhi: Sage.

Peterson, C. and Seligman, M. (2001). *Values in action inventory of strengths (VIA-IS) Manual*. Department of Psychology, University of Pennsylvania.

Peterson, C., Seligman, M. E. P. and Vaillant, G. E. (1988). Pessimistic explanatory style in a risk factor for physical illness: A thirty-five year longitudinal study. *Journal of Personality and Social Psychology*, 55, 23-27.

Radley, A. (1994). *Making sense of an illness*. London: Sage.

Rosenman, R.H., Brand, R.J., Sholtz, R.I. and Friedman, M. (1976). Multivariate prediction of heart disease during 8.5 years follow up in the Western collaborative group study. *American Journal of Cardiology*, 37, 903-10.

Rothbaum, F., Weisz, J. R. and Snyder, S. S. (1982). Changing the world and changing the self: A two process model of perceived control. *Journal of Personality and Social Psychology*, 42, 5-37.

Ryan, R. M. and Deci, E. L. (2001). On happiness and human potentials: A review of research on hedonic and eudiamonic well-being. *Annual Review of Psychology*, 52, 141-66.

Scheier, M. F. and Carver, C. S. (1985). Optimism, coping and health: Assessment and implications of generalized outcome expectancies. *Health Psychology*, 4, 219-47.

Scheier, M. F., Weintraub, J. K. and Carver, C. S. (1986). Divergent strategies of optimists and pessimists. *Journal of Personality and Social Psychology*, 51, 1257-64.

Schleifer, S. J., Eckholdt, H. M., Cohen, J. and Keller, S. E. (1993). Analysis of partial variance (APV) as a statistical approach to control day to day variation in immune assays. *Brain Behavior Immunology*, 7, 243-52.

Schleifer, S. J., Keller, S. E., Bond, R. N., Cohen, J. and Stein, M. (1989). Major depressive disorder and immunity: Role of age, sex, severity and hospitalization. *Arch. General Psychiatry*, 46, 81-87.

Seligman, M. (2002). *Authentic happiness*. New York: Free Press.

Selye, K. (1976). *The stress of life*. New York: McGraw-Hill.

Sen, Amartya. (1999). *Development as freedom*. New York: Knopf.

Sharma, S. (1988). Stress and anxiety. In J. Pandey (Ed.), *Psychology in India: The state of the art*, Vol. 1 (pp. 191-247). New Delhi: Sage.

Sharma S. (1999). Social support, stress and psychological well-being. In G. Misra (Ed.), *Psychological perspectives on stress and health* (pp. 126–46). New Delhi: Concept.

Sharma, S. and Misra, G. (2010). Health psychology: Progress and challenges. In G. Misra (Ed.), *Psychology in India, Vol. 3–Clinical and health psychology* (pp. 265–316). New Delhi: Pearson Education.

Siegel, B. S. (1986). *Love, medicine and miracles*. London: Arrow Books.

Singh, Rajbir, Yadava, Amrita and Sharma, N. R. (Eds). (2005). *Health psychology*. New Delhi: Global Vision.

Sloan, R. P. and Bagiella, E. (2001). Religion and health. *Health Psychology*, 20, 228.

Snyder, C. and Lopez, S. (2002). *Handbook of positive psychology*. New York: Oxford University Press.

Svoboda, R. E. (1992). *Ayurveda: Life, health and longevity*. New Delhi: Penguin Books.

Swami Rama, Ballentine, R. and Swami, Ajay (1976). *Yoga and psychotherapy*. Honesdale, PA: Himalayan Institute.

Taylor, S. E. (2006). *Health psychology*. New Delhi: Tata Mcgraw Hill.

———. (1983). Adjustment to threatening events. *American Psychologist*, 38, 1161–73.

Temoshok, L. (1987). Personality, coping style, emotions and cancer: Towards an integrative model. *Cancer Surveys*, 6, 545–67.

Thakar, G. and Misra, G. (1999). Job and well-being: The experience of employed women. In G. Misra (Ed.), *Psychological perspectives on stress and health* (pp. 211–37). New Delhi: Concept.

Uchino, B. N., Uno, D. and Holt-Lunstad, J. (1999). Social support, physiological processes, and health. *Current Directions in Psychological Science*, 8, 145–48.

Vaillant, G. E. and Mukamal, K. (2001). Successful aging. *American Journal of Psychiatry*, 158, 839–47.

Verma, S. K. and Verma, A. (1989). *Manual for PGI general wellbeing measure*. Lucknow: Ankur Psychological Agency.

Weiner, B. (1985). 'Spontaneous' causal thinking. *Psychological Bulletin*, 97, 74–84.

Westbrook, M. T. and Viney, L. L. (1982). Patterns of anxiety in the chronically ill. *British Journal of Medical Psychology*, 55(1), 87–95.

Williams, S. J. and Calnan, M. (Eds). (1996). *Modern medicine: Lay perspectives and experiences*. London: UCL Press.

WHO. (1978). *Alma–Ata declaration*. Geneva: World Health Organization (WHO).

Wortman, C. B. and Brehm, J. W. (1975). Responses to uncontrollable outcomes: An integration of reactance theory and the learned helplessness model. In L. Berkowitz (Ed.), *Advances in experimental social psychology* (Vol. 8). New York: Academic Press.

Zimmerman, Francis. (1987). *The jungle and the aroma of meats: An ecological theme in Hindu medicine*. Berkeley: University of California Press.

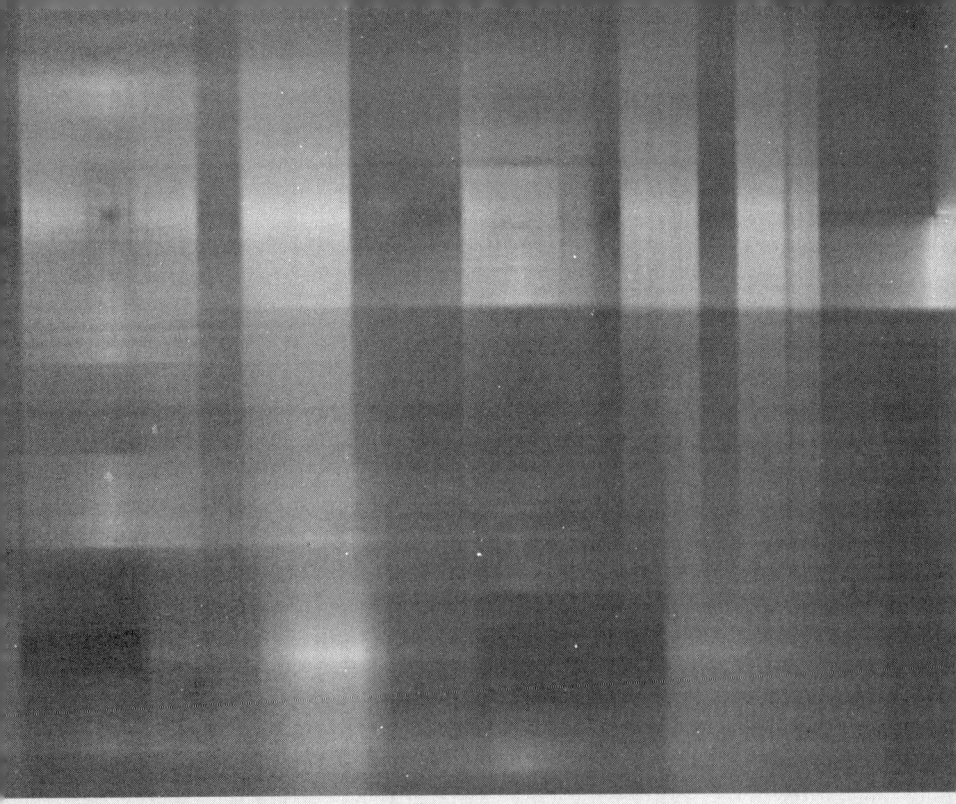

Part I

CONCEPTUAL FOUNDATIONS

Introduction

The notion of health has evolved in a variety of traditions and cultural contexts. Social scientists, medical practitioners and common man arrive at their own understanding of what it means to be healthy (Capewell, 1994; Singh, Misra, Varma and Mishra, 1999). However, the desirability of a longer lifespan is something that seems common to everyone. All of us want a healthy life. Several thousand years ago, the Vedic seers had beautifully described the longing for hundred years (*Jivem sharadah shatam*) but only a life which is active, vibrant and full of dignity. Such an active life is possible only when a person is healthy. Health has been rightly considered as the main pathway for attaining all the life goals including right conduct (*dharma*), worldly pursuits (*artha*), fulfilling the desires (*kama*) and liberation (*moksha*) (*Dharmarthakammokshanam arogyam mulamuttamam*). The folk tradition also treats health with a high premium. In the modern period, health is certainly a priority concern for most countries.

The Indian perspective on health has flourished with the ideas of harmony, evolution and connectivity across life forms. It is embedded in the ecology in which a person or group is embedded. It is broad enough to incorporate the whole range of existential concerns as reflected in the Upanishadic concept of Pancha Koshas (Annamaya, Pranamaya, Vigyanmaya, Manomaya and Anandmaya), which articulates human existence in terms of a multi-layered organization. In this scheme, the idea of 'being' is of a conscious being and not of a reactive organism. It operates following the principles of complementarity, inter-dependence, sharing and reciprocity between self and other (which includes the environment also). The idea of Being (Consciousness!) as Sachidanand reminds us about the essentially blissful nature of Self that remains hidden because of our ignorance. In this sense, health becomes a journey of self-discovery. We need to recognize ourselves and see the true nature of being. It is the ignorance (*avidya*) that blurs vision of our blissful true nature and puts us in a state when one remains perturbed, sick or ill. In other words, when you are not healthy, you are not in your (true) self. Being healthy or non-healthy is thus a statement about your location or position. The way one is positioned and the stance that is taken in viewing the world and self decide how healthy he or she is. A healthy person is one who is auto-locus (*swastha*) and not located elsewhere (*parastha*). A healthy or *swastha* person, however, is not egocentric; rather, such a person is in tune with the inner and outer environment. It denotes 'a state of being rooted in one's self. And "self" implies the consciousness of soul principle operating on various planes: physical, vital and mental and also in communion with the cosmic consciousness' (Basu, 2000, p. 2).

Ayurveda, the Indian science of life has twin goals, i.e., preservation and promotion of health and prevention and management of disease. Thus, it attends to the needs and requirements of the healthy as well as of the people who are suffering from diseases. Ayurveda also holds that a person is a *jiva* or *rashi purusha* which is a composite of body, sense organs, mind and self. Thus, a holistic view is maintained that takes into account a dynamic functional unit.

Any discussion of health from the view of Ayurveda will remain incomplete without a reference to the concept of Tridoshas consisting of *vata*, *pitta* and *kapha*. They refer to primordial bioactive substances operating at the cellular and sub-cellular levels. They pervade throughout the body and their qualities can be accelerated or inhibited both by external and internal influences, leading to decrease or increase of a specific attribute. *Vata* (movement) is composed of ether and air. It governs the mode of movement within the body and therefore can be seen as the force which directs nerve impulses, circulation, respiration and elimination. *Vata* works as a promoter of biological activity that is responsible for rotating the *doshas*. *Pitta* (bile) is composed of fire and water and represents the process of transformation or metabolism. It is also responsible for metabolism in the organ and tissue systems, as well as cellular metabolism. *Kapha* (inertia) is predominantly a combination of water and earth elements. *Kapha* is responsible for growth and adding structure, unit by unit. Another function of the *kapha dosha* is to offer protection. Cerebral spinal fluid protects the brain and spinal column and is a type of *kapha* found in the body. The bodily organization is often treated in terms of these *doshas*. The mental organization is viewed in terms of three *gunas*, i.e., *satwa*, *rajas* and *tamas*.

According to Charaka, a disease can be tackled in three ways, i.e., *samsodhan*, *samsamana* and *nidan parivarjana*. *Samsodhan* refers to diffusing the pathology and expulsion from the body of pathology, which consists of morbid *doshas* and accumulated toxic metabolic substances. It tries to purify, clean the internal environment and considers body as a whole. To this end, the techniques of *panchakarmas* are used. These techniques include *vaman* (emesis), *virechan* (purgation), *vasti* (enemeta), *nasya* (errhines) and *raktamoksana* (aphaeresis).

Samsamana is palliative therapy involving the use of drugs and diet. They not only pacify the *doshas* but also create hostile environment for the diseases. Diet can contribute to (*pathya*), or can be counter to health. The digestion is related to the nature of food. One must eat only when previous food is digested and person is hungry. Excess food or poor processing of the consumed food results in toxic elements. One should avoid incompatible (e.g., milk-salt) and adulterated food.

Nidan parivarjana means avoiding and checking/controlling the etiological factors that lead to the disease state. The premise is that absence of etiology shall prevent the disease and help in treating the person. There is provision of Sadvritta that includes proper daily conduct.

The idea of health has become a prime concern for everyone. However, beyond a general comprehension, the common man, the practitioners and the policymakers often confine to different loci of focus while attending to the health issues. This section tries to explore the different facets of health in a historical perspective. As will be clear from the chapters included in this section, the concept of health and emphasis on different aspects (e.g., physical, mental, social, spiritual) of health has evolved in specific historical and socio-cultural contexts. The various disciplines that claim to deal with health and illness like clinical psychology, psychiatry, abnormal psychology and medical anthropology have positioned themselves with different vantage points. While health psychology as an emerging field of study deals primarily with health care with an explicit emphasis on health promotion, it would be worthwhile to examine the changing concerns about health.

In the first chapter, Srinivas Murthi has traced the journey of the notion of mental health in the modern world. Organized in four sections, focusing on mental illness and mental health, prevention and promotion of mental health and the Indian perspective of mental health, and development of mental health programme, respectively, this chapter helps in understanding the shifting concerns and activities in this area of study. It is noted that the early emphasis was more on diseases and not so much on health. The recognition of health as individual responsibility rather than a service was a major shift that took place in 1980s. The WHO initiative to treat health in a more inclusive way that encompasses freedom from illness as well as a positive state including spiritual aspects is a real breakthrough. Murthi considers PHC as a genuine beginning of relating health services to societal needs as the first element of a continuing health care process. Reminding of the early work of Govindswamy in 1950s, Murthi notes that restoration, prevention and upgrading (positive health) constitute the scope of mental health.

Historically, however, abnormal behaviour has been treated as act of devil or criminal. Then there was a move from evil to ill, which resulted in considering the mental patients not bad but mad/insane. It was Freud who, with his emphasis on the intrapsychic forces, changed the focus from illness to wellness. Later on, behaviourism drew attention towards the role played by the external environmental factors. As Murthi says, the study of the factors affecting the human mind from 'above' was replaced with those from 'within' and later 'without'. The beginning of anti-psychiatry movement led to recognition of the social origins of mental illness and health. Also, the effects of life events and the role of social support in ameliorating the health problems were indicated. Attention was paid to the altered states of consciousness (trance) which showed that people with training and under special circumstances can function at different levels of brain organization. The psychological states following disaster experience is another area, and psychoneuroimmunology has emerged as the most recent area that links neuropeptides and psychosomatic network. There is a clear move from a medical to a biosocial view of health and illness. The last quarter of twentieth century witnessed a shift from illness to prevention and promotion of mental health.

Finally, Murthy outlines the distinctive features of the Indian view of mental health. He notes that the Indian approach defies mind/body duality and is holistic to the core. As such, it recognizes spiritual health too as an essential component of mental health. Murthi builds his arguments on the basis of textual sources, cross-cultural considerations of personality dynamics, traditional concepts of therapy and place of family in therapeutic interventions. In the contemporary period, the emphasis is more on the mental health development programmes, involving the individual, the family and the community. Thus, there is a shift from a purely medical model to social model. The present scenario creates a challenge as well as extends opportunities to the researchers and professionals in the area of health.

The need to study health behaviours is becoming more and more crucial as the contemporary man in the developed as well as the Westernized parts of the developing world is increasingly engaging in describing the everyday experiences by using the terms 'stress', 'hassle', 'burnout', 'anxiety', 'depression' and 'tension'. The second chapter of this section is a chapter by Madan Palsane and David Lam that examines stress and coping within a cultural perspective. They note that many differences and similarities exist in the etiology, perception and effects and coping with stress across cultures as modernization and urbanization have been the key players in shaping the modern life. However, stress is an individual as well as a socio-cultural issue. The development and change in people's motivational structure is central to it.

In contemporary societies, breakdown of support network and increase in self-centredness has contributed to increase in the level of stress. The American society is often termed as 'achieving society' in which economic and material pursuits figure very prominently. In such a scenario, competition and maximizing one's benefits at any cost becomes the main concern. This results in absence of satisfaction and increase in the degree of conflict and frustration. This situation leads to stress as an epidemic. The urban achievement-oriented people from the eastern part of the world are but counterparts of the Western individual. Incidentally, they are the people, though in a small minority, on whom majority of research is conducted.

It is noted that within the domain of Euro-American psychology, 'stress' has been treated as a stimulus, as a response and also as the interaction of person and the situation. In the Indian tradition, suffering and *dukha* are considered as an inherent part of the life world. This leads to awareness 'that a man can mend his ways and stand up anew as it is impossible to conceptualize life as stress-free: no stress no life'. Suffering occurs at the lower level of existence, at the level of our material existence—the human body. It does not occur at the level of self or *atman*. Stress may be self or environment generated. The genesis of stress lies in the desire that leads to misery and afflictions (*kleshas*). In the course of our life experiences, we become conditioned with certain events and stimuli. This leads to a reservoir of *karmas* (*karmashaya*). In the Chinese culture, there is emphasis on developing one's humanity (*jen*), which is the best way to prevent suffering. Illness (*yin*) is darkness and wellness (*yang*) is light. The key concepts in the Indian tradition relevant to stress are *dharma*, detachment, impulse control, transcendence and rebirth. The afflictions that create pain and suffering can be removed by many ways. In particular, three main path ways are: action (*karma*), knowledge (*jyan*) and devotion to God (*bhakti*). All of them offer ways of coping with stress and live a healthy life.

Living stress-free life and enjoying well-being is unmistakably a goal cherished by everyone. Within the discipline of psychology, this issue has received attention in the context of discussions about the process of adjustment. This is the theme of the third chapter in which Durganand Sinha has tried to bring into focus the essence of the notion of well-being—an obvious but often obscure way to characterize the desirable state of human life or its existential condition. Bodily health and rich material conditions are often insufficient for the experience of well-being, since it ignores the mental, psychological and social aspects of human life. Since well-being of the people is always an underlying concern in all the policies and plans, it is necessary to spell out its details. As a concept, it belongs to a family of concepts that characterize effective functioning of people within their life circumstances. While literally it means a desirable, satisfactory state, Sinha draws attention to the process of adjustment and a person's ability to satisfy one's needs. He contrasts adjustment with maladjustment and recognizes that well-being or normal psychological adjustment is a relative state of affairs. It is relative to the situation as well as to the values prevalent in a particular culture or subculture. The maladjustive patterns of behaviour are the first indicators of the absence of psychosocial well-being in a person. Drawing from Sushrut, the first surgeon of ancient India, Sinha turns attention to the notion of health as a state of delight or a feeling of spiritual, mental and physical well-being. Referring to Charak, he draws an important conclusion that well-being/health is not merely possession of certain characteristics but cultivation of certain positive qualities.

In the Indian context, internal equipoise/equilibrium that relates to individual's internal functions or maintaining harmony, balance and internal self-regulation is frequently emphasized. In this context, Sinha relies on the notion of homeostasis. He argues that achieving a state of balance (*sama*), even on social and psychological planes, is equally valuable. In his view, the health status depends on the states of equilibrium of *Doshas*, *Dhatus*, *Agni* and *Mal*. For want of clarity let us define the components. *Doshas* (*Vata*, *Pitta* and *Kapha*) are already discussed earlier. *Dhatus* are body tissues that support, sustain and nourish the body. *Agni* refers to the metabolic enzymes. *Mal* stands for the metabolic by-products and waste products. When the state of disequilibrium occurs due to inadequate association of season, action and sensory modalities people experience ill health. In contrast, adequate association leads to health and well-being.

Referring to Buddhism and *Samkhya* philosophies, he finds the virtue of following the middle path (*madhyam marg*) or avoiding the extremes. Referring to *Bhagavadgita*, Sinha illustrates the characteristics of an equipoised person (*sthitaprajya*) who experiences total well-being. He also refers to the notion of 'competence' and 'quality of life', and notes that economic resources are not positively and linearly related to the experience of psychological well-being. It is non-linear and treats the satisfaction of social and community level needs as important. Some of the key aspects of the Indian notion of well-being include control over the senses, not being overwhelmed by the experiences of success or sorrow, maintaining harmony orientation and being in tune with the environment.

The concern with well-being has become more and more critical in the contemporary period, particularly in the discussions of positive psychology. In this context, the contribution of Srivastava and Misra extends the debate on well-being. The apparent signs of discomfort and distress in the people and increasing degree of striving for happiness have become the major concerns. The search for pleasure has been on since Vedic period till date. It constitutes a significant dimension of human experience and emotional life. Individual need satisfaction is important in the West. Myers and Diener (1995) mention that self-esteem, optimism, extraversion and a sense of personal mastery or control are important for happiness. This list shows the salience of egocentric tendencies. In contrast, the East has a different orientation. No time of life is notably happiest and most satisfying. Subjective well-being increases as one moves up on the economic ladder; once societies arrive there, the level of happiness plateau briefly and then begins to turn downward as values and expectations change. Subjective well-being follows a curvilinear path.

It has also been noted that optimism is necessary to avoid depression, but strangely enough, optimism has been declining with economic development. Srivastava and Misra (Chapter 5) note that there are three positions in this regard: all economic growth contributes to well-being, some economic growth contributes to well-being and some economic growth detracts from well-being. The construal of happiness is related to the goals set by the people. Commitment to goal and success often contribute to happiness, which in turn contributes to positive experiences, health and control. But it is not very stable. The Indian view holds that happiness is relative and context-specific. Also, life is considered to be a play of pleasure and pain. Minimization of needs is necessary for happiness and the collective concern has to be given due importance. Being poor is not necessarily something that makes people unhappy. Happiness is in the state of being equidistant to poverty and affluence. The concept of social quality of life does reflect this component. Keyes (1998) views it as a construct comprising of social actualization, social acceptance, social integration, social contribution and social contribution.

It seems that the idea of health at personal as well as the collective level requires an assumption about good life, an idea about body and an image of human existence. It refers to a desirable ideal state that has positive impact on people's quality of life. These assumptions are inter-related and signify the value of cultural meanings and practices that are shared by the people. From the Indian cultural perspective, human existence is not coterminous with body; instead, body serves some higher cause. It is an instrument/apparatus to perform certain functions and it has to be duly attended to in order to perform those functions. Also, it is realized that a person is placed in a nested hierarchy of worlds that correspond with one's existential reality. The most important proposition is that self and environment are composed of similar material ingredients (*prakriti*). The mental and physical both comprise of the five basic elements (*pancha mahabhutas*: earth, water, fire, air and ether). This suggests for an inclusive concept of health that does regard environmental health and personal health both at an equal footing. Finally, health is treated as a continuous journey and not a station. Thus, being healthy is a process as it signifies living healthy. It is present at the moment when one is able to live a balanced and harmonious life. It involves the realization that self and other/environment are not in conflict but are in communion and together grow by facilitating each others' functioning.

In the introductory chapter, it was pointed out that restoration, maintenance and growth are three key aspects of health. Attention is usually paid more to the first, less frequently to the second and least frequently to the third. In the contemporary world, we need to attend to all the three functions. Health is an asset which is most precious, vulnerable and works as a life force. Therefore, everyone wants to maintain, preserve and enhance it. But what can be done and how—its strategies—depend upon the way we construe health, well-being and happiness. Our ideas determine what we would like to do for it. Since health psychology strives to promoting health, this section shall make an effort to delineate the various facets of health. Taken together the four chapters included in this section, try to encompass the whole range of health concerns—from disease and stress to health, well-being and happiness.

REFERENCES

Basu, S. (2000). *Integral health*. Pondicherry: Sri Aurobindo Ashram.
Capewell, S. (1994). Are health and illness defined by society or by doctors?. *Proceedings of Royal College of Physicians Edinburgh*, 24, 181-86.
Keyes, Coery Lee M. (1998). Social well-being. *Social Psychology Quarterly*, 61, 121-40.
Myers, D. G. and Diener, E. (1995). Who is happy? *Psychological Science*, 6, 10-19.
Singh, T., Misra, G., Varma, S. and Mishra, R. C. (1999). Concept of health and illness in four systems of medicine: Some policy implications. In G. Misra (Ed.), *Psychological perspectives on stress and health* (pp. 66-84). New Delhi: Concept.

2

Evolution of the Concept of Mental Health: From Mental Illness to Mental Health

R. SRINIVASA MURTHY

The evolution of the concept of mental health is linked to the large developments in the understanding of human behaviour. Starting from explanations of supernatural causation, we have arrived at understanding the states of mind and mental health from a holistic point of view. Rapid advances in the understanding of the human brain and individual and group behaviour open up new possibilities for non-medical and wider psychosocial actions towards promotion of mental health. Indian mental health professionals now have the advantage of structuring mental health programmes with these new understandings.

INTRODUCTION

The WHO constitution defines health as a state of complete physical, mental and social well-being and not merely the absence of disease or infirmity. However, WHO, in the first 30 years (1948–1978), focused largely on specific illnesses (tuberculosis, malaria) and not so much on 'health' (William, 1988a, pp. 7–23). The Alma Ata conference in 1978, (WHO, 1978) is a landmark in the development of the concept of health. The conference viewed health as an individual's responsibility rather than a service to be delivered to individuals (William, 1988b, p. 185). The concept of primary health care is revolutionary both in terms of conceptual clarity and details included for achieving the goal.

Primary Health Care is essential health care based on practical, scientifically sound and socially acceptable methods and technology, made universally accessible to individuals and families in the community through their full participation and at a cost that the community and country can afford to maintain at every stage of their development in the spirit of self-reliance and self-determination. It forms an integral part both of the main focus, and of the overall social and economic development of the community. It is the first level of contact of individuals, the family and community with the national system bringing health care as close as possible to where people live and work, and constitutes the first element of a continuing health care process (WHO, 1978).

Further, the Alma Ata Recommendation includes promotion of mental health as one of the eight components of primary health care. This shift in emphasis from illness to health is important, as the term 'mental' connotes illness rather than well-being. This article traces the evolution of concepts of mental illness and mental health, categorization of mental health issues, recent developments in the prevention of mental and psychosocial disorders, current approaches to mental health programme development and concludes by outlining the future of mental health care with special reference to India.

SCOPE OF MENTAL HEALTH

The scope and importance of mental health has been known to range from the care of the ill to the promotion of mental health by professionals. One of the earliest Indian psychiatrists to clearly outline the broad scope was Govindaswamy. In as early as 1948, he stated:

> The field of mental health includes three sets of objectives. One of these has to do with mentally ill persons. For them the objective is the restoration of health. A second has to do with those people who are mentally healthy but who may become ill if they are not protected from conditions that are conducive to mental illness, which however are not the same for every individual. The objective for those persons is prevention. The third objective has to do with the upgrading of mental health of normal persons quite apart from any question of disease or infirmity. This is positive mental health. It consists in the protection and development at all levels of human

society of secure, affectionate and satisfying human relationships and in the reduction of hostile tensions in persons and groups. (Govindaswamy, 1970; as quoted in Rao 1970)

UNDERSTANDING MENTAL ILLNESS AND MENTAL HEALTH

For the last 500 years, the Western approach to 'deviant' or 'abnormal' behaviour has been influenced predominantly by religion and science.

Till about the seventeenth century, all abnormal behaviour was seen as an act of the 'devil', i.e., 'against God'. Hallucinations were seen as communications with Satan. Consequently, the 'ill' were seen as 'evil' and Christianity approved specific sanctions to kill them or punish them. The book *Malleus Maleficarum* by Johann Sprenger and Heinrich Kraemer, 1487, illustrates this (Alexander and Selesnick, 1967). The descriptions of 'witches' were of mentally ill persons, and it is both a book of pornography and a textbook of psychopathology (Alexander and Selesnick, 1967, p. 67; Deutsch, 1937).

The next phase considered all abnormal behaviour as 'criminal', i.e., anyone whose behaviour was socially unacceptable was classified as 'bad' and they were put in jails along with other criminals. There was no attempt to view their behaviour from other angles.

With the advent of modern scientific thought, the focus shifted from 'evil' to 'ill'—in a way, people are not 'bad', but 'mad' or 'insane'. This shift, however subtle, was significant. The healing hand of humanism replaced the rigors of religious punishment. The ill were looked after in more humane surroundings, at that time called asylums. A statement in the early nineteenth century reflects this humane approach:

> Moral treatment consists in removing patients from their residence to some proper asylums, and for this purpose a calm retreat in the country is preferred, for it is found that continuance at home aggravates the disease, as the improper association of ideas cannot be destroyed ... hospitals are the only places where insane persons can be at once humanely and properly controlled. (Deutsch, 1937, pp. 91-92)

However, this advancement, though important, was double-edged as institutions became places of human exploitation and abuse. These aspects were most aptly brought out by Clifford Beers, an inmate of asylums for many years. His work, *The Mind that Found Itself* (1921), is significant, as it affected the social consciousness of the community and helped promote better care for the mentally ill. As a reaction to the ills of the asylums, the 'mental-hygiene movement' was started; a major progression from 'illness' to 'wellness'. This public awareness also started the preventive psychiatry movement.

At the turn of the twentieth century, there were other major developments in mental health. The most significant was the contribution of Sigmund Freud. He presented behaviour and mental functions as 'understandable' and evolved a coherent theory of personality called 'psychoanalysis'. He gave the world a new conception of both infancy and adolescence, and characterology, and evolved a system of treatment where the origin of the disease would be revealed. He unlocked the mysticisms of the past, revealed unknown mental mechanisms and established a new prophylaxis in a new combination of the practical and theoretic.

This contribution of Sigmund Freud shifted the focus from the 'illness' to 'wellness' and the isotonic views of behaviour to understandability of behaviour rooted in childhood experiences and parent-child relationships. Around the same time, others like Carl Jung, Alfred Adler, Otto Rank presented variations in the same theme. Psychoanalysis as theory and treatment method took mental illness from institutions to outpatients and homes. The child guidance movement of the early 1920s envisaged healthy development of all individuals by preventive measures through proper parental guidance. However, looking back at this point in time, one result was the highly 'ego centred' approach to individual development. This was considered a major breakthrough at that time, but as new thoughts emerged in the second half of twentieth century, this view point proves to be of limited value (Henderson, Pryrone and Duncan-Jones, 1981). There are growing concerns about 'individualism' as a goal for individuals and communities. The necessity to consider needs beyond fulfilment is a new stream of thought that reduces the Freudian emphasis on the specific individual personality, rooted mainly in childhood experiences.

In other words, what happened was that the mental health profession had to overcome the handicaps of 'odium theologicum' and later 'odium sexicium'. The study of factors affecting the human mind from 'above' was replaced with those from 'within', and later, 'without'. The highly subjective and internalized approach of psychoanalysis was replaced by the behaviouristic school of thought, which stresses the role of environment as a determinant of behaviour and maintains that observable behaviour is the essential basis of psychological investigation.

The next major contribution to understanding behaviour was the work of B. F. Skinner and J. B. Watson—the behaviouristic schools of thought. Based on learning theories, this was a mixture of biological and social theories. This contrasted with the totally intrapsychic theories of psychoanalysis. An important outcome was 'behaviour therapy' as a method of treatment, with specific applicability to a variety of human emotional problems (Watson and Rayner, 1920; Skinner, 1953; Rachman, 1963).

The antipsychiatry movement started in the West. The background is a complex outcome of institutional care, human rights and anti-professional feelings. Clare traces it as follows:

> The 'antipsychiatry' movement has sprung up, the main principle of which appears to be that mental illness is a reductive smear that obscures and defiles the despairing cries of the downtrodden and exploited against an alienating and dehumanized society. Psychiatric intervention is portrayed as a violent assault perpetrated under the guise of treatment, and the psychiatrist is deemed to be an agent of the dominant political order, and an agent of repression and of power. Antipsychiatrists demand the abolition of existing psychiatric institutions and insist that psychiatrists either acknowledge their true role as society's police or become agents of personal and social change. (Clare, 1976, pp. 2-3)

In India, there has been no such movement against psychiatry, partly reflecting the limited number of institutions and professionals.

In the last 30 years, there has been a shift to the social origins of mental health and illness. If fact, this line of thought is still in a developmental phase. The dominant theories are of life stress, social support, social network and family life (Brown, Birley and Wing, 1972; Henderson et al., 1981; Holmes and Rahe, 1967; Mechanic and Aiken, 1986). It is interesting to note that there is much discomfort to view the 'social roots' of mental health and mental illness. This is most probably due to the high premium placed by Western thought on individual independence as the only desired goal for all.

The association of life events and illness onset has been part of the folklore. Recent studies indicate that these observations may be another indication of folklore being folk wisdom (Holmes and Rahe, 1967). However, systematic studies of impact of life events are of recent origin. The collective evidence arising from: (*a*) those exposed to intense stressful situations like wars and disaster, and (*b*) those experiencing single life events like bereavement, suggests that illnesses occur against a background of accumulating life events. The life events can be either positive (for example, birth of a child, promotion or moving to a new house), or negative (bereavement, legal problems). The studies show an association between a wide range of health problems and experienced life stresses. An area that has been studied systematically is the impact of bereavement (Dyke and Kaufman, 1983). A large number of studies have demonstrated that the death of a loved one is a precipitatory event for many mental and somatic diseases. There is evidence that conjugal bereavement is associated with excess mortality. In one study, there was a seven-fold increase in mortality in the first year of bereavement. There is not only an increase in suicide rates but increased occurrence of accidents, infectious diseases, heart diseases, depression, cancer and alcoholism. There is accumulating evidence about the changed endocrinological and immunological functions during bereavement, pointing to the possible mechanisms involved in the vulnerable status (Hall, 1990).

A related aspect to the theory of stress is the topic of 'social supports and social networks'. Durkheim, more than a century ago, recognized its importance in understanding the risk of suicide. He maintains:

> There is a preservation of individuals, both men and women, by marriage, but after a certain age the preservation is less due to marriage itself than to children. After a certain age, according to the statistics, married women without children do not enjoy the coefficient of preservation, but on the contrary suffer a coefficient of aggravation. Hence it is not so much marriage that protects as family and children. In childless wives there is aggravation. (Aron, 1980)

This recognition of the modifying role of social supports and available social network has received considerable attention in the last 10 years. In a way, this is a reaction to the breakdown of the family supports. The initial studies found a higher mortality among those with fewer social ties (Mechanic and Aiken, 1986). The course and outcome of mental disorders, especially schizophrenia (Brown, Birley, and Wing, 1972, pp. 241-58) has been studied in detail as to its relationship to family interactions (Rasi, 1986). Similarly, studies of persons with neurosis and its relationship to social supports has demonstrated the close relationship with the non-availability of supports and coping skills to occurrence and chronicity of specific mental disorders (Henderson et al., 1981). An interesting outcome has been the development of family intervention by psychoeducational programmes and the demonstration of these family interventions in the reduction of relapses in chronic schizophrenic patients. This has added a new dimension to mental health care (Leff et al., 1985, pp. 594-600).

In the last decade, this research has opened a variety of new possibilities for intervention and prevention of chronicity by measures other than drugs and other physical interventions. This area has specific relevance to developing countries in general, and India in particular, as the family and social networks are still intact and largely functioning. The next set of variables that are emerging as important are related to lifestyles.

Till recently, a number of altered states of mind were considered as psychological in origin. Recent evidence (Ervin et al., 1988, pp. 267-84; Simons, Ervin and Prince, 1988, pp. 249-66) is providing insights that can explain the states of mind from a biological perspective. I would use two examples to illustrate this link.

Trance is a common phenomenon in a number of countries. Trance and possession occur both in religious settings and in situations of psychosocial distress. Traditionally, they were viewed from the supernatural angle. About 100 years ago, with the advent of psychoanalysis, they were explained as 'dissociation' and came under the group of 'hysterical phenomenon'. A study reported in 1988, throws fresh light on this phenomenon. The study was carried out at the Thaipusam Festival in Kuala Lumpur, Malaysia. During this three day festival, worshippers fulfil a vow made in times of illness or other trouble to offer special worship to Lord Muruga. As part of their worship, many enter an analgesic trance and allow their bodies to be pierced by special hooks and needles (Simons et al., 1988, pp. 249-66). The study carried out the determination of Endorphin-like Immunoreactivity (ELI), urinary corticosteroids and creatinine in the urine during the training period and the day of worship from novice trancers, experienced trancers and the musicians. The major physiological findings of this study were:

> Trance onset is characterised by increased muscle tone and striking exacerbation of physiologic tremor and pupillary dilatation, early in training, trances are characterised by poorly organised motor hyperactivity and occasionally the display of intense emotion. With experience, the motor patterns become more coherently organised with few affective displays. In both cases, trances are accompanied by amnesia. This state is suggestive of other situations in which limbic system dominates the behavioral program. The response to the termination stimulus (of deep pain) is an abrupt hypotonia, unconsciousness and areflexia as might be seen at the end of a seizure ... with progressive training (or past experience) there was dampening of the major physiologic signs. At the same time, the dance patterns become well organised and individually specific, as if there were increasing cortical involvement in this primarily limbic activity ... Biochemically, corticoids and ELI, as peripheral indicators of the stress state, show orderly differences

within groups. In the initial sessions, the experienced trancers had lower values than did the novices, and for both groups there was a systematic decrease in excreted values over the period of training. (Ervin et al., 1988, pp. 267-84)

The investigators conclude, on the basis of the preliminary findings:

The physiologic signs of the trance state, are consistent with the hypothesis that central opiate mechanisms are indeed involved. Further, the entire behavioral, autonomic and endocrinologic syndrome is consistent with a state of cerebral organisation dominated by the limbic system, as indicated by the euphoria and analgesia characteristic of basolateral amygdala activation, and the amnesia consistent with spread of activation to the hippocampus. That the amygdala is a key locus of control or cortisol and beta-endorphin secretion is consistent with this overall hypothesis. In conclusion, we propose that the individual entering trance arrives with a set of culturally defined expectations and learned techniques for narrowing and focussing attention as in hypnosis ... this special state of organisation of the brain may underlie a wide spectrum of trance states.

The importance of these initial observations, though tentative at this point of time, is the recognition that individuals with training, and under special circumstances, can function at different levels of the brain organization. The need to enter altered states of mind periodically in a healthy manner could have implications in understanding problems like drug dependence.

The other area where a biological basis is being explored is that of the psychological states following disaster experience. The initial results of studies of the universal pattern of post traumatic stress disorders were characterized by panic attacks, blunted affective feelings, hyperreactivity and need to recount the events repeatedly. The biological studies suggest that there are changes in the form of increase in the secretion of Corticotrophine-releasing Factor (CRF), which alerts the body for emergencies and hyperactivity of the opiod system of the brain which can blunt the feeling of pain. These can explain the clinical features of being startled by the most innocuous stimuli, troubled sleep, irritability, pain, recurrent nightmares and flashbacks that repeat the original disaster experience among the disaster survivors.

These new insights support the view that there is a wide range of research effort linking the neuropeptide and psychosomatic network where the mind and body constantly chatter back and forth using a vocabulary

Evolution of the Concept of Mental Health • 65

of biochemicals. This has also initiated a new discipline called 'psychoneuroimmunology' (Hall, 1990).

In recent times, these developments are contributing towards a biosocial model for the understanding of common mental disorders. The emerging model of vulnerability, destabilization and restitution has practical value in understanding of mental disorders as well as treatment of the disorders (Goldberg and Huxley, 1992). These new understandings have implications beyond theory:

> There is now a explosion of knowledge about mental disorder, and it at last becomes possible to discern the outlines of a model for mental disorder which takes account of findings in both social psychiatry and molecular biology. However, we have not made corresponding progress in refining the administrative and architectural requirements for meeting the needs of the mentally ill, and in most countries of the world services for the mentally ill, survive on the crumbs left from the banquet of general health care. At times of scarce resources, our services are very easy to prune. The liberation of others—clinical psychologists, nurses and social workers—from domination by the medical profession has occurred in many countries, and has been the enemy of a united service which offers the best to patients, and which commands adequate resources from society. (Goldberg and Huxley, 1992, p. 163)

PREVENTION AND PROMOTION OF MENTAL HEALTH

During the last decade, the focus has shifted from mental disorders to mental health. World Health Organization's publication, *Prevention of Mental, Neurological and Psychosocial Disorders* in 1986 is a milestone. The document concluded:

> Mental, neurological and psychosocial disorders constitute an enormous public health burden. A comprehensive programme directed against their biological and social causes could substantially reduce suffering, the destruction of human potential and economic loss. It would require the commitment of governments and coordinated action by many social sectors. (WHO, 1986)

The new knowledge, that can be applied towards the above goals, from various sources has been summarized (WHO, 1986) as follows:

1. In the event of acute loss, there is evidence that group and individual support can diminish risk for physical and mental health problems. Self-help and mutual aid groups can improve health with minimum cost to the health services.
2. Cultural factors are among the principal determinants of human behaviour. A knowledge of cultural and religious beliefs and practices can be applied in health services by all levels of personnel. Ways of preserving values that promote mental health should be identified by systematic studies.
3. Retarded mental development and behaviour disorders among children growing up in families that are unable to provide suitable stimulation can be minimized by early psychosocial stimulation of infants, and by day care programmes of good quality with active parent participation.
4. Many patients who consult primary health care either have no ascertainable biological abnormality or, if they have one, complain disproportionately about their discomfort and dysfunction. In this group, unless the psychosocial source of physical symptoms is recognized, the people affected are likely to be inappropriately investigated and treated. The inclusion of basic mental health skills like listening and support reduces the cost of treatment and improves the outcome.
5. Alcohol consumption contributes heavily to physical and mental health problems like cirrhosis of liver, difficulties at work and home, traffic accidents and family disruption. In women, it can lead to a foetal alcohol syndrome.
6. Individual lifestyles can influence the risk of disease. Examples are excess animal fat in diet, insufficient physical exercise, psychosocial stress and smoking.
7. Self-help groups organized by the public can effectively reduce the chronicity of alcohol dependence, increase the financial ability of handicapped and function as pressure groups to affect policy changes.
8. Schools can be an important starting point for promotion of mental health. A particularly promising way of preventing substance abuse among early adolescents is to encourage them to acquire behavioural skills necessary to resist the pressure to use cigarettes, drugs and alcohol.
9. Early recognition of sensory and motor handicaps and the use of prosthetic devices to minimise handicaps can prevent both cognitive underachievement and social maladjustment.

Evolution of the Concept of Mental Health • 67

10. Teachers can identify and care for children with sensory or motor handicaps, or with mental health problems that have not been detected by the parents or the health personnel.
11. Family breakdown interferes with the development of children. Improving the status of women has a definite impact on the development of children.
12. Community attitudes towards chronic mentally ill persons can determine the course, outcome and level of functioning of the ill individuals. It is important to examine the specific ways in which societal response and clinical interventions affect the phenomenology, severity and chronicity of major mental disorders.
13. There are numerous techniques, drugs and treatment styles which are used by traditional healers. These should be studied to incorporate elements which have proved useful, such as group psychotherapy through rituals.
14. In the case of severe neuropsychiatric disorders like schizophrenia and epilepsy, it is clearly demonstrated that early recognition and proper and complete treatment can prevent chronicity and help cure.
15. A large number of measures can be taken to prevent mental handicaps in the community. Some important ones are:

   (i) prenatal and perinatal care
   (ii) programmes for child nutrition
   (iii) immunization of children
   (iv) family planning
   (v) iodization of salt (in specific areas)
   (vi) active immunization of pregnant women against tetanus
   (vii) active resuscitation of the newborn
   (viii) cervicograph
   (ix) prevention and early treatment of infections
   (x) preventing pregnancies of older women (beyond 35 years)
   (xi) long-term follow-up of low birth weight babies
   (xii) maternal nutrition and correction of anaemia in pregnant women

16. Information sharing with the families of the disabled is necessary to enhance family coping skills.
17. In the total mental health activities, the following community resources have important contributions to make to prevent mental disorders, care of the mentally ill and promotion of mental health:

(i) ill persons
(ii) families of ill individuals
(iii) child care workers
(iv) health workers
(v) medical officers
(vi) school children
(vii) teachers
(viii) volunteers and NGOs
(ix) community leaders/religious leaders
(x) police

18. Urbanization places individuals in an 'at risk' position for mental health problems, due to enhanced stress, decreased social supports and loss of traditional patterns of life. Urgent measures to support individuals, families and social policy making are required to limit the adverse effects.

THE INDIAN VIEW OF MENTAL HEALTH

Before reviewing the development of the 'modern' concepts, it would be appropriate to consider the Indian concept of mental health. Indian psychiatrists have described how mental health has been an important part of Indian philosophy and social thought. Wig (1990, pp. 71-80) has summarized this as follows:

> Indian culture has always attached great significance to spiritual life. The term spiritual is, of course, not identical with the term mental, but both recognise the value of inner mental life and experiences. In India, the term health is usually not confined to physical state: in any Indian definition of health there is always reference to mental harmony and potential for spiritual growth. The present day term mental health is European in concept and origin. There is no exact equivalent of the term mind in Indian languages, because the differentiation of 'body' and 'mind' has never been important in Indian philosophy, as it has been in modern European thought. Thus, when we speak of 'mental health' especially positive mental health, not merely the absence of mental disorder, the average Indian will always perceive in it an underlying reference to spiritual development. Understood in this way 'mental health' is very important for him, is something to which he attaches great value: he is willing to spend time and

resources in pursuit of it. This holistic approach to health in general and mental health in particular to a large extent, reflects the current concept of mental health.

Indian philosophy attaches great importance to the spiritual dimension of life. The ultimate goal of life is self-realization or realization of one's inner nature. Material things are regarded as illusions, and are hence impermanent. There are repeated references in the religious texts to the need for detachment from material things and for a search for the spiritual meaning of life (Wig, 1990, p. 73). A number of Indian mental health professionals have focused on the various aspects of Indian concepts of mental health (Wig, 1990, pp. 71-79; Neki, 1977, pp. 94-112; Satyanand, 1965; Sinha, 1990; Vahia et al., 1973, pp. 557-65; Ramu, Venkataram and Janakiramaiah, 1988, pp. 41-46).

Four themes can be identified in this area. First, the recognition of the rich knowledge available in the classical texts of India. Govindaswamy (1970; as quoted in Rao, 1970) noted the following:

> Many psychological doctrines and results of modern research have been anticipated and commented upon with great, insight by the ancient sages of India. They have stated categorically that in the ultimate analysis. selfishness on the psychological side and starvation on the physical side are responsible for disorganisation in the individual and society alike. This fact stands as true today as when it was enunciated centuries ago, and forms the pivot around which psychiatry revolved. Hughings Jacksons' conception of levels in the nervous system, their integration in health and dis-organisation in disease is in a very general manner was anticipated in the Sankya System. Problems of consciousness are dealt with in a penetratingly analytical manner in Mandukya, Chandogya and Prasna Upanisads. The Yoga Vaishastha, Sankara's Vivekachudamani, the commentaries on various Darsanas by Kumarila Bhatta and Appayya Dikshitar are rich storehouses of learning for the student of psychological medicine. The Buddhist works on philosophy are equally important and comparatively more objective in character ... it must however be stated that to the ancient sages, the problems of personality and of mind, as we understand them, were only aspects of the general problem of ultimate reality and treated as such, hence the impression that Indian Psychology is subjective, mystic and philosophical, but there is nothing to prevent students of modern medicine and psychology to study in a purely objective manner, such a study is imperative if India has to assume in future, the role of the leader of world psychiatry.

The second set of observations have focused on the cross-cultural consideration of dynamics in terms of personality functioning. Specific reference can be made to the contributions of Neki (1977, pp. 93-112) with regard to the concept of 'dependence-independence'. He has referred to the limitations of using dependence-independence as developmental bipolarity and suggested the value of dependence as a concept. He has pointed out, 'though independence may be prized as a socio-political ideal, as goal of individual development, it is not much cherished. In fact the Indian culture tends to foster dependence right from birth'. He has also referred to the implications for therapy, especially psychotherapy.

Carstairs and Kapur (1976) have examined the prevalence of mental disorders in different social groups in South India. There are references to the role of social stress, modernization and occurrence of mental disorders. Similar observations have been made by Chakraborty (1990) from Calcutta.

The third area where contributions have been made is the area of using traditional concepts for therapy. A very important contribution has been the work of Vahia et al., (1973, pp. 557-65) using psychophysiological therapy based on the concept of Patanjali for the treatment of neurotic and psychosomatic disorders. Over the course of nine years, about 250 patients were treated with the above therapy and compared with drugs, or both. The results indicate that the Patanjali system is useful in treating psychoneurosis and bronchial asthma. Another area has been the use of concepts of the *Gita* in psychotherapy.

The growing problem of drug dependence has prompted professionals to consider the role of Yoga and meditation for prevention of drug abuse and therapy of dependent individuals.

The fourth area has been in relation to the place of family in therapy. Number of investigators have pointed out the enduring bonds of Indian family and its value in the care of mentally ill persons (Surya, 1970, pp. 381-92; Narayanan, 1977; Bhatti, 1980; Srinivasa Murthy, 1991).

In international literature, the first phase saw the family as the causative factor for the illness. The second phase focused on the interaction of the patients and family. The current phase takes into consideration the 'trauma' of living with a chronically mentally ill member.

However, the situation in India has been different. Due to strong family bonds, the families of the mentally ill have continued to be their primary care providers. This has been utilized to a great extent to provide education and skills, both in active treatment as well as in rehabilitation. However, as we are heading towards a change in the family structure, especially in the rural areas, there is a need for active consideration of mechanisms and measures to keep the family as an important resource in mental health care. This would require the mental health professionals (especially the non-medical group) not only to consider families as partners (rather than as adversaries or substitutes), but also to develop appropriate approaches and mechanisms to work with families.

MENTAL HEALTH PROGRAMME DEVELOPMENT

India represents a mixture of the old and new. In the area of mental health, there is both the 'preying on the gullible'/'moments of madness' (Balse, 1971; *India Today*, 1981a, 1981b) and innovative approaches to mental health care.

A review of the course of mental health care programmes in the country reflect the above developments in understanding mental illnesses and mental health, as well as broadening the areas of activity of mental health professionals. Following the Bhore Committee Report, the period of 1947–1960 was characterized by enhancing the number of mental hospitals (Bhore, 1946). This was followed by the general hospital psychiatric unit movement (1960–1975) (Wig, 1978, pp. 1–3). Since 1975, the community mental health programmes have been the main thrust area for the development of services in developing countries (WHO, 1974; 1975; 1990; Srinivasa Murthy, 1983, pp. 16–29). The community mental health movement has so far focused on the care of mentally ill persons, utilizing community resources, specially the medical infrastructure (Wig et al., 1981, pp. 275–90; Srinivasa Murthy and Wig, 1983, pp. 1486–90; Isaac, 1988; Srinivasa Murthy, 1987, pp. 37–40). It is only in the last few years that efforts have been directed towards work with the educational infrastructure (Kapur and Cariappa, 1978; Kapur, Cariappa and Parthasarathy, 1980) and the welfare infrastructure to develop promotive and preventive mental health programmes. The last 15 years of policymaking in India have also been one of decentralization and deprofessionalization (GOI, 1982; DGHS, 1990; GOI, 1989). The central point of the developments has been the utilization of community resources for mental health care. These are in line with the developments in the Western countries (Sartorius et al., 1990). In this context, the mental health professionals have a unique opportunity to develop broad-based and complete mental health programmes, utilizing the current concept of mental health. This requires the professionals not only to accept work outside the institutions, but also beyond the needs of the ill persons and consider the opportunities for prevention of mental disorders and promotion of mental health. This also requires a greater role for the non-medical mental health professionals and better utilization of cultural resources in terms of beliefs, practices and institutions like family and community groups.

The development of mental health from mental illness has been reviewed in this article. These changes emphasize the role of the individual, the family and the community. At a larger level, there is recognition of an important role for the government, in terms of its policies, which can influence the mental health status of the individual. Specifically, policies regarding alcohol availability, housing, industrialization, urbanization, working women, welfare measures for the elderly, environmental degradation, can contribute positively or negatively towards the decreasing or increasing of mental morbidity and suffering. It is essential that mental health professionals sensitize policymakers and politicians to these aspects of their decisions.

The major shift that has occurred in the last 100 years from mental illness to mental health is an issue which has major implications for social work in India. As pointed out earlier, the shift has been from a purely medical to a biosocial model (Goldberg and Huxley, 1992). The interventions range from policies at the society level, specific drug treatment, support in crisis, utilization of different community resources and psychosocial interventions in the form of social support (case work, etc.). In addition, at the national level, there is a shift from the institutions to the community, from professionals to non-professionals, from vertical programmes to integration, public involvement and education to destigmatize mental health care.

All these changes offer new opportunities for social workers. *First*, they would be able to initiate a number of mental health activities. *Second*, they can coordinate with other mental health professionals, both in institutions and in the community. *Third*, they can initiate community level action in the areas of crisis interventions, alcohol policy, services for children of working mothers, street children, migrant populations, so that the adverse effects are minimised. *Fourth*, they can work with planners, policymakers, politicians and the press to sensitize the larger society to a holistic view of mental health. There is a special scope for Indian social workers in the areas of strengthening the family, harmonizing intergenerational relationship, utilizing cultural beliefs and practices towards promotion of mental health. *Lastly*, research and evaluation should form a very important aspect of all these efforts, as mental health issues cannot be understood in global terms alone but in local and specific situations. It is noted that in India, very often, good ideas have a premature death while relatively mediocre ideas have received unqualified support. Social workers can develop both the methodology of evaluation and training personnel for research efforts. It is this challenge that social workers face in India while fostering mental health.

In conclusion, it may be said that the development of the concept of mental health has been a reflection of the larger developments about the understanding of the mind as well as the total health of individuals and communities. We are in an advantageous position to develop programmes to match both the dictates of society as well as the individual. Mental health professionals working in developing countries feel that this is a unique opportunity.

> The major advantage for the psychiatrist in a developing ... country is the very paucity of previous provision for the mentally sick. Thus he does not have to expend his energies in frustrating attempts to dismantle an inert and cumbersome administrative infrastructure; nor does he have to concern himself with finding a method of absorbing large numbers of solidly built prison-like mental hospitals into a more efficient and humane psychiatric programme—there is little need for him to struggle with large armies of personnel in various categories, each ... unwilling to change from the security of the well defined roles to meet the challenge of the present and the future ... (he has) at least a fairly clean canvas to develop (his) themes. (German, 1975, pp. 409–20)

The development of the concept of mental health from mental illness has two features, namely, a steady evolution of the concepts of causation and a broadening in the scope of mental health and mental illness—a moving away from a highly individual orientation to a larger social system orientation. This point in time, in terms of understanding and scope is not an end point. The advances in biological and social science will bring forward better ways of understanding mental disorders and developing care programmes. The challenge lies in continuously trying to channelize different viewpoints and mobilize divergent efforts in order to promote and nurture physical and mental harmony. The challenge offers opportunities for innovation. Here lies the road to the future.

Acknowledgements

My sincere thanks and gratitude to Professor N. N. Wig, New Delhi, for the continuous stimulation and support in writing this chapter. The critical suggestions of Dr Ajai R. Singh, Bombay, have added depth to the concepts and coverage. Dr Sheild Srenivasan and Ms Katy Gandevia have specifically helped me by their comments to enhance the coverage and critical evaluation of the different developments reviewed.

References

Alexander, F. G. and Selesnick, S. T. (1967). *The history of psychiatry: An evaluation of psychiatric thought and practice from prehistoric times to the present.* London: Allen and Unwin.
Aron, R. (1980). *Modern thoughts of sociology.* Harmondsworth: Penguin.
Balse, M. (1971). A million Indians suffer from mental sickness—How does psychiatry help them. *The Illustrated Weekly of India,* 12 September.
Beers, C. (1921). *The mind that found itself.* New York: Doubleday.
Bhatti, R. S. (1980). Psychiatric family ward treatment. *Family Process,* 19, 193-200.
Bhore, J. (1946). *Health survey and development committee report.* New Delhi: Government of India.
Brown, G. W., Birley, J. L. T. and Wing, J. K. (1972). Influence of family life on the course of schizophrenic disorders: A replication. *British Journal of Psychiatry,* 121, 241-58.
Carstairs, G. M. and Kapur, R. L. (1976). *The great universe of Kota: Stress change and mental disorders in an Indian village.* London: Hogarth.
Clare, A. (1976). *Psychiatry in dissent.* London: Routledge.
Chakraborty, A. (1990). *Social stress and mental health—A social psychiatric field study of Calcutta.* Delhi: Sage.
Deutsch, A. (1937). *The mentally ill in America.* New York: Columbia University Press.
DGHS. (1990). *National mental health programme—A progress report (1982-1990).* Nirman Bhavan, New Delhi: Directorate General of Health Services (India).
Dyke, C. V. and Kaufman, C. I. (1983). Psychobiology of bereavement. In L. Temospok, C. V. Dyke and L. S. Zegans (Eds), *Emotion in health and illness.* New York: Grune and Stratton.
Ervin, F. R., Palmour, R. M., Pearson, B. E., Prince, R. A. and Simons, R. C. (1988). The psychobiology of trance-II. *Transcultural Psychiatric Research Review,* 25, 267-84.
German, G. A. (1975). Trends in psychiatry in Black Africa. In S. Arieti and G. Chrizanowski (Eds), *New dimensions in psychiatry: A world view* (pp. 409-28). New York: Wiley.

GOI. (1982). *National mental health programme for India.* New Delhi: Ministry of Health and Family Welfare, Government of India.
———. (1989). *National mental health programme for India*—Progress Report (1982-1988). New Delhi: Ministry of Health and Family Welfare, Government of India.
Goldberg, D. and Huxley, P. (1992). *Common mental disorders—A biosocial model.* London: Routledge.
Hall, S. S. (1990). Spanning the Chasm. *SPAN,* July, 2-7.
Henderson, A. S., Pryrone, D. G. and Duncan-Jones, P. (1981). *Neurosis and the social environment.* Sydney: Academic Press.
Holmes, T. A. and Rahe, R. H. (1967). The social readjustment rating scale. *Journal of Psychosomatic Research,* 11, 213-15.
India Today. (1981a, September). Preying on the gullible, 16-30.
———. (1981b, October). A moment of madness, 16-30.
Isaac, M. K. (1988). Bellary district mental health programme. *Community Mental Health News,* Issue 11 and 12. ICMR-CAR on Community Mental Health. Bangalore: NIMHANS.
Kapur, M. and Cariappa, I. (1978). Evaluation of training programme for school teachers in student counselling, *Indian Journal of Psychiatry,* 20, 289.
Kapur, M., Cariappa, I. and Parthasarathy, R. (1980). Evaluation of an orientation course for teachers on emotional problems amongst school children. *Indian Journal of Clinical Psychology,* 7, 103.
Leff, J. P., Kuipers, L., Berkowitz, T. and Sturgeon, D. (1985). A controlled trial of social intervention in the families of schizophrenic patients: Two year follow up. *British Journal of Psychiatry,* 146, 594-600.
Mechanic, D. and Aiken, L. (1986). *Applications of social sciences in clinical medicine and health policy.* New Brunswick: Rutgers University Press.
Narayanan, H. S. (1977). Experience of group and family therapy in India. *International Journal of Group Psychotherapy,* 1, 517.
Neki, J. S. (1977). Dependence: cross-cultural consideration of dynamics. In S. Arieti and G. Chizanowski (Eds), *New dimensions in psychiatry: A world view* (pp. 93-112). New York: Wiley.
Rachman, S. (1963). Introduction to behaviour therapy. *Behaviour Research Therapy,* 1, 3-15.
Ramu, M. G., Venkataram, B. S. and Janakiramaiah, N. (1988). Manovikaras with special reference to Udvega (Anxiety) and Vishada (depression). *NIMHANS Journal,* 6, 41-46.
Rao, S. K. Ramachandra (1970). Lectures and writings of Dr M. V. Govindaswamy. In S. K. Ramachandra Rao (Ed), Bangalore.
Rasi, S. V. (1986). The detection and modification of psychosocial and behavioural risk factors. In L. H. Aiken and D. Mechanic (Eds), *Applications of social science to Clinical medicine and social policy.* New Jersey: Rutgers University Press.
Sartorius, N., Goldberg, D., de Girolamo, G.O., Costa de Silva, J.A., Lecrubier, Y. and Wittchan, H. U. (Eds). (1990). *Psychological disorders in general medical settings.* Toronto: Hogrefe & Huber/WHO.

Satyanand, D. (1965). *Positive mental health.* New Delhi: Indian Council of Medical Research.
Simons, R. C., Ervin, F. R. and Prince, R. H. (1988). The psychobiology of trance-I. *Transcultural Psychiatric Research Review,* 25, 249-66.
Sinha, D. (1990). *Psychology in a third world country.* New Delhi: Sage.
Skinner, B. F. (1953). *Science and human behaviour.* New York: Macmillan.
Srinivasa Murthy, R. (1983). Treatment and rehabilitation of the severely mentally ill in developing countries: Experiences of South East Asia. *International Journal of Mental Health,* 12(3), 16-29.
———. (1987). Recent developments in community mental health care in India. In *Collaborative studies on severe mental morbidity* (pp. 37-40). New Delhi: Indian Council of Medical Research.
———. (1991). Family and schizophrenia—A resource reconsidered. *Paper presented at the SCARF Workshop on Family and Schizophrenia,* 9 August.
Srinivasa Murthy, R. and Wig, N. N. (1983). A training approach to enhancing mental health manpower in a developing country. *American journal of psychiatry,* 140, 1486-90.
Surya, N. C. (1970). Ego structure in the Hindu joint family: Some considerations. In W. Caudill and T. Lin (Eds), *Mental health research in Asia and the Pacific* (pp. 381-92). Honululu: East-West Center.
Vahia, N. S., Doongagi, D. R., Jeste, D. V., Ravindranath, S., Kapoor S. N. and Ardhapurkar, I. (1973). Psychophysiologic therapy based on the concepts of Patanjali. *American Journal of Psychotherapy,* 27, 557-65.
Watson, J. B. and Rayner, R. (1920). Conditional emotional reactions. *Journal of Experimental Psychology,* 3, 1-14.
Wig, N. N. (1978). General hospital psychiatric units—Right time for evaluation. *Indian Journal of Psychiatry,* 20, 1.
———. (1990). Indian concepts of mental health and their impact on the care of the mentally ill. *International Journal of Mental Health,* 18(3), 71-80.
Wig, N. N., Srinivasa Murthy, R. and Harding, T. W. (1981). A model for rural psychiatric services—Raipur Rani experience. *Indian Journal of Psychiatry,* 23, 275-90.
William, G. (1988a). WHO—The days of the mass campaigns. *WHO Health Forum,* 9, 7-23.
———. (1988b). WHO: Reaching out to all. *World Health Forum,* 9, 185-99.
WHO. (1974). *Community action for mental health care.* New Delhi: SEARD, SEA/Ment/22.
———. (1975). Organisation of mental health services in developing countries. *Technical Report Series* No. 564, Geneva: World Health Organization.
———. (1978). *Primary health care.* Geneva: World Health Organization.
———. (1986). *Prevention of mental, neurological and psychosocial disorders.* Geneva: World Health Organization.
———. (1990). *Preventing chronic diseases.* Geneva: World Health Organization.

3

Stress and Coping from Traditional Indian and Chinese Perspectives

M.N. PALSANE AND DAVID J. LAM

INTRODUCTION

The purpose of writing on Asian perspectives of stress and coping is to increase our understanding of the socio-cultural variations in stressful phenomena. Differences exist in the incidence, causes, perceptions and effects of stress, and in ways of coping. There are similarities as well in relation to stress processes, and the modernization and urbanization of many countries in Asia.

It is not a straightforward matter to place Western and Eastern ideas on stress and coping in a comparative perspective. This is because when we read the Western (mostly American) literature, we are dealing with some defined concepts beginning with Hans Selye and perhaps coming up to Richard Lazarus. Most books deal with more or less a uniform list of topics and problems.

The Eastern perspective is much less specific than the Western. First, the Eastern perspectives vary from Middle Eastern to Far Eastern societies and cultures. Second, and more importantly, there is a rich tradition of religion and philosophy in this regard which cannot be overlooked by any serious student of stress and coping. This has been stated by Evans, Palsane and D'Souza (1983) in the following words:

Concepts developed in technologically advanced regions in a Judeo-Christian cultural setting need to be empirically tested before they are accepted as applicable in a developing country with vastly different objective daily life conditions and a philosophy of life emanating from the religious-cultural traditions of Hinduism.

Similarly, Hong and Lam (1992) have pointed out that stress-related concepts, as applied in an Eastern setting such as Chinese society, must be understood not only in the context of individual functioning, but also as a socio-cultural issue.

The long historical development of civilization may be looked at from a motivational angle with implications for stress. Theoretically, if we accept the story of Adam and Eve as the beginning of civilization, the roots of the altruistic motive or consideration for others may have begun at this stage. In other words, the self-centredness of Adam and Eve became attenuated. As the family, clan, tribe and society developed, this process continued. In the recorded part of history, religious and philosophical writings emphasized consideration for others and curbing of self-centredness. The history of civilization, thus, is a history of expanding the sense of self. Man[1] could identify with a larger body of humankind. With the onset of the industrial revolution, the focus on time and motion increased. The man of the industrial age thinks in terms of the instrumentality of every moment, action and thing. This has also extended to himself, his family, society, country and, for that matter, his religion. He has thus reverted to self-centredness. This development and change in motivational pattern have implications for stress. It is well known that susceptibility to stress is reduced with the expansion of meaningful social networks.

The breakdown of religion, associated with the breakdown of values and increased self-centredness, has perhaps led to a greater degree of stress. This may be on account of increased competition, insecurity, anomie, alienation and breakdown of family and other social networks. Evidence for this is available in the comparison of modern Western societies with traditional Oriental ones.

CONTEXTUAL DIFFERENCES IN THE STUDY OF STRESS

Looking at stress conceptually, we can see that the West and the East talk about totally different things. This is because culturally, the two definitions

---

[1] Use of the masculine also signifies the feminine.

and even terminologies are different. To understand this, we have to look at the social and cultural history to know the context. First let us look at the West (America) where the phenomenon of stress came to the limelight. The American society has a short history. It comprises migrants from different countries. The psychology of migrants reveals that they have high aspirations, strong motives to pursue their goals against all odds, dissatisfaction with the status quo and zeal for adventure. Young people in Asia today, keen to go to the United States (US), view it as a land of unlimited opportunities. A society made up of more or less this type of population has shaped itself into what David McClelland called the 'achieving society'.

The phenomena of migration as well as achievement in an achieving society are largely in terms of economic and material pursuits. For high achievement orientation coupled with individualistic goals, pragmatism is a suitable philosophy of life. The social system and culture promote competition at the cost of cooperation. Interactions between spouses, parents and children, friends, employers and employees are largely governed by the social exchange principle of cost and benefit. Everyone is out to maximize his or her benefits, perhaps at the cost of others. The reality of competition is that everyone cannot win. Or rather, when one wins, several lose. The possibilities of conflict and frustration are greater in such a culture than in less competitive societies. The spirit of adventure and achievement orientation push individuals further into new vistas of enterprise. Scientific progress, technological and industrial advancements are largely a result of such a temperament. Exploitation of the environment and material progress have gone hand in hand. Here one is reminded of the character 'Pokhom' in the famous story of Leo Tolstoy—*How Much Land Does a Man Require?* In the absence of satisfaction, and in the face of conflict and frustration, stress takes the form of an epidemic.

The foregoing is a simplified description of the stress phenomenon as it may exist in American society. It should help in understanding why the perspective and the facts are different in the East.

As against the 'new world' of America, the Asian world is old. Asian societies and cultures have a long history. Social structures have evolved different religions to provide philosophies of life in the course of social evolution. These philosophies have provided stable social structures and a set of functional values, yet they have also made them stagnant. Even in this so-called age of science, the appeal of religion is very strong and can at times destabilize large countries. Naturally, superstition takes precedence over reason and there is tremendous resistance to change. With high density of population and low literacy level, the inertia against change sets large sections of the population apart from the few who have had the benefits of Western education and therefore have become the change agents of modernization. There is, therefore, an urban achievement-oriented Eastern counterpart of the Western individual, but this is a minority in these countries. The exceptions are countries such as Japan, Hong Kong, Singapore and, perhaps, South Korea and Taiwan, where modernization has been more pervasive.

Stress and coping in the Eastern perspective will have to be studied in two ways. One approach is more like that used in the West as it applies to the minority urban populations, on whom some studies are available, using similar conceptual frameworks. However, more important than this approach is the orientation to this problem in traditional societies and populations. This is of necessity more theoretical in the absence of empirical data.

Modern Concepts of Stress and Coping

The individual and the environment can be viewed as parts of a larger system of nature. Alternatively, they can be juxtaposed against each other in interaction, where the person is seen as making adjustments to various demands, whether internal or external. The life process itself implies this interaction, and the adjustment and dynamism involved. Stress results when there is an imbalance in this process of adjustment, and the demands on the individual exceed his or her capacity and resources to meet the demands. This is the current Western view of stress, and coping is the effort an individual exerts in order to meet the extra demands.

When considered in relation to the concepts of stress and coping, adjustment appears to overlap with coping behaviour. According to Lazarus (1976), coping is synonymous with adjustment in the sense that both are problem-solving processes in the face of demands and difficulties. Adjustment 'is an even broader concept referring to all reactions to environmental and internal demands'. Coping, on the other hand, is restricted to 'what the person does to handle stressful or emotionally charged demands' (Lazarus, 1976). Coping behaviour in this sense is a subset of adjustment behaviour.

It is necessary to understand these semantic distinctions while dealing with Eastern or Asian thinking. The reason is because the situations facing the individual, and the levels of solution to the problem differ from

Western to Eastern cultures. For example, in the West, there is emphasis on treating or curing a disease, while in India and China, there is emphasis on treating a patient, sometimes with the entire family being involved in the process of treatment (Kakar, 1982).

The term 'stress' is used in at least three different ways. First, it refers to the stimulus or stressor such as noise, accident and economic loss. Second, it indicates the response to stress such as increased blood pressure level, emotional upset, and impaired performance. The third meaning takes into account the interaction between the stressor and the individual and how the individual evaluates the stressor situation in relation to his resources to counteract. The appraisal of stress gives rise to the emotion of anxiety as a response to the threat. Within the Western framework such threats can range from minor to major, involving either trivial issues such as reaching a destination on time, or major ones such as death of a spouse. Some have short-term implications while others may have more long-term ones. (For a more detailed and technical account of this, see Evans and Cohen, 1987.)

SUFFERING IN ASIAN THOUGHT

While discussing the Eastern definitions of these concepts we have not come across any parallel term for stress. Related terms are suffering, pressure, anxiety, misery, pain, which may be represented by the Sanskrit term *dukha*. It is a mistake to consider these as synonymous with stress. The thinking in India in particular, and the religions and philosophies of the East in general, centres on the phenomenon of suffering, the term we shall adopt instead of *dukha* for convenience. Suffering is seen as a life process. According to Bowker (1970, p. 203), 'Suffering was ... seen as a result of a conflict inherent in creation. Duality ... is apparent in almost all the particulars of creation', and as S. Radhakrishnan (1979) has described it: '[C]osmic process is one of universal and unceasing change and is patterned on a duality which is perpetually in conflict, the perfect order of heaven and the chaos of the dark waters. Life creates opposites, as it creates sexes, in order to reconcile them.' According to the Buddhists, 'Birth is attended with pain, decay (aging) is painful, disease is painful, death is painful, painful is separation from the pleasant and any craving that is unsatisfied, that too, is painful' (Rhys Davids, 1973, p. 148).

In the Islamic tradition, suffering is inherent in the life process and is in the hands of God. God is conceived as omnipotent and compassionate and inflicts suffering on people either to punish them for their sins or to test their faith in him. The sufferers are expected to be patient and try their best to accept the suffering as God-given, maintain their faith in God and, at the same time, endure and overcome it with their best efforts. The suffering as usual is in the nature of everyday life problems such as temptations, dissatisfaction, hunger, poverty, conflict and hostility (Bowker, 1970).

The Japanese, following Zen Buddhism, believe that suffering is an essential part of existence, it stems from desires, and controlling desires through the path of discipline can mitigate suffering. Greed, hate, delusion and pride are considered important causes of suffering and are rooted in individual self-centredness. Transcendence is advised not in terms of pursuit of the supernormal, but in terms of compassion for others overcoming self-centredness. Understanding the true nature of self as well as suffering is the key to overcoming the latter; following the middle path and avoiding the extremes of indulgence or asceticism is recommended as the lifestyle to take suffering in one's stride.

In a similar vein, the Chinese philosopher Mencius wrote about not only why suffering was common but also how it led to beneficial outcomes. In the *Kao Tzu*, his Sixth Book, he said,

> Heaven, when it is about to place a great responsibility on a man, always first tests his resolution, wears out his sinews and bones with toil, exposes his body to starvation, subjects him to extreme poverty, frustrates his efforts so as to stimulate his mind, toughen his nature and make good his deficiencies.

Thus, these trials and tribulations, whether inflicted by heaven or earth, ultimately lead to the awareness that a man can 'mend his ways' and 'stand up anew'. Expressed in modern Western language, Mencius' ideas are that stress and its by-products serve to strengthen a person's psychological hardiness and overall fitness. In this sense, life without stress would be no life at all, or as Mencius put it, 'We realize that anxiety and distress lead to life and that ease and comfort end in death.'

In Western literature one can find similar thinking where stress is equated with an effort at adaptation to change, which is a life-long process, and where complete freedom from stress is considered possible only after death. However, the operational part of the concept of stress in the West is largely distress or negative aspects of adaptation and its outcomes. In the East, pleasure as well as pain are considered stressful and part of suffering. This is because existence is viewed differently. The analysis of behaviour at the level of body–mind is considered less significant and existence is viewed meaningful only at the higher transpersonal level of self, *atman* or soul, which in turn is equated with Brahman, the ultimate reality. All the rest is illusion (*maya*). Suffering belongs to the lower levels of existence—at the levels of body and mind. Existence at these levels is also considered inevitable before one is able to liberate oneself from suffering and the cycle of rebirth involving perpetual suffering.

Suffering is viewed differently in the West and the East. There is a greater degree of acceptance or tolerance of suffering in the East than in the West. This may have to do with locus of control. People in the East with faith in God, fate, rebirth and the like, accept misfortune as given, which has to be suffered. From a religious perspective, some even consider suffering as necessary for purifying the soul as a way to salvation or liberation, and therefore voluntarily undertake fasts and other privations.

Another related term is misery. According to Jadunath Sinha (1986, p. 221), 'Bharatmuni mentions distress, mental anguish, etc. as the determinant causes of misery. Dhananjaya and Viswanatha define misery as loss of mental vigour owing to poverty, misfortune, and the like. Dhanika defines misery as powerlessness or depression of the mind due to poverty, vomiting, etc.' The conditions and symptoms are quite comparable to those related to stress in modern literature. As we discuss the causes of suffering, coping and remedies, our understanding of Eastern thought in these contexts will be enhanced.

CAUSES OF SUFFERING OR ADVERSITY

It is a common practice among stress researchers to give a taxonomy of stresses: life stress, family stress, minor hassles of daily life, severe chronic strains, occupational and organizational stress, environmental stress, socio-cultural stress, physiological stress, etc. (see Evans and Cohen, 1987 for a systematic treatment). Though these are not exhaustive categories, they help in mapping the important fields of stressors. Specific manifestations of misery or suffering are unimportant in traditional Indian thought; they are only symptoms. More important are the causes that give rise to suffering (*dukha*).

While discussing types of pain (used in the sense of suffering), the Indian ancient philosophers talked about three categories and their origins (Sinha, 1986). The first category of 'self-generated pain' is caused by factors within the individual. This includes physical pain and results from the imbalance of the body humours. Mental pain results from desires, anger, greed, delusion, fear, envy, dejection and non-perception of certain objects. The second category, called 'environment-generated pain', is caused by other individuals, the animate and inanimate world. The third category, 'supernatural pain', is caused by ghosts and spirits. Apart from the classification used, the antecedents of stress are comparable to those in the different fields listed above. The third category, however, belongs to the imaginary world, which confirms the modern notion that stress lies not so much in the environment, but in the mind of man.

Just as modern psychology links frustration to the intensity of desires (Cofer and Appley, 1964), traditional Indian literature also lays great emphasis on desires in the causation of suffering, misery and pain (Caraka, 1949; Radhakrishnan, 1979; Sankaracharya, 1972). The traditional scriptures relate the intensity of desires to suffering. The text on the holistic system of Indian medicine reads, 'Desire is the cause of worries and harbours miseries. Reduction of the desires leads to relief from all the miseries' (Carakasamhita, 1949).

The *Bhagavadgita* (Radhakrishnan, 1979, ch. 2, pp. 125-26, verse 62-63) describes the chain of behaviour in two verses implicating desires with stress and its consequences:

> When a man dwells in his mind on the objects of sense, attachment to them is produced. From attachment springs desire and from desire comes anger.
>
> From anger arises bewilderment, from bewilderment loss of memory; and from loss of memory, the destruction of intelligence and from the destruction of intelligence he perishes.

These verses reflect the sequence of association, desire, frustration and anger, confusion, memory, intellectual failure and survival. Written more than 2,000 years ago they have empirical validation even today.

The text on the Indian system of medicine, *Carakasamhita* (Caraka, 1949, pp. 993-94), also asserts: 'The derangement of understanding, will and memory, the onset of adverse season and effect of past action, and contact with unwholesome sense-objects—these should be known as the causes of suffering.'

Similar ideas are expressed in Yoga philosophy. The science and philosophy of Yoga are widely recommended and used in spiritual pursuits as well as modern clinical practice. Apart from physical and breathing exercises, the study of its underlying philosophy and comprehensive package of practices lead to tremendous psychological benefits.

According to the Yoga philosophy, individuals develop a false sense of ego by identifying themselves with things around them. Desires in which there is ego involvement become more strong. Likes and dislikes, attractions and repulsions develop in terms of these strong needs with ego involvements. In Patanjali's *Yogasutras*, these ego involvements, attractions and repulsions are called afflictions (*kleshas*). This is an important concept in Yoga and provides an explanation of suffering (Rao, 1983). 'The lack of awareness of reality, the sense of egoism or ` I-am-ness', attractions and repulsions towards objects and the strong desire for life are great afflictions or causes of all miseries in life' (Taimni, 1961, p. 130). Thus *kleshas* are viewed as primary causes of suffering.

The above quotation lists five *kleshas*: ignorance (*avidya*), egoism (*asmita*), attraction (*raga*), repulsion (*dvesa*), and lust for life (*abhinivesa*). *Avidya* is the most important. The Sanskrit term *avidya* is often erroneously translated as ignorance. Though it is ignorance, it is of a different kind. Woods (1914) has correctly translated it as 'undifferentiated consciousness'. Owing to the lack of fundamental differentiation, *avidya* may also be understood as mistaken knowledge, the mistake lying particularly in the acceptance of something non-self as the self (Kulkarni, 1972). The individual mistakes the mind and body as his true self instead of the real transcendental self and this mistake gives rise to the other four afflictions. Before discussing these other afflictions, it is necessary to elaborate on the concept of *avidya*.

In Indian philosophy and religious thought, the self, also called the soul or *atman*, is treated differently than the mind and the body. Whereas the mind and body have their roots in matter or worldly experience, the self is identified with the transcendental and larger common self called *brahman*, a cosmic or universal principle. Because of *samskaras*, the conditioning through experience, this self becomes attached to objects in the environment including one's body. The mind is a result of these experiences. Some philosophers have denied the existence of matter and have called it illusion (*maya*), while others have viewed it as separate from the soul and assigned it a subordinate place. The mind and body belong to this subordinate level according to Yoga. *Avidya* implies that the self degenerates through experiences and mistakes the mind and body as his true self. It is a kind of fixation at a lower level of existence.

Having identified with the body and the mind, the self develops an identity which is his ego, or the property of 'I-am-ness'. Whereas in the form of transcendental self or *brahman*, one is infinite in size, shape, properties, etc., in the form of body and mind, one becomes limited and bound. The ego is bound by attachments in terms of objects that satisfy its needs and those that are obstacles to need fulfilment. The afflictions of attraction (*raga*) for objects of need satisfaction, and repulsion (*dvesa*) for those which obstruct need satisfaction, are further outcomes of the false sense of ego due to mistaken identity. This process of indulgence in false satisfaction of desires leads to increased desires and needs which in turn increases lust for life (*abhinivesa*).

It is necessary to understand at this stage how suffering is inherent in the life process. Associations with material objects and other beings are part of the experience of living. It is inevitable that attachments, repulsions, and a sense of ego will develop from birth. *Kleshas* are, therefore, not to be avoided but understood and transcended. The concept of universal self appears essentially as a grand rationalization to avoid fixation with desires, satisfactions or frustrations. Taylor (1983) has emphasized the need for creating illusions about oneself, meanings and control in one's efforts at adaptation, and to a limit, this is healthy. Most religious systems have attempted to provide a basis for such illusions that are not only socially acceptable but also valued. Idiosyncratic illusions, on the other hand, may not only be maladaptive but also warrant labelling as abnormal. The ideas about the supernatural and transcendental belong to the category of socially acceptable rationalizations, which have served the purpose of protecting common man from stresses of many kinds. Eastern religions and philosophical traditions have created very elaborate systems of ideas and literature, myths and beliefs over a long history of civilization in this region, so that even today sections of the population who follow these ideas seem to do better with their stress management efforts.

The cause of suffering is also linked with rebirth and this is another important theme of rationalization. For all intentional actions of an individual during his life, there is positive or negative credit and he is rewarded or punished in proportion to these. Actions with expectancy of rewards bear fruits which thus accumulate credits. Actions are supposed to be done as duties prescribed for one's role and status without an expectancy of outcome, which is difficult. These accumulated credits are called *karmasaya* or *karma (samcita)*. In Chinese philosophy, they are sometimes called 'accumulated blessings'. This account is carried forward life after life. Salvation (*moksha*) is attained only after the individual suffers in proportion to the past accumulated *karma*, and does not accumulate any *karma* by denouncing expectancy of outcomes. Even positive credit leads to rebirth and is an obstacle to salvation. Thus, rebirth is considered a form of suffering. Freedom from suffering is not attaining heaven by doing good deeds, but liberation from the cycle of rebirth. Total detachment in action is needed to bring the eligibility for heaven or hell to zero. The soul or self merges with the larger self, *brahman*, and attains *moksha*.

In China, the ancient philosopher Confucius (cited from de Bary, Chan and Watson, 1960) wrote extensively about the virtues of being a 'gentleman'. One of these virtues was freedom from stress. In chapter 12 of his *Analects*, he said, 'the gentleman has neither anxiety nor fear.... When he looks into himself and finds no cause for self-reproach, what has he to be anxious about what has he to fear?' The emphasis was on self-cultivation which thereby led to stress resistant qualities.

Being a gentleman implies improving oneself in a variety of areas. However, for the purpose of our discussion, the following quote from chapter 14 of the *Analects* is instructive: 'The way of the gentleman is threefold.... Being human, he has no anxieties; being wise, he has no perplexities; being brave, he has no fear' (see de Bary, Chan and Watson, 1960, ch. 11).

CONSEQUENCES OF SUFFERING

'(Mental) pain, despair, nervousness and hard breathing are the symptoms of a distracted condition of mind' (*Yogasutra*, 1-31 in Taimni, 1961). The distraction of the mind is not simple distraction, but is a result of destabilization of the mind (*citta*) due to afflictions (*kleshas*). There is a sense of helplessness leading to despair and nervousness. Nervousness here is described not only in psychological terms but also in terms of trembling and shaking. There is disturbance in the breathing process as well. Thus, suffering leads to serious psychological and physical symptoms and dysfunction.

In traditional Chinese thought, suffering can have short-term as well as long-term consequences. The short-term effects include most of the symptoms now associated with stress-related illnesses, namely, weakened nerves (neurasthenia), irritability, and tension on the psychological side, and exhaustion, poor appetite, headache, upset stomach and the like on the physical side. The long-term effects, on the other hand, are more positive, provided one is able to cope with the suffering and emerge even stronger than before. We have already discussed Mencius' viewpoint of how stress, or suffering, leads to life whereas comfort, or the absence of suffering, leads to death. Many Chinese people believe that present suffering is preordained from a previous life, and that the forbearance of suffering serves to repay an earlier debt and thus is not to be avoided. We can say that present suffering prevents further suffering later. This notion is reflected in the Chinese saying that 'a hundred forbearances become golden'.

In Confucian thought, developing one's humanity (*jen*) is the best way of preventing suffering, whether on an individual level or in society as a whole. Conversely, 'without humanity a man cannot long endure adversity' (*Analects* ch. 4, cf. de Bary, Chan and Watson, 1960). Humanity is cultivated by practising five virtues—courtesy, magnanimity, good faith, diligence and kindness. It should be noted that most of these virtues are interpersonal in nature.

Treating the short-term consequences of suffering is one of the functions of traditional Chinese medicine. In this system, illness results when the forces of *yin* (darkness) and *yang* (light) are out of balance. For example, certain forms of suffering may lead to depression in a person which is a *yin* illness, while other forms of stress may produce aggression or overeating, which are *yang* disturbances. *Yin* and *yang* forces mediate between the causes of suffering, or stressors, and the consequences of suffering, or stress responses. Attaining a healthy balance between *yin* and *yang* thus minimizes the ill-effects of stress.

In terms of the Indian medical system, the body has three constituents: *vata*, *pitta* and *kapha* (wind, bile, and mucus). The mind has three constituent *gunas* (properties), that is, *sattva or the potential consciousness or light*; *rajas*, activity or dynamism; and *tamas*, dullness, massiveness, inertia and darkness (Safaya, 1976). Normality consists of balance of these physical and mental constituents. Lapses of discipline in terms of derangement of understanding, will and memory result in suffering, which in turn produces an imbalance in these constituents, producing pathology of a physical or mental kind. The quotation from the *Bhagavadgita* cited earlier in connection with the causes of suffering, and linking desires to attachments, anger, confusion, lapses of memory and intelligence is pertinent here also. The frustration of desires leading to anger causes stress and results in performance deficits in memory and intelligence and even death. These ancient ideas are finding empirical confirmation in present day literature on stress.

MEDIATORS OF SUFFERING

The Indian tradition has, from time to time and through different religions and health customs, emphasized the following:

1. *Dharma* (right conduct) as highest value.
2. Detachment.
3. Impulse control.
4. Belief in rebirth and *karma* principle.
5. Transcendence.

These are not the only concepts, but they are the important ones in relation to stress and suffering. They are not independent but inter-related.

Dharma (right conduct) is prescribed as the highest value or goal to be pursued, the others being *artha* (economics, politics and civics), *kama* (life of sex, pleasures and aesthetics), and *moksha* (salvation) (Kane, 1962). Though *moksha* is the ultimate goal, it is attained incidentally on following *dharma*. Commonly *dharma* is translated as religion but it is better translated as correct conduct, not in terms of moral or ethical principle, but in terms of essential human nature in the context of other things. Just as the sun and the moon, animals and trees exist and function following some laws, so does the human being. Keeping within the limits of these laws is *dharma*. If there is a dispute or difference in interpretation, the reference has to be made to the laws of nature. Keeping close to nature safeguards the health of the system of nature as well as its various components. Stress may be generated if the components cross their limits. Even today, research indicates that people who follow religion and certain disciplines of nature suffer less from stress (Cox, 1981).

The principle of detachment involves one looking at pleasures as well as suffering with equanimity. Not being too involved in objects of pleasure, and not being too concerned about avoidance of suffering is seen as part of one's essential nature. Attachments develop due to association and conditioning. They have to be overcome. Detachment tones down the emotional damage to physical and mental health. In other words, detachment is the basis for emotional stability, a quality highly valued in modern mental health science. Pande and Naidu (1986) have demonstrated this effect by studying effort versus outcome orientation and the stress–strain relationship.

Impulse control is related to the theme of desires. As mentioned earlier, desires are the root cause of misery. Impulse is the result of desire and goal object perception. By the systematic practice processes is a matter of practice over time.

> Conscious training through concentration and meditation teaches the individual how to control his thoughts and voluntarily eliminate unwanted

ones, just as movements and muscle tensions can be eliminated by relaxation procedures. This reduces the causes of arousal and the concomitant bodily disturbances that accompany certain thoughts. (Palsane, 1987, p. 175)

But these measures help one overcome the symptoms only, and that too on a temporary basis. On a long-term basis the solution lies in developing the philosophy and practice of life consistent with what has been already said in relation to the causes of suffering and a stress resistant personality style.

Taylor (1983) has proposed a theory of cognitive adaptation. The belief system which mediates cognitive appraisal is an effort to adapt at the cognitive level. In this sense, the elements of Taylor's theory find support in the practices that are advocated by Indian tradition. Taylor has stated that 'the adjustment process centers around three themes: A search for meaning in the experience, an attempt to regain mastery over the event in particular and over one's life generally, and an effort to restore self-esteem through self-enhancing evaluation'. In many religious rituals, the person has to go without food, water, sleep or material resources. The most common ritual is fasting for a short or long time. For example, in Jainism, a person may fast from one day to 10 days. Children are also encouraged to fast for a day. It is important to examine this from Taylor's perspective.

In the first place, fasting is a deprivation and is a threatening event in the sense of survival. In the context of religion, fasting has a social sanction and meaning which is acquired by people in the process of socialization. Even those alien to the ritual of fasting, develop meaning in it for religious or health reasons. Second, by gradually adopting the ritual, one gains control over hunger or food deprivation, and the accompanying symptoms. By engaging in one or more rituals of this kind, one gains a sense of control and mastery over oneself, one's life and one's destiny. Last, the more one pursues such socially valued goals, the more one goes up in the esteem of others and also in one's own esteem. Religion is an organized system of beliefs and practices for the promotion of this kind of cognitive control over suffering. In this sense, the Eastern religions have always emphasized the role of privations in what they called purifying the body and spirit. Essentially these practices have deep psychological significance in terms of meaning, control and self-esteem. In this way they serve as long-term strategies for developing a stress-resistant personality style or lifestyle.

Coping with suffering is thus different in the Eastern perspective and consists of more long-term strategies involving the development of a philosophy of life as well as a lifestyle.

In Western literature on coping, two methods are mentioned: (a) direct action or task-oriented coping, and (b) palliative or defence-oriented coping. Evidence for both modes can be found in the Oriental traditions. In the *Bhagavadgita*, Lord Krishna, while counselling Arjuna to resolve the crisis involved in the conflict and war with his cousins, relatives and *gurus*, propounded both the task-oriented as well as defence-oriented approaches. He was advised to engage in the battle wholeheartedly as a matter of moral duty (*dharma* as a member of the warrior class), ignoring the result in terms of any losses on either side. The results were decided by God and these took their own course. This belief about detaching the outcome from action was a rationalization for engaging in an unpleasant action like war.

Under the influence of religion, Indian society has become fatalistic, complacent and stagnant. Such attitudes act as obstacles to economic and technological development which is needed for improving the quality of life of the masses. But this attitude of satisfaction with whatever one has may have served to protect the mental health of this society in the face of large-scale poverty and deprivation.

Ritual is an important aspect of all religions. Rituals are either individually or collectively performed. When individually performed like worship, prayer, and *mantra* recitation (*japa*), they reinforce the belief system underlying such performances. The element of faith becomes strong and that faith is beneficial for remedial work (faith healing). When rituals are collectively performed, it is a manifestation of the social network. It counteracts anomie and alienation. The collective rituals in certain cases among Hindus at the time of death and thereafter, serve to bring back the bereaved family members into the mainstream of activity (occupational therapy) and provide them emotional stability.

Similar to rituals, social customs with respect to marriages, death, childbirth and any number of other occasions, bring together not only relatives and friends, but also casual acquaintances and neighbours. This kind of social sharing helps carry out activities such as celebrations easily. Also, it helps in maintaining the supportive social network. Active social sharing at such a level is beneficial in terms of social cohesion, social control, social facilitation and norm sending, thereby discouraging social disorganization. This, in turn, may provide a socially healthy environment for individuals so they can build stress resistance as well as counteract it more effectively.

For example, the extended family is an old institution in Chinese as well as Indian society. It used to be common for a large extended family to live under the same roof. Such a family would include the family patriarch, his wife (or wives), his male children and their wives, his unmarried female children (the married female children typically lived with their husbands' families), and his grandchildren. Occasionally the patriarch's unmarried brothers or sisters would also be included. Such extended social networks provide social support not only on special occasions but also on a daily basis. The forms of support provided include informational, emotional and material. However, it must be mentioned that extended families often create stresses of their own. Role strain, such as between a woman and her mother-in-law or among siblings, are common sources of stress.

Another important part of the Oriental traditions is meditation. This may be a part of religious rituals or independent of religion. There are a number of techniques of meditation, including practice in the recitation of *mantra*, withdrawal of attention from objects of thought or senses, concentration and free-floating thought process. Different kinds of meditations serve different purposes and suit different people accordingly. Yogic, Zen and Sufi systems are some such traditions.

In addition, the philosophy of Taoism gave rise to a tradition of meditation in China. The following brief selections from the *Tao-Te Ching* (cf. Chan, 1963) make reference to the concept of meditation as practised by a number of Chinese people, then and now:

> Attain complete vacuity.
> Maintain steadfast quietude (verse 16).
> Act without action.
> Do without ado (verse 63). (see Chan, 1963)

In fact, Taoism as developed by Lao Tzu and elaborated by Chuang Tzu contributed to the popularity of Zen Buddhism in China in the seventh and eighth centuries. The aim was to achieve enlightenment, impartiality, universality and harmony with nature. Meditation was not perceived as a method to cope with stress as such, but as a general way of being.

Yoga takes many forms like *karma yoga* or yoga of action, *bhakti yoga* or yoga of devotion, *jnana yoga* or the yoga of knowledge, and *raj yoga* or the eight-stage yoga of Patanjali. Though the last one is universally popular, individual differences require choice of emphasis among the first three. The fourth one is an elementary level for any yogic pursuit. In the yoga of action, a person engages in his business or action as a matter of duty without expecting any outcome and this engagement itself is the life goal for him. In the yoga of devotion one does everything as a representative of God and surrenders himself completely to him; he is temperamentally emotional with a marked degree of love and compassion. In the yoga of knowledge, a person uses his high intellectual ability in understanding the truth; his tremendous awareness, insight and wisdom make him a philosopher.

These three ways are the common modes or inclinations of human functioning representing action, emotion and thought. People achieve their life goals through an emphasis that varies along these three dimensions. The same approach is also used in dealing with obstacles producing stress or suffering in the achievement of life goals. Persons resort to one or more of these ways according to their temperament while coping with stress.

REFERENCES

Bowker, J. (1970). *Problems of suffering in religions of the world*. Cambridge: Cambridge University Press.

Caraka. (1949). *Carakasamhita*, Vol. III with translation in Hindi, Gujarati, and English. Jamnagar: Shri Gulabkunverba Ayurvedic Society.

Chan, W. T. (Trans.). (1963). *The way of Lao-Tzu (Tao-te ching)*. Indianapolis: Bobbs-Merrill.

Cofer, C. N. and Appley, M. H. (1964). *Motivation: Theory and research*. New York: Wiley.

Cox, T. (1981). *Stress*. London: Macmillan.

de Bary, W. T., Chan, W. T. and Watson, B. (1960). *Sources of Chinese tradition*, Vol. I. New York: Columbia University Press.

Evans, G. W. and Cohen, S. (1987). Environmental stress. In D. Stokols and I. Altman (Eds), *Handbook of environmental psychology*. New York: John Wiley.

Evans, G. W., Palsane, M. N. and D'Souza, R. (1983). Life stress and health in India. *Indian Psychologist*, 2(2), 62-78.

Evans, G. W., Shapiro, H. H. and Lewis, M. A. (In press). Specifying dysfunctional mismatches between different control dimensions. *British Journal of Psychology*, 83, 34-45.

Hong, Y. Y. and Lam, D. J. (1992). Appraisal, coping, and guilt as correlates of test anxiety. In K. Hagrvet and T. Backer Johnsen (Eds), *Advances in test anxiety research*, Vol. 7 (pp. 277-87). Lisse: Swets and Zeitlinger.

Kakar, S. (1982). *Shamans, mystics and doctors: A psychological inquiry into India and its healing traditions*. Bombay: Oxford University Press.

Kane, P. V. (1962). *History of Dharmasastra*, Vol. V, Part II. Pune: Bhandarkar Oriental Research Institute.

Kulkarni, T. R. (1972). *Upanishads and Yoga*. Bombay: Bharatiya Vidya Bhavan.

Lazarus, R. S. (1976). *Patterns of adjustment* (3rd ed.). Tokyo: McGraw-Hill Kogakusha.

Naidu, R. K. (1986). Belief, trust, impulse control and health. *Journal of Social and Economic Studies*, 3(4), 370-77.

Palsane, M. N. (1987). Yoga as psychotherapy. In M. L. Gharote and M. Lockhart (Eds), *The art of survival*. London: Unwin Paperbacks.

Palsane, M. N., Bhavsar, S. N., Goswami, R. P. and Evans, G. W. (1986). The concept of stress in the Indian tradition. *Journal of Indian Psychology*, 5(1), 1-12.

Pande, N. and Naidu, R. K. (1986). Effort and outcome orientations as moderators of stress-strain relationship. *Psychological Studies*, 31(2), 207-14.

Radhakrishnan, S. (1979). *Bhagvadgita*. Bombay: Blackie.

Rao, S. K. R. (1983). The conception of stress in Indian thought: I. The theoretical aspects of stress in Sankhya and Yoga systems, and II. The practical involvement in Gita and Ayurveda. *NIMHANS Journal*, 1(2), 115-31.

Rhys Davids, T. W. (Trans.). (1973). *Buddhist Sutras* (translation of Dhamma-Chakkappavattana-sutta). Delhi: Motilal Banarsidass.

Rothbaum, F., Weisz, J. R. and Snyder, S. S. (1982). Changing the world and changing the self: A two-process model of perceived control. *Journal of Personality and Social Psychology*, 42(1), 25-37.

Rotter, J. B. (1966). Generalised expectancies for internal versus external control of reinforcement. *Psychological Monographs*, 80, 1-28.

Safaya, R. (1976). *Indian psychology*. New Delhi: Munshiram Manoharlal.

Sankaracharya. (1972). *Srisankaragranthavali*, Samputa 11 (Yogataravali) (4th ed.). Srirangam: Srivanivilasa-Mudranalaya.

Shejwal, B. R. (1984). *A study of life events stress and some of us personality correlates*. Doctoral dissertation, University of Poona, Pune.

Sinha, Jadunath. (1986). *Indian psychology: Vol. II, Emotion and will*. Delhi: Motilal Banarsidass.

Srivastava, A. K., Naidu, R. K. and Misra, G. (1986). *Impulse control, stress and performance*. Unpublished paper (Personal communication).

Taimni, I. K. (1961). *The science of yoga*. Adyar, Madras: The Theosophical Publishing House.

Taylor, S. E. (1983). Adjustment to threatening events: A theory of cognitive adaptation. *American Psychologist*, 38(11), 1161-173.

Woods, J. H. (1914). *The Yoga system of Patanjali*. Cambridge, MA: Harvard University Press.

4

Concept of Psycho-social Well-being: Western and Indian Perspectives

DURGANAND SINHA

An invocation that is popular even today among people aptly reflects the universal and perennial concern for the well-being of the entire mankind. It runs as:

> Sarve Bhavantu Sukhinah Sarve Santu Niramayah,
> Sarve Bhadrani Pashyantu Makashchitdduhkhabhagbhavet.

(Let everyone be prosperous, let everyone be without disease and let no one think of unhappiness of anyone.)

The sloka embodies the essence of what could be regarded as the characteristics of the state of human well-being. The Hindu scriptures, especially *Carakasamhita* are replete with passages reflecting similar concern for the man and steps to ensure his health and welfare. Though the importance of the well-being is accepted by everyone, it is rarely that effort has been made to analyze systematically and scientifically its various constituents, and outline the indicators that would give an accurate idea of the state of his well-being. Except for a very small circle of people, mostly scholars and a few administrators and policy makers, very little serious effort has been made to define well-being, and indicate how to assess reliably that a person is enjoying such a state. Popularly, whenever we talk of well-being, the factors of health and material condition of the individual and the community inevitably come to the fore. It is thought that a person is happy if he is free from ailments and is in good health and when his family possesses enough means to meet his physical needs and other demands. But equating well-being with health and economic condition alone is taking a very partial and narrow view of man that ignores mental, psychological and social aspects of his existence. Though physical and material aspects are important, we cannot meaningfully talk of well-being without taking into account the individual's entire existential condition. In view of the primary importance of health, nutrition and economic status, the focus has naturally been on the physical and material aspects. But his psychological and social development, the kinds of adjustment he learns to make with various aspects of his environment and the unfolding of his personality as a whole are equally important. Therefore, apart from designing and initiating policies and programmes to ensure his well-being, it is also essential to have a clear idea as to what well-being actually means, and develop a set of indicators.

Since a lot of confusion and ambiguity prevails in this area, it is necessary to define and elucidate the concept of 'well-being' and delimit its meaning in the context of other related concepts. In psychological as well as popular parlance, the concepts that are used frequently when talking about well-being are welfare, adjustment, adaptation, balance, equilibrium, homeostasis, competence and health. In recent years, the expression 'quality of life' has also come in. Well-being seems to share certain elements from each of these inter-related concepts.

Well-being is an expression commonly used in popular parlance, and does not usually find a place in technical literature. Therefore, it is all the more essential to define it and delimit its meaning. In its widest sense, and as defined in Oxford Dictionary, 'well-being' is equated with 'welfare' which in turn is conceptualized as 'satisfactory state, health, prosperity'. It denotes a desirable state of affairs of the individual that ensures proper development of his potential so that he is able to meet the various demands of his environment, and satisfy his needs in a socially acceptable manner. The technical concept that comes closest to it is that of 'adjustment'. Ruch and Warren (1958, p. 590) in their textbook *Psychology and Life* define the 'adjustment process' as 'the continuous process of attempting to overcome inner and outer obstacles to the satisfaction of biological and social needs'. It implies a continuous process of interaction between the individual and his environment. Some sort of maladjustment of the organism to its particular environment is a basic requirement. The environment is made up of not only physical objects but other individuals, social institutions and situations which not only provide objects and means of satisfying the various needs of the individual, but often serve as obstacles to their satisfaction. Some of the normal processes of the individual get thwarted. The disturbing factors may be the agents outside the organism (extra-organic) or, in some instances, intra-organic. Maladjustment is an organism–environment fact, not just the one or the other. Expressed in Lewinian terms, B=f (PE), i.e., the behaviour is a function of both the person and the environment in dynamic inter-relation. Adjustment is equated with those responses which denote harmonious and effective relationship with the environment whereby psychological growth is promoted. In Wolman's dictionary (Wolman, 1973), it is defined as 'harmonious relationship with environment involving the ability to satisfy most of one's needs and meet most of the demands, both physical and social, that are put upon one'.

It is to be noted that in this definition, the aspect of ability for satisfying one's needs has been emphasized. In other words, as a result of interactions with his environment, the individual *learns* or acquires certain skills and abilities which are instrumental in meeting the demands of his environment and in satisfaction of his needs. According to Thompson (1965), psychological adjustment denotes the ways that individuals modify their behaviour patterns to reach goals or incentives that satisfy their psychological and physical needs. It is obvious that well-being implies that the environment provides the necessary inputs for the proper development of those skills and abilities through which he is able to satisfy his basic and psychological needs, and thereby achieve a degree of adjustment. A state of maladjustment would denote absence of such conditions or presence of factors that prevent the satisfaction of his needs and thereby militate against his well-being. As such, the concepts of adjustment and well-being are very similar.

Most individuals are able to adjust to their natural environments within the normal range. It, however, does not imply that normally adjusted individuals are able to fulfil all their needs and reach all of the goals they project for themselves or that they never suffer from various degrees of frustration. Most of the striving behaviour eventuates in the attainment of reasonably adequate goals which are acceptable to society at large, and that denotes a state of psychological well-being. But frustrations due to non-fulfilment of one's goals are also matters of common experience.

Thompson (1965) has spelt out at some length the psychological processes that are associated with a satisfactory state of well-being. The person who makes majority of his adjustments within normal range has learned to do the following: (*a*) deny or delay immediate need satisfaction for long-term gains, (*b*) perceive difference between socially acceptable and unacceptable goals that promise to satisfy his needs, (c) select goals that are realistic and within his grasp, (d) select goals for satisfying his needs that maximize his psychological abilities, for example, compensation mechanism whereby he *substitutes*, if necessary, his goals that cannot be satisfied, (e) vary his behaviour, (f) satisfy majority of his psychological needs on 'reality level' rather than resort frequently to fantasy, (g) develop tolerance for frustration, and making goal-oriented rather than ego-defensive reactions to frustration, (h) tolerate a reasonable amount of anxiety so that his behaviour is not disrupted, (i) seek variety of goals to satisfy his psychological needs so that development of monomanias and socially unacceptable eccentricities in behavior patterns is prevented, (j) accept natural and social outcomes of his behaviour and plans for future accordingly, i.e., profit from experience, re-evaluate the situation and try another approach, (k) develop warm personal relationships with a reasonable number of associates, (l) face future, re-direct his behaviour in terms of past experience, and not be psychologically paralyzed by guilt feelings over past failures, inadequacies and behaviour transgressions, and (m) self-report that he feels 'happy', 'adequate' and so on. It is also to be noted that successful adjustment invariably implies capacity to handle stress or stressful situation. The individual is able to cope with it without much cost. He reacts to it in positive ways. Rather than being overwhelmed by stress, it enriches rather than damages him. In fact, in one of the ancient Indian verses, it is said that an adjusted individual is not too disturbed either by sorrow or by joy. The mechanism of coping is well illustrated in a line of a folk song that is popular in North East India, immortalized by the famous writer Phanishwarnath Renu in his popular story *Teesari Kasam* (Third Vow): *Phate kaleja gavo geet, dukh sahne ka ekahi reet* (When your heart is broken in sorrow, singing is the only way of bearing it).

Looking from the reverse angle, absence of well-being would mean that the individual makes maladjustive responses to the environment so that his needs are not satisfied, and when faced with problem-solving situations, conflicts and frustrations, he reacts in what is often termed as ego-defensive ways which hardly enable him to cope successfully with his problems. He experiences unhappiness, anxiety, frustration, depression and so on which are all indicative of absence of psycho-social well-being. It is to be noted that in course of his life, every individual experiences every day many such frustrations, anxieties and stresses. Apart from daily hassles, many of these frustration may have far-reaching consequences. But most people are able to tolerate and cope with them. Instead of being overwhelmed by intensive anxiety which is debilitating and saps the available energy of the individual so that he is unable to solve the problems, a healthy, adjusted and normal person bounces back from those frustrations, disappointments and disabling states, and continues on his path of goal-oriented behaviour. To use an analogy, the individual is like gold which when put into fire comes out shining and more brilliant.

These dynamic qualities of normal psychological adjustment illustrate the complexity of the problem. Well-being is related to all aspects of psychological growth of the individual—physical, perception, language skills, intelligence, sociability and social sensitivity, emotional maturity, learning, enduring aspects of personality and cultural values. Normal adjustment and psycho-social well-being is very much related to cultural and social values of a particular society. Further, a person may be considered well adjusted in one situation (for example, in his home) but poorly adjusted in another (for example, at his work). This relativity of psychological adjustment is to be borne in mind when diagnosing on the basis of limited sample of his behaviour whether the individual is adjusted or maladjusted. Thus, well-being or what could be termed as normal psychological adjustment is a relative state of affairs—relative to the situation as well as to the values of a particular culture or subculture. Well-being would often differ in connotation from one culture to another. Basic theoretical and cross-cultural issues in defining well-being are encountered. While there are quite a few 'universals' in identifying and assessing a person's well-being, one has to view him in a particular socio-cultural and economic context, and spell out the factors of well-being in specific socio-cultural setting.

Psycho-social well-being or 'good' health in that both are desirable state of affairs, are well recognized, but difficult to define. The latter is often negatively defined as absence of ill health or as the relative absence of physiological malfunctioning in an organism. It has been taken to consist in freedom from any subjective feelings of discomfort or disability and from any objective disturbances of functions. According to this approach which has till lately been popular in psychology in conceptualizing 'normality', 'mental health' and so on, one can understand health by studying conditions of its absence, i.e., when things had gone wrong with the adjustive organism. Thus, one of the ways to understand well-being would be to locate and identify the maladjustive patterns of behaviour like *aggressive* responses (when he breaks, destroys, objects, injures himself or others and resorts to verbal aggression), *withdrawal* responses (he goes frequently into fantasy, becomes uncommunicative), *rationalization* (frequently shifting blame for his inadequacies to another person, displays 'sour grapes' mechanism), *regression* (goes back to infantile level of behaviour like temper tantrums, loss of motor or language skill) and *psychosomatic disturbances* (development of anorexia, loss of appetite, headaches, diarrohoea, and other physiological malfunctionings). These may be the first indicators of absence of psycho-social well-being in a person.

Health in recent times has been conceptualized in more positive terms. According to the constitution of the WHO, health is a state of complete physical, mental and social well-being, and is not merely the absence of disease or infirmity. This is very close to the definition of health in various treatise of Indian medical science. Sushrut, the ancient proponent of the traditional system of medicine, defined health as *prasannan-mendriyamanah swastha*. That is, health is a state of delight or a feeling of spiritual, physical and mental well-being (Sharma, 1981, pp. 239-40). In the sloka (chapter 16, verse 41), aspect of *sama* (in right or natural quantity) has been emphasized. Essential features of a healthy person is that he possesses *in right quantity* (neither too little nor too much) the defects or weaknesses (*samadosah*), digestive quality (*samagni*), semen (*samadhatu*) and whose bodily functions are normal (*malakriyah*). In *Carakasamhita* the ancient work on the Indian system of medicine, which is rightly designated as the *Ayurveda* (the treatise on life), the characteristics of happy and unhappy life (*sukhswarup* and *dukhswarup*) have been elaborated.

> Life is said to be happy if the person is not afflicted with any somatic and psychic disorder, is particularly youthful, capable with strength, energy, reputation, manliness and prowess, possessing knowledge, specific knowledge and strong sense organs and sense objects, having immense wealth and various favourable enjoyments, has achieved desired results of all actions and moves about where he likes; contrary to it is unhappy life. (chapter 30, sloka 22)

Further, life is said to be beneficial (*hitayu*) if the person is a well-wisher of all creatures; is abstaining from taking other's possession; is truthful and calm, is taking steps after examining the situation; is free from carelessness; is observing the three categories (virtue, wealth and enjoyment) without their mutual conflict; is worshipping the worthy person; is devoted to knowledge; is understanding and has serenity of mind; is keeping company of elderly persons; has controlled all the impulses of attachment, aversion and envy, intoxication and conceit; is engaged in various types of gifts; is constantly devoted to penance, knowledge and peace; has knowledge and devotion to metaphysics; is keeping eye to both the worlds; and is endowed with memory and intelligence. Opposite of it is non-beneficial life (*ahitayu*) (chapter 30, sloka 24).

It is worth observing that health was conceived in very wide sense which comprised the total well-being and happiness. It was not only equated with the possession of health and absence of ailments, but cultivation of certain psychological qualities, personality characteristics and intellectual and moral values like memory, intelligence, freedom from inner conflicts, absence of carelessness, devotion to knowledge, control of impulses, envy, and conceit, serenity, truthfulness and the like were considered as its essential constituents. Since the foundations of these behavioural characteristics and dispositions are laid early in childhood, many of these require to be emphasized in the socialization and education of the child if he is to develop into a healthy and well-adjusted human being.

In traditional Indian conceptualization of the state of well-being, mental health appears to be regarded as an essential aspect of health. In any case, the concept of mental health is nearer to that of psycho-social well-being. The former is often defined in terms of adaptation to the environment and internal equipoise or equilibrium. Wolman (1973) defines it as 'a state of relatively good adjustment, feelings of well-being and actualization of one's potentialities and capacities'. It is an essential element of *sukhaswarup* or happy life. It is to be noted that any attempt at defining it inevitably has reference to socio-cultural environment. In some environments, stresses and demands upon the individual warp him and induce mental illness, no matter how healthy he would have been under happier environment. Thus, in understanding well-being one has to take account of the nature of the environment in which the individual functions.

There are a few other related concepts which require some elucidation. The physiological concept of adaptation (often restricted to sensory sphere) or its biological meaning of structural or behavioural changes in the organism or of its part, so that it fits more perfectly to the altered conditions in environment and having survival value, has been used in a more general sense and, in certain ways, defines well-being. In this sense, adaptation means any beneficial modification in the organism or the system that is necessary to meet the environmental demands. The emphasis is on the capacity to modify oneself to cope with changed circumstances, which is an integral aspect of well-being.

Homeostasis is another relevant concept. In its original form, it connotes internal form of self-regulation for maintaining an internal bodily balance or adjustment. As Cannon (1932) in his famous treatise *The wisdom of the body* points out,

> Organism, composed of material which is characterized by the utmost inconstancy and unsteadiness, have somehow learned the method of

maintaining constancy and keeping steady in the presence of conditions which might reasonably be expected to prove profoundly disturbing ... somehow the unstable stuff of which we are composed had learned the trick of maintaining stability.

From internal self-regulatory mechanism, the connotation of homeostasis has been expanded to comprise the process of psychological and even social adjustment. As Freeman (1948) has observed, when the tendency of the organism or the individual is to maintain its normality against internal and external disrupting agencies, the alterations made by him in his relations to physical and social surroundings are the phenomena are called psychological. Psychological adjustments are homeostatic phenomena writ large. Thus, from physiological homeostasis as exemplified by maintenance of body temperature or oxygen–carbondioxide balance and so on which are largely automatic, the concept has acquired a psychological connotation to include perceptual, intellectual functioning of the individual and even social relationships. It is a compensatory adjustment to meet any threat to personality (Drever, 1952) or a state of balance the individual maintains during the process of living. The balance is continually upset and recreated through complex interactions. Therefore, homeostasis is a dynamic equilibrium, because the individual is constantly taking corrective/adjustive action to restore the equilibrium.

The organism has learned to achieve a state of balance even on psychological and social planes, which is to be taken as an important component of individual's psycho-social well-being. In fact, individual's constant effort for such an equilibrium, which of course is dynamic and ever changing, is a useful way of describing many of the varieties of interactions between the individual and his world.

As it has already been observed, in traditional Indian treatise on medicine, similar idea of maintaining balance has been constantly emphasized in the context of health and ill health. Having various qualities in right or natural quantities (*sama*) is considered essential for health. *Asantulan* (imbalance) is the cause of illness:

> *Vikaro dhatuvaisamyam, samyam prakritiruchayte, Sukhsamgraka-ogyam, vikaro duhkhameva cha.* (chapter 9, sloka 4)

(Any disturbance in the equilibrium of *dhatu*—*vata, pitta* and *kapha*—is known as disease, and on the other hand, the state of their equilibrium is health). (Sharma and Dash, 1976)

This aspect of avoidance of extremes and thereby maintaining an equilibrium is considered vital to man's health:

Ati sarvatra varjayet
(Excess is to be avoided everywhere.)

This is true not only with regard to bodily functions, pleasures of senses, but with the total life and conduct. In Buddhist philosophy also, avoidance of extremes and adoption of middle (*madhyama*) path has been emphasized all through, which implies maintaining a kind of equilibrium.

In Sankhya philosophy, however, the idea of equilibrium has been greatly elaborated. The world is constituted by the three *gunas* or qualities called the *sattva* or the element of pleasure and illumination, *rajas* or priniciple of activity which on the affective side is the cause of all painful experiences and is of the nature of pain (*dukha*), and *Tamas* or principle of passivity that clouds our intellect thereby producing ignorance, confusion and bewilderment (*moha*). *Tamas* by obstructing activity induces sleep, drowziness and laziness, and produces the state of apathy or indifference (*vishada*). The relation among the three *gunas* constituting the world is one of the constant conflict as well as cooperation. These three always go together, and the nature of things as well as the state that the individual experiences is determined by the predominant *guna*. It is on the basis of preponderance of one or the other *guna* that one becomes intelligent, active or indolent, and experiences various degrees of well-being or otherwise. It is the state of *samyavastha* or equilibrium of the three that holds the secret to an individual's well-being.

According to Sankhya, our life on this earth is a mixture of joys and sorrows, pleasures and pains. There are many pleasures of life, and though many creatures have a good share of them, many more are the pains and sufferings of life, and *all* living beings are subject to them. There are three kinds of pain that go against our well-being, namely, the *adhyatmika*, *adhibhautika* and *adhidaivika*. The first is due to intra-organic causes like bodily disorders and mental affections which include bodily pains, pangs of fear, anger, greed and so on. The second is produced by extra-organic natural causes such as snake-bite, pain on being hit by objects, murder and so on. The third kind of suffering is caused by extra-organic supernatural causes such as pain inflicted by ghosts, demons and so on.

All men desire to avoid every kind of pain, and attain a state of enjoyment and well-being for all times by putting an end to all sufferings. But, on this earth we cannot have pleasure only and exclude pain altogether.

Therefore, during one's earthly existence the best a person can do is to maintain a kind of balance or equilibrium which is itself a state of well-being. However, for complete freedom from all pain and suffering and experiencing a state of absolute well-being, attainment of liberation is essential. It is only after the removal of our ignorance and gaining knowledge into the nature of reality that liberation (*mukti*) can be attained. The Sankhya philosophy like other Indian systems of knowledge has laid down the necessary steps for removal of ignorance and ending all sufferings.

The idea of avoidance of extremes and maintaining a kind of balance or equilibrium in all human functioning is repeatedly considered in *Bhagavadgita* to be the characteristic of a person who is wise and can enjoy a state of psychological well-being. Of the numerous verses stating the idea, a selection of them is given here. Along with the emphasis on equipoise, a number of psychological qualities have been indicated which are regarded as essential for well-being. The characteristics that have been emphasized are that a calm man is the same in pain and pleasure (chapter II verse 15: *samadukha-sukhatndhiram*); he is equipoised in success and failure: *sidhyasidhyoh samo* (chapter II, verse 48); he is content with what comes to him without effort, is unaffected by conflict, and is free from envy; he is even-minded in success and failure and is not bound even while acting: *Yadrichchhalavasantustho dvandvatito vimatsarah, samah sidhavasiddhou cha kritvanapi na nibadhyate* (chapter IV, verse 22). Further, he hates no creatures and is friendly and compassionate towards all (*advesta sarvabhutanam mitram karuna eva cha*), and who is free from the feelings of 'I' and 'mine', even-minded in pleasure and pain (*nirmamo nirahan-karah samdukhasukha kshami*), forbearing, ever content, steady in meditation, self-controlled and possessed of firm conviction (chapter XII, verses 13 and 14: *santustam satatan yogi yatatma dhriranischaya*); he is such as cannot be agitated by the world (*lokan-nodvijate*) or is free from joy, envy, fear and anxiety (chapter XII; verse 15: *harsdmarsabhayodvegaimukto*); he is free from dependence (*anapekshah*), pure and prompt (*shuchirdakha*), unconcerned and untroubled (*udasino gatavyathah*), renouncing every undertaking (*sarvarambhaparityagi*) (chapter XII, verse 16). In the next three verses, a few more characteristics have been enumerated: he neither rejoices nor hates (*na hrisyati na dvesthi*), neither grieves at the parting of beloved object nor shows longing for it (*na shochati na kanksati*), he renounces both good and evil (*shubhashubha parityagi*) and is full of devotion (*bhaktiman*); he who is same for friend and foe and in honour and dishonour (*samah shatrau cha mitre' cha tatha manapamanayah*), he is same in cold and heat and is free from all attachment (*shitosnasukhadukhesu samah sangavivarjitah*); for him censure and praise are equal, is silent, content with anything, homeless, steady minded and full of devotion (*tulyanindastutirmauni santusto yenakenachit aniketah sthirmatirbhaktimanme*).

The qualities and the psychological characteristics outlined above are of course ideal. However, they give an idea of the psychological, moral, and spiritual characteristics of an individual that would ensure his total well-being. It would be too much to expect the presence of such qualities in the average person. But when considering what constitutes well-being, these cannot be ignored, and should be regarded as normative and indicative of those features in man which are valued in the society.

Another concept which is relevant and integral to well-being is that of competence. It refers to individual's capacity to control and master his environment. It is the skill to deal with the environment in such a way as to satisfy his needs as well as maintain a state of balance or equilibrium within himself and with the environment. Which one of these two aspects of competence is emphasized varies from culture to culture. In the West generally, competence in the sense of exercising control over environment is stressed so that one has the capacity to utilize the available resources for his own well-being. In India and in some other eastern cultures, this aspect of control and exploitation of environment for one's own good is underplayed, and competence is regarded more as a capacity to develop and maintain a harmonious relationship with environment which is vital to individual well-being. It is more a question of being *in tune* with one's environment. Analogy of jungle fighting could be advanced to bring out the difference in emphasis. In one case it would mean remove the *jungle to fight* (as the US army seems to have tried in Vietnam), and the other approach would be to *fight in the jungle* (as the Vietnamese guerrilla fighters had done). In fact, it is related to the whole question of model of man that is prevalent in the culture concerned. As has been pointed out (Sinha, 1981, p. 7), the model of man in the West is one of 'man *and* the environment'. A kind of dichotomy between the two is implied. As far as the Indian tradition goes, the model is 'man–environment' or 'man–society', i.e., a kind of symbiotic relationship between man and his society or the environment where you cannot separate one from the other. Unlike in the West where well-being implies to a great extent mastery and control over environment and exercising control over others, in the Indian ethos, it consists to a great extent in establishing harmony with the environment and unfolding of one's own potential therein. Unfolding of potentialities of the self is emphasized more and mastery over external environment is considered only secondary to one's well-being. For well-being, one is expected to develop a relationship with environment that is not distracting or disturbing. It is implied in the expression *nirlipt* or non-involvement, and in the definition of a well-developed wise man given in *Bhagavadgita*: that he is not unduly perturbed in sorrow, and in happiness he is not overwhelmed.

In recent years, a related concept that has entered both scientific discussions and popular conversations is that of *quality of life*. It is considered to be a composite measure of physical, mental and social well-being as perceived by each individual or group of individuals, and of happiness, satisfaction and gratification involving mainly such non-esoteric life concerns as health, marriage, family, work, housing, financial situation, educational opportunities, self-esteem, creativity, competence, belongingness, and trust in others (Andrews and Withy, 1976; Campbell and Converse, 1970). It generally covers overall satisfaction as well as satisfaction in the component areas. Being somewhat polymorphous, it tends to cover a variety of areas such as physical and psychological complaints, feeling of well-being, personal functioning and general limitations (Nagpal and Sell, 1985). Thus, the quality of life can be evaluated by taking a number of aspects of a person's life and assessing person's subjective feelings of happiness or unhappiness about the various life concerns.

Like all other indicators of well-being, it has both objective and subjective components. The former relates to things like education, employment status, financial resources and comforts of modern living, i.e., what is generally known as standard of living. In an United Nations publication, a parallel expression is used, 'level of living' (United Nations, 1961) which is said to consist of nine components: health, food consumption, education, occupation and work conditions, housing, social security, clothing, recreation and leisure, and human rights. All these characteristics are supposed to influence human well-being. Further, it is felt that mere availability of goods and services to the individual or the community does not, in itself, determine his satisfaction and well-being but also his expectations and perceptions of reality which is often referred to as the subjective component of quality of life or subjective well-being, or well-being as *experienced* by each individual. It is believed to be a function of the degree of congruence between the individual's wishes and needs on the one hand and environmental demands and opportunities on the other.

It is, however, to be noted that the relationship between economic resources and objective components of well-being and his subjective well-being is not linear, but curvilinear and complex. It is generally observed that up to a certain level of living, the major determinant of well-being is the 'fit' or matching between objective or situational characteristic and the individual's expectations, abilities, and needs as perceived by the individual. At a lower level, every increase in amenities is likely to result in a direct increase in subjective well-being. But beyond a certain point, the relationship is not so direct, and any prediction becomes difficult. Beyond that threshold even an increase in economic resources, housing or leisure time need not necessarily be accompanied by high level or an increase in individual satisfaction or well-being.

Quite frequently the problem of well-being is viewed within the framework of Maslow's theory of hierarchy of needs. Man's most vital needs are concerned with his *survival*. His social needs relate to his *security* and the community comes in later, while the higher order ego-related needs concern his self-fulfilment and are designated as *self-actualization*. It has been contended that there is a general tendency to ignore higher order needs until those relating to his survival have been satisfied. But once this is done, higher order needs become more salient. Thus, as a policy the first essential step towards man's well-being is to guarantee the satisfaction of the basic needs that ensure his survival, health and physical welfare. Once that is achieved, it is not enough merely to be concerned with reducing morbidity and mortality and protecting his health. At that stage, the entire spectrum of his well-being and quality of life undergoes a transformation, and there is an increasing emphasis on psychosocial aspects of living. Therefore, any social policy on human well-being has to take into cognizance sooner rather than later the satisfaction of his social and community needs and ensuring a sense of self-fulfilment.

Thus, there is certain amount of difference not only about the concept itself but also in what is regarded as well-being among various cultural and subcultural groups. By and large in the conceptualizations made in the West, the ability to satisfy one's needs, avoidance of frustrations and stress and exercising certain amount of control on the environment are emphasized. Even with regard to the concept of homeostasis, it is the disturbance caused in the bodily state, and thwarting or blocking of one's needs that lead to a state of disequilibrium which the organism/individual tends to avoid. Since it is the environment that provides the inputs that lead to need satisfaction, the strategy that inevitably suggests itself is one of conquering or exploiting it to enhance the satisfaction of personal and social needs. Even social environment is sought to be influenced and shaped so that it satisfies various psychological and social needs of the individual. In the Indian tradition, the approach is entirely different. Firstly, control over the senses is considered essential. While total denial of needs is not implied, what is emphasized through and through is the maintenance of *balance* between extremes of satisfaction and denial, as also the adoption of a path of moderation. Secondly, realizing the inevitability of frustration, failure as well as success, sorrows and joys, it is repeatedly emphasized that not being overwhelmed by either is the essence of one's well-being.

Lastly, adjustment does not so much consist of controlling and exploiting the environment as in maintaining a harmonious relationship with it. Here, the key concept is *being in tune* rather than conquering the environment. Thus, the values in child rearing that are likely to be emphasized, and the behavioural qualities inculcated in the child through socialization and education for the sake of his well-being are likely to differ from culture to culture depending upon the world view and the nature of man–environment relationship that is conceptualized. Therefore, in spelling out indicators for psycho-social well-being, cross-national and inter-community differences in conceptualization of well-being have to be kept in mind.

REFERENCES

Andrews, F. M. and Withy, S. B. (1976). *Social indicators of well-being—American's perceptions of life quality.* New York: Plenum Press.

Campbell, A. and Converse, P. (1970). *Monitoring the quality of American life: A proposal to the Russell Sage foundation.* Ann Arbor: Survey Research Centre, University of Michigan.

Cannon, W. B. (1932). *The wisdom of the body.* New York: Norton & Co.

Drever, J. (1952). *A dictionary of psychology.* Harmondsworth, Middlesex: Penguin Books.

Freeman, G. L. (1948). *The energetics of human behaviour.* Ithaca, NY: Cornell University Press.

Nagpal, R. and Sell, H. (1985). *Subjective well-being.* New Delhi: World Health Organisation Regional Office for South-East Asia.

Ruch, F. L. and Warren, N. (1958). *Psychology and life.* Chicago: Scott, Foresman & Co.

Sharma, P. (1981). *Charaka samhita* (English translation). Varanasi: Chaukhambha Orientalia.

Sharma, R. K. and Dash, B. (1976). *Charaka samhita.* Varanasi: Choukhambha Sanskrit Series Office.

Sinha, D. (1981). Social psychology in India: A historical perspective. In J. Pandy (Ed.), *Perspectives on experimental social psychology in India.* New Delhi: Concept Publishing Co.

Thompson, D. D. (1965). *Child psychology.* Bombay: Times of India Press.

United Nations. (1961). *International definition of measurement of levels of living: An interim guide.* U.N. Publication 61, IV. 7.

Wolman, B. B. (Ed.). (1973). *Dictionary of behavioural sciences.* New York: Van Nostrand Reinhold.

5

Cultural Perspectives on Nature and Experience of Happiness

ASHOK K. SRIVASTAVA AND GIRISHWAR MISRA

The ultimate aim of all human activity can broadly be described as an ongoing quest for greater happiness. To be happy is the very core of all human motivation. In almost all societies, people rank the quest for happiness as one of their most cherished goals in life (Diener and Oishi, 2000). Fordyce (1987) conducted several hundred polls with students and adults to know 'what is the most important thing in life'. The most common response was 'happiness', which was followed by 'love', 'success', 'good health' and 'my religion'. In a survey (Diener and Lucas, 2004) across 48 nations, people desired high levels of happiness and fearlessness for their children. Considering the importance of happiness, the Government of Bhutan has already declared itself concerned with gross national happiness (Bond, 2003). In the Indian context, a questionnaire was administered to 817 people aged 25–55 years, residing in eight major cities (*Outlook*, 2005). About 75 per cent respondents reported that they were happy. About 99 per cent respondents believed that their parents were happier in comparison to them. More than half reported that peaceful state of mind provided them happiness (52 per cent), which was followed by health (50 per cent), success at work (43 per cent), family (40 per cent), money (38 per cent), love (33 per cent), etc.

People in general across the world report that they would need following, in order of priority, for their lives to be completely happy: material living conditions, happy family life, personal or family health, interesting job and personal characteristics such as emotional stability, self-discipline, etc. (Easterlin, 2004). Rice and Steele (2004), in a recent study, have shown that the aspects of culture that influence subjective well-being are passed from people who lived centuries ago to their contemporary descendents and also travel with people as they emigrate to faraway lands. The societies seem to have normal baseline levels of well-being that are culturally determined, which do change but the rate of change is slow (Inglehart and Klingemann, 2000).

The experience of happiness shows considerable degree of individual and group variations. Some people have the capacity to be remarkably happy, even in the face of adverse circumstances or hard times. They appear to have a talent for happiness, see the world around them through rose-coloured glasses, make out the silver lining even in misfortune, live in the present and find joy in the little things from day-to-day circumstances and events. In contrast, there are persons who, even in best of times, seem chronically unhappy, peering at the world through grey coloured glasses, always complaining, accentuating the negative, dwelling on the down side of the trivial and sublime and generally deriving little pleasure from life. Thus, anecdotal evidence and everyday experience alike suggest that one of the most salient and significant dimensions of human experience and emotional life is happiness.

Happiness as a state of mind may be universal, but its meaning and conceptualization vary across cultures. The cultural syndrome of individualism–collectivism seems to be prominently related to happiness. Studies (Diener, Diener and Diener, 1995; Schyns, 1998; Veenhoven, 1997) have shown that people in individualist cultures tend to report higher satisfaction and happiness with their lives than in collectivist cultures. In individualist cultures, happiness is often seen as a reflection of personal achievement. Being unhappy may mean that one has not made the most of one's life. Individualists are more likely to see themselves as separate from other people (autonomous self), and thus, individuals' needs, goals and desires are weighted heavily. In contrast, the collectivists often see the self as intertwined with other people (interdependent self), and relations with others are emphasized. In collectivistic cultures, behaviour and emotions are dependent on norms and duties of the community or group (Kitayama and Markus, 1994; Triandis, 1994). It may, therefore, be appropriate to assume that meaning of happiness would vary in individualistic and collectivistic cultures. It has been argued (Kitayama and Markus, 2000) that happiness in individualistic cultures is bound to be subjective, personal or individual in scope, while it is more relational, intersubjective, communal and collective in scope in collectivistic societies. Kinnier, Kernes, Tribbensee and Van Puymbroeck (2003) examined what eminent people have said about the meaning of life. Ten themes were identified from the writings of 195 eminent people. About 17 per cent of the sample endorsed the view that life is 'to enjoy or experience, enjoy the "moment", "the journey"'. The second theme, life is 'to love, help, or serve others; to show or experience compassion', was endorsed by 13 per cent of the sample. Mohandas Gandhi and the Dalai Lama were among the people who endorsed the second theme. Gandhi said, 'My consolation and my happiness are to be found in service of all that lives, because the Divine essence is the sum total of all life' (Durant, 1932, p. 84). Studies (for example, Chang, 1996; Kitayama, Markus and Kurokawa, 2000; Lu, Gilmour and Kao, 2001; Lu and Shih, 1997) further reveal that the conception of happiness in East Asia refers to harmony of interpersonal relationships, achievement at work and contentment with life. It particularly refers to a tranquil state of mind achieved through harmony with other people, with society and with nature.

This chapter clarifies the meaning of happiness and other related concepts. It further analyses the nature of happiness as understood and practised in the West. In view of the variations in the nature of self in the Western and Eastern cultural contexts, the unique characteristics of happiness in the Indian context are discerned.

MEANING OF SUBJECTIVE WELL-BEING (SWB), HAPPINESS AND SATISFACTION

The terms happiness and SWB have been used interchangeably in research literature to indicate a psychological construct, the meaning of which everybody knows but the definition of which nobody can give (cf. Argyle, 1987; Myers and Diener, 1995). Robert Lane (1991), a political scientist, considers that SWB consists of happiness and satisfaction with life as a whole. SWB is generally agreed to be more than the absence of negative affect or cognition. Diener (1984) listed three hallmarks of the construct: (*a*) it resides within the experience of the individual; (*b*) it includes positive measures; and (*c*) it involves global assessment of all aspects of a person's life. SWB was defined as 'a person's evaluative reactions to his or her life—either in terms of life satisfaction (cognitive evaluations) or affect (ongoing emotional reactions)' (Diener and Diener, 1995, p. 653). Ryff and Keyes (1995) proposed that well-being has six aspects: self-acceptance, positive relations with others, autonomy, environmental mastery, purpose in life and personal growth.

Happiness is often presented as synonymous with SWB. It has both objective and subjective meanings. In the objective sense, happiness is living in good conditions, such as material prosperity, peace and freedom. In the subjective sense, happiness is a state of mind. This context refers to momentary feelings as well as a stable appreciation of life. Veenhoven (2000) defined happiness '... as the degree to which someone evaluates positively the overall quality of his or her present life as a whole' (p. 267). In other words, happiness is about how much one likes the life one lives. According to Lyubomirsky (2001), happiness refers to 'the experience of joy, contentment or positive well-being, combined with a sense that one's life is good, meaningful and worthwhile' (p. 239).

The concept of happiness denotes an overall evaluation of life on multiple criteria. The object of evaluation is life in its entirety and not a specific domain of life, such as the family life. The enjoyment of family life adds to the appreciation of life, but does not constitute it. The appraisal of life can concern different periods of time: how life has been, how life is now and how life will probably be in the future.

It is assumed that the term life satisfaction carries the same meaning and is often used interchangeably with happiness. An advantage of using the term life satisfaction over the word happiness is that it emphasizes the subjective character of the concept. Though happiness and satisfaction are related, sometimes they are not the same. For example, in a study (Campbell, Converse and Rodgers, 1976) it was found that Americans younger than 35 years were most happy and those over 75 years were the least happy group. Yet, the satisfaction expressed by the older group were higher than the satisfaction expressed by the younger group. It was argued that young may be happy, but they are yet to realize their goals. Therefore, they may be less satisfied than the older group who may find in their later years that they are better off than they had anticipated and thus feel satisfied with their lives. The life satisfaction, thus, may be viewed as cognitive conceptualization of happiness or SWB, which may involve judgements of fulfilments of one's needs, goals and wishes. Happiness is an affective construct and life satisfaction is a cognitive one. Measures of happiness and life satisfaction share a maximum of 50–69 per cent common variance. The degree of life satisfaction involves one's evaluation of one's life or life accomplishments against some standard. Happiness, on the other hand, is more emotional. People simply report they are happy. This is an emotional response, a gut reaction, without knowing why they feel the way they do.

Assessment of Happiness: The study of SWB began with the development of valid and reliable measures of the concept in the 1960s and 1970s.

The most common measures involve asking people how satisfied or happy they are with their lives. These self-report measures usually correlate highly with each other and with other non-self-report indicators of well-being, such as informant data, memory measures and physical behaviour. A large number of self-report measures have been developed (for details, see Sirgy, 2002).

RESEARCH ON HAPPINESS IN THE WEST: AN OVERVIEW

The scientific study of happiness started in 1960s in USA with a view to chart mental health. Two major books were published during this period by Gurin, Veroff and Feld (1960), and Broadburn (1969). At that time, happiness was also a topic in an innovating cross-national study on human 'concerns' by Cantril (1965). Happiness was a central theme in several American Social Indicator studies during the 1970s. Landmark books were published by Campbell, Converse and Rodgers (1976), and Andrews and Withey (1976). The theme was studied in other countries as well: in the Nordic countries by Allardt (1976) and in Germany by Glatzer and Zapf (1984). In the 1980s, a first large-scale longitudinal survey on happiness was completed in Australia by Heady and Wearing (1992). Reviews of researches have been published by Veenhoven (1984), Argyle (1987), Myers (1992), Diener et al. (1999) and Lyubomirsky (2001).

Reviewing the research literature related to happiness more than three decades ago, Wilson (1967) had concluded that the happy person is a 'young, healthy, well-educated, extroverted, optimistic, worry-free, religious, married person with high self-esteem, job morale, modest aspirations, of either sex and of wide range of intelligence' (p. 294). In the four decades since Wilson's review, researchers now know a great deal more about the correlates of SWB. This type of research indicates that happy people are simply those with the most advantages—for example, a comfortable income, robust health, a supportive marriage and lack of tragedy or trauma in their lives (see Argyle, 1999; Diener et al., 1999; Eysenck, 1990; Myers, 1992, for review). However, researchers in recent years are now less interested in simply describing the demographic characteristics that correlate with it. The reason is that objective circumstances, demographic variables and life events do not predict more than 8–15 per cent of the variance of happiness (Andrews and Withey, 1976; Argyle, 1999; Diener, 1984). Therefore, in recent years efforts have been directed towards understanding the processes that define and underlie happiness. This trend represents a greater recognition of the central role played by people's goals, beliefs coping efforts and dispositions.

According to Myers and Diener (1995), four traits consistently characterize happy people: *self-esteem, optimism, extraversion* and *a sense of personal mastery or control*. Happy individuals have social, outgoing personalities, as well as positive feelings about themselves, their sense of mastery and the future. These attitudes can be self-fulfilling, leading happy people to experience more positive events and more fulfilling social relationships, which can further enhance well-being. Furthermore, happy people's positive attitudes and judgements may lead them to perceive life experiences in a way that sustains their positive moods. Since SWB is commonly defined as an aggregate of life satisfaction and the balance of affect, it is not surprising that happy individuals demonstrate both high satisfaction with their lives (Myers and Diener, 1995, for review) and frequent positive moods. The happy people are satisfied with their lives, in general as well as with specific life domains, such as work, friendship, marriage, health and the self (Argyle, 1987; Diener et al., 1999). Not surprisingly, loneliness is negatively correlated with happiness, especially in older adults (Lee and Ishii-Kuntz, 1987), and positively correlated with depression (Seligman, 1991).

Who Is Happy?

When asked about their happiness, people across the world paint a rosier picture (Inglehart, 1990; Myers, 1993). Myers and Diener (1996) have aggregated data from 916 surveys of 1.1 million people in 45 nations. They calibrated SWB onto a 0-10 scale (where 0 is the low extreme, such as very unhappy or completely dissatisfied with life, 5 is neutral, and 10 is the high extreme). The average response was 6.75.

Much against the belief that there are unhappy times of life, such as times of adolescent stress, middle age crisis or old age decline, repeated surveys across the industrialized world reveal that no time of life is notably happiest and most satisfying (Myers and Diener, 1995). Similarly, despite the well-known gender gaps in misery—men more often act in antisocial ways or become alcoholic, women are more often ruminate and get depressed or anxious—men and women are equally likely to declare themselves very happy and satisfied with their lives. Extroverted persons are likely to declare themselves to be happier.

Wealth and Happiness

Majority of the people do not agree to the proposition that money can buy happiness. But they do agree to the fact that a little more money can make them little happier. Americans believe that more money can improve their quality of life (Campbell, 1981). 'The modern American dream seems to have become life, liberty and the purchase of happiness' (Myers, 2000, p. 58). In economics, the generally asked question is whether increase in material prosperity is accompanied by increases in SWB. Krugman (1998) wrote, 'in the end, economics is not about wealth, it's about the pursuit of happiness' (p. 24).

The question that arises is: Does being well-off indeed produce—or at least correlate with—happiness? Diener (2000) reports that there is some tendency for wealthy nations to have more satisfied people. The Swiss and Scandinavians, for instance, are generally prosperous and satisfied. However, in nations among Gross National Product (GNP) of more than $8,000 per person, the correlation between national wealth and well-being evaporates. The countries like Germany and Japan with GNP higher than $24,000 per person report moderate level of happiness. Happiness tends to be lower among the very poor. Once comfortable, however, more money provides diminishing returns on happiness. Human capacity for adaptation helps explain a major conclusion of SWB research: objective life circumstances have a negligible role to play in a theory of happiness (Kammann, 1983). Compared with their grandparents, today's young adults have grown up with much more affluence, slightly less happiness and much greater risk of depression and assorted social pathologies. Myers (2001) calls it the *American Paradox*. The more people strive for extrinsic goals such as money, the more numerous their problems and the less robust their well-being (Kasser and Ryan, 1996). Lane (1996) argued that while SWB increases on the way up the economic ladder to modernity, once societies 'arrive', their level of happiness plateau briefly and then begin to turn downward as values and expectations change. SWB follows a curvilinear path: where the affluence effect meets the economist fallacy, there is a downturn in felicity. Optimism is necessary to avoid depression, but optimism has been declining with economic development.

To the poor, though money is important, but it is their desire to have a say in matters related to them that made them happier. For example, in a study, The World Bank (cited in Wolfensohn, 2004) conducted a study of 60,000 poor people in 60 countries to know their views about poverty.

The $1 a day or $2 a day that they live on was almost the last thing mentioned. What mattered was voice, an ability to contribute to their future, women not wanting to be beaten up and an opportunity for their kids. That is, there was a yearning for participation in these countries; a yearning to be heard; a profound value in knowing what is happening around them.

Goodwin (1997) has proposed three models about the relationship between economic growth and human well-being. The first model assumes that all economic growth contributes to the well-being (Figure 5.1).

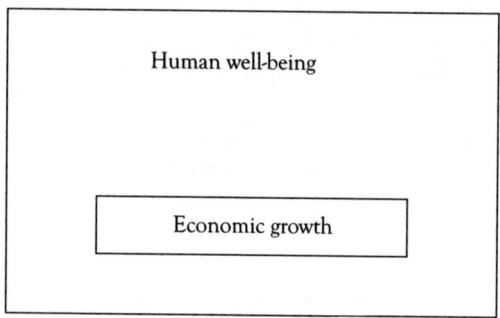

Figure 5.1: All Economic Growth Contributes to Well-being

Source: Goodwin (1997).

This model considers satisfaction of consumer wants and preferences to contribute to human well-being. It gives no value to the experience of human beings in their economic role as producers, regulators, merchandisers, etc. (let alone other human roles, such as citizens, parents and others).

The other two models assume that economic growth is a smaller set than human well-being. In these models the two concepts are not only portrayed as overlapping sets, but also some part of economic growth lies outside of human well-being (Figures 5.2 and 5.3).

Figure 5.2 indicates that all aspects of economic growth that lie outside the larger set are neutral in their effect on human well-being. Figure 5.3, however, depicts a different belief: some aspects of economic growth not only do not contribute to, but actually detract from the more general human well-being. Some examples of the third type could be: economic growth causing pollution, giving rise to selfishness or breakdown in the community, shooting of criminal activities, etc.

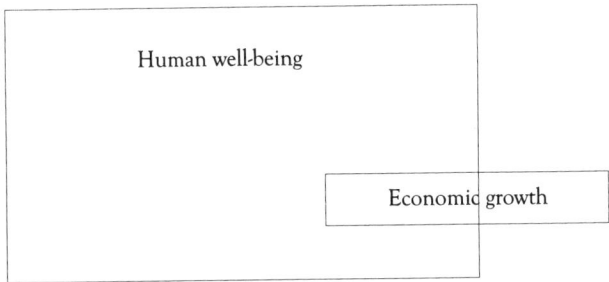

Figure 5.2: Some Economic Growth is Neutral with Respect to Well-being
Source: Goodwin (1997).

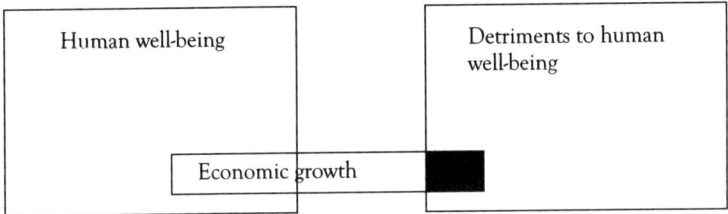

Figure 5.3: Some Economic Growth May Detract from Well-being
Source: Goodwin (1997).

Construal of Happiness

One reason for the low correlation between objective circumstances, life events and happiness has been that people do not experience events or situations passively; rather, they are 'cognitively processed' (Scarr, 1988, p. 240)—i.e., construed and framed, evaluated and interpreted, contemplated and remembered (Bruner, 1986; Ross, 1990)—so that each individual may essentially live in a separate subjective social world. Thus, understanding of cognitive and motivational processes is essential for understanding the dynamics of happiness, i.e., why some people are happier than others. Research efforts have focused on exploring hedonically relevant psychological processes, such as social comparison, self-evaluation and person perception that distinguish between the chronically happy and unhappy individuals.

People select and construct different social worlds through their own acts. Research evidence suggests that comparison with how one's peers are doing (Diener and Fujita, 1997; McFarland and Miller, 1994), with one's experiences in the past (Tversky and Griffin, 1991) and with one's desires and ideals (Carver and Scheier, 1998) influence whether the present makes one happy.

It has been reported that content and structure of the goals that people choose, as well as the amount of personal goal-related progress they perceive, shape the experience of well-being. Western literature shows that happiness and satisfaction are enhanced when people's goals are: (a) *intrinsic*—i.e., concerned with community contribution, emotional intimacy and personal growth (Kasser and Ryan, 1993; 1996); (b) *self-concordant and congruent with one's motives and needs* (Sheldon and Elliot, 1999); (c) *feasible and realistic* (Diener and Fujita, 1995); (d) *valued by one's culture* (Cantor and Sanderson, 1999; Suh, 2000); and (e) *not conflicting* (Emmons, 1996). Furthermore, people appear to be relatively happier when they: (a) choose to pursue success, rather than to avoid failure (Elliot and Sheldon, 1997); (b) are highly committed to their goals (Cantor and Sanderson, 1999) and believe that they are making progress towards them (Csikszentmihalyi, 1990).

People's appraisal of ordinary and extraordinary life events have also been found to be associated with different levels of well-being. For example, happier and more satisfied people are relatively more likely to be characterized by optimistic strategies and biases expressed in the response to life's victories and defeats. Happy people perceive and frame life circumstances in positive ways (DeNeve and Cooper, 1998), expect favourable life circumstances in the future (Scheier and Carver, 1993; Seligman, 1991), feel control over one's outcomes (Bandura, 1997) and confidence about one's abilities and skills (Lyubomirsky and Lepper, 2000). In addition, inclination to encode into memory the negative aspects of events (Seidlitz and Diener, 1993) and to dwell and reflect excessively on oneself and on one's problems (Lyubomirsky et al., 1999) have been inversely related to well-being.

The theoretical models of coping with stress describe cognitive and motivational processes that people use—whether actively and consciously or through habit—in ways that appear to diminish distress and to enhance happiness. For example, studies reveal relatively higher level of well-being among the people: (a) who show positive illusions, i.e., bolstered perception of themselves, their futures and the extent of their control (Armor and Taylor, 1998); (b) who derive positive meaning from negative events

(Folkman, 1997); (c) who use humour (Martin and Lefcourt, 1983; Nezu, Nezu and Blissett, 1988), and spirituality and faith (Folkman, 1997) in coping with adversity; (d) who do not engage in repetitive, self-focused rumination (Nolen-Hoeksema and Morrow, 1991), and who use social comparison in adaptive ways (Ahrens, 1991).

Comparing Happy and Unhappy People

Happy individuals appear to be less sensitive to social comparison information than the unhappy ones. Unhappy individuals are deflated rather than delighted about their peer accomplishments and triumphs and are relieved rather than disappointed in the face of their colleagues' and acquaintances' failures and undoing (Lyubomirsky and Ross, 1997). Thus, happiness and unhappiness are the *phenomenon of viewing the glass as half full or half empty*, respectively. Chronically happy and unhappy individuals have also been found to differ in the ways in which they respond to life events and daily situations. Happy people perceive, evaluate and think about the same events in more positive ways than do unhappy ones. Further, happy people tend to recall both positive and negative life events more favourably and adaptively—for example, by drawing humour or didactic value from adversity or by emphasizing recent improvement in their lives (Lyubomirsky and Tucker, 1998). Happy individuals are relatively better equipped to manage life's stresses, downturns and uplifts.

Is Happiness a Stable Trait?

Though happiness is a relatively stable condition, it is *not a once-and-forever thing*. Adaptation is susceptible to change over time as events, conditions, key transactions and processes in a person's life unfold. This view indicates that as happiness can erode under conditions of adversity, favourable conditions or processes, both natural and engineered, can enhance it. The challenge lies in identifying factors or conditions that advance or restrict happiness, which can be used to shape informed effort to promote it. The factors that shape happiness become more numerous and complex, and assume different strengths as the person gets older. Whereas for the infants, happiness is defined largely by the behaviour within a delimited family micro-system, in later childhood it is defined within the broader mesosystems that reflect interfaces within the family, peers and school related factors. In adulthood, happiness is importantly shaped by the society's complex, albeit often overlooked, macro-systems that underlie formal and informal social structures. Thus the happiness challenge will, in the aggregate, need to embrace person-related, transactional-contextual and environmental-societal determinants (Cowen, 1991).

In sum, a happy person in the Western world seems to be the one who possesses health and wealth, and lacks tragedy in social lives. The studies, however, show that economic growth after a certain point becomes detrimental to human well-being. The experience of happiness is a complex phenomenon, which depends upon comparison with others, past experiences, goals and ideals, biases, etc. It seems that happy individuals are less sensitive to social comparison information and are better equipped to manage life's stresses.

THE INDIAN VIEW OF HAPPINESS

Happiness is one of the great and pervasive themes of Indian thought. As Halbfass (1997) noted, 'Its meaning and ambiguities, its relevance for the human condition, its pursuit and its transcendence have been the subject of intense philosophical, psychological and soteriological inquiry and debate' (p. 150). The Indian tradition, in general, has recognized the natural desire of all human beings to be happy at every stage and in every aspect of life. Well-being of others (*paropkar*) has been given significant place in social life. The *Charaka Samhita*, the ancient work on the Hindu system of medicine, described the concept of *sukhswarup* (happy life). In daily life, the younger ones' greetings are responded with the blessings as 'khush raho' (be happy) by the elders. The Sanskrit equivalent of happiness, that is '*sukham*' (*su* = plenty, *kham* = space) indicates that the state of happiness is a natural state of (limitless) space. According to *Bhagavadgita*, a happy state indicates larger accommodative mental space within a person (Menon, 1998). Bharata, in his *Natya Shastra*, identified eight *rasas* (aesthetic relish) with their corresponding eight *bhavas* (common human emotions). *Hasya* (comic) is one of the important *rasas* with its corresponding *bhava* of *hasa* (mirth) (Paranjpe, 2009). A number of terms indicating the happy state of the individual such as *sukha, ananda, ullasa, priti* or *santosh, prasanna, mast, harsh, khusi, lalita*, as well as their semantic cognates and their counterparts in the terminology of unhappiness and pain (*dukha, aprasanna, vishad, klesha, paritap*, etc.) have been used and discussed in a number of ways.

The classical Vaisesika system recognizes happiness or pleasure (*sukha*) as one of 24 qualities (*gunas*) of human beings, which occur in the presence of pleasant or desirable things. It generates such symptoms as gratification, affection, brightness of the eyes, etc. (*anugrahabhisvanganayandiprasadajanaka*). In case the pertinent objects are not actually present, their recollection or anticipation may produce *sukha*. However, the kind of *sukh* enjoyed by wise people (or seers) is altogether different which is manifested even if there is no actual object of enjoyment, nor any recollection or anticipation is present; it is based entirely on knowledge, inner space, contentment and a special kind of good *karma* (or deeds) (*vidyasamasamtosadharmavisesanimitta*) (Halbfass, 1997). The opposite of *sukha* is *dukha*, which is associated with undesirable objects and bad *karma* (*adharma*) and produces such feelings as anger (*krodh*), distress (*upghata*) and depression (*dainya*). The Vaisesika discriminates 'happiness of the wise' from the 'regular' *sukha*. The latter refers to an affective response to an external stimulant based on gratification of desires (*anugraha*). The former refers to a dispositional happiness based on the inner resources of a person, which is characterized by transformation or transcendence. It is argued that humans should search for inner source of happiness, called *satchitanand* (*sat* = being truthful, *chit* = being aware or conscious of and *anand* = bliss).

The Indian tradition in general recognizes the scheme of four 'human goals of man' (*purusartha*). These goals are: *dharma* (religious duty), *artha* (political and economic success), *kama* (pleasure, especially of erotic kind) and *moksha* (liberation). In this list, *kama* seems to correspond most directly to *sukha* (*moksha* to absence of pain). However, a closer look would indicate that the acquisition of power and wealth (*artha*) and the accumulation of religious merit (*dharma*) do imply the potential to enjoy pleasure and well-being at a later time. This later time may even be located beyond the limits of our current existence. For example, *dharma* is the means to secure the rewards of heavenly well-being or the enjoyment of a pleasant rebirth. According to Hindu philosophy of *prarabdha karma* (accumulated deeds), the happiness or sorrow one gets in the present life is a consequence of both of actions performed by him in the present life and his actions in the past lives. It is, therefore, possible that right actions in this life may be accompanied by sorrow and wrong ones by happiness as a result of consequences of actions in past lives (Chaturvedi, 2001). The Kautilya's *Arthashastra* propagated a normal balance in life between *dharma*, *artha* and *kama*, without giving undue prominence to any one of them. However, it considers wealth or *artha* to be the first and most necessary of these objects of human life. It further states that wealth and pleasure (or *kama*) are the only objects of human pursuit (Jolly and Schmidt, 1923).

The *swastika* is the most auspicious symbol in Hindu traditions. For every holy occasion (for example, birth, marriage or any joyous occasion), *swastika* symbol is drawn or painted, carved or sculpted at the place of worship. *Swastika* stands for universal welfare. '*Swasti*' means well-being of one and all, '*ka*' means symbol. Thus, *swastika* indicates happiness, safety, fertility and prosperity. The four corners of the *swastika* represent four *purusharthanas* (aims of life), namely, *dharma*, *artha*, *kama* and *moksha*, and the perfectly symmetrical shape indicates the balance. The four stages in a man's life—*brahmacharya* (celibacy), *grihastha* (housekeeper), *vanaprashta* (seclusion) and *sanyasa* (renunciation)—are also said to represent the four corners of *swastika*, and the life being the one connecting them in a brilliant embrace (Kamat, 2003).

Relational Nature of Happiness

The Indian view of self maintains self-other continuity, transcendental self, tolerance for dissonance and coexistence of separate elements and emphasizes on mind training and self-control (Misra, 2010) and operates with abstract generalization and universal categories. Also, the Indian perspective on reality and human functioning is holistic, recognizes coherence and natural order across all life forms, emphasizes self-discipline and gives *dharma* as the sacred moral code.

Peace of mind and being free of worries has been emphasized as aspect of self in India (Roland, 1984). The individual feels good and happy by acting as is expected of him/her by the family and friends, sacrificing his/her interests for the in-group, displaying affection towards in-group and maintaining harmony with in-group. Marriott (1976) argued that Hindu conceptions assume that the self, a dividual, is an open entity that is given shape by the social context. This has been beautifully described by Kakar (1978). Miller, Bersoff and Harwood (1990), in a carefully controlled study on moral reasoning, found that Indians regard responsiveness to the needs of others as an objective moral obligation. It has been argued that the Indian child is encouraged to develop an adult self which is more responsive to family and community demands and responsibilities, and more dependent on family status, prosperity and approval. Indians thus develop a more 'familial self'. Salve (2000) argues that living in the present is an essential key to happiness and stress-free life. To him, 'Discarding all prejudices, ideologies, presumptions and assumptions, living in the present moment and giving the credits of the final results to the Almighty, one can definitely experiences bliss—a state that is beyond happiness' (Salve, 2000, p. 14).

The recognition of encompassing nature of happiness becomes more evident in the following prayer:

> *Sarve bhavantu sukhinaha, sarve santu niramayah*
> *Sarve bhadrani pasyantu, ma kaschid dukhabhaga bhavet.*

(May all be happy, may all be free from disease, may all perceive good and may not suffer from sorrow.)

Since Vedic period a more inclusive view of life and existence, in which interdependence with earlier animate and inanimate world gets a legitimate place, has been stressed upon which emphasizes interconnectedness across all life forms and conditions. Kautilya's *Arthashastra*, a tratise on policy, also advocates that a king's happiness lies in the happiness of the people, and his welfare is related to the welfare of the people. The king should not give priority to his own interests; rather, he should consider the interest of the people. The *Chhandogyopanishad* argues that happiness lies in the vastness, greatness; happiness is not found in smallness; undoubtedly happiness lies in greatness; therefore, one should always try to know that greatness (*Yo vai bhuma tatsukham; Nalpe sukhmast; Bhumaiva sukham; Bhuma twewa vijigyasitvyah*).

The Indian philosopher Sri Aurobindo believed that true happiness lies in finding and maintenance of a natural harmony of spirit, mind and body. Happiness comes from the soul's satisfaction, not from the vital's or the body. Only when egoism dies and God in man governs his own human universality can this earth support a happy and contended race of beings. The happy heart is smiling, peaceful, wide-open and without a shadow. Mahatma Gandhi emphasized minimization of human needs and greed for attaining happiness.

Complementarity in Happiness and Unhappiness

A story in India goes like this:

> Once a rich man wanted to be happy. He was in search of a wise man who could guide him on how to be happy. Some villagers assured him that a Sufi mystic who lived in the forest would be able to help him. The man found the mystic sitting peacefully below a tree. He stopped his horse and told him that he was unhappy. The mystic said that to find happiness he would have to hand over his jewels. The man gave him a bag of diamonds. Taking the jewel bag the mystic ran away. Thinking that he has been robbed, the man chased the mystic but failed to catch him. Desperate for his diamonds he returned to the forest. To his surprise he found the mystic sat in silence

with his eyes closed at the same spot and the bag lay in front of him. Grabbing it, he danced with joy. The mystic opened his eyes and asked the man if he was happy to recover his riches. The man fell at his feet. The mystic added: You have to know suffering; only then you know what happiness is. (in Shashin, 2004, p. 18)

Human life consists of a mixture of both happiness and sorrow or misery. In fact, in the Indian tradition, the search for knowledge begins with the realization of suffering (*dukh*), and *moksha* was treated as liberation from suffering and culminates in Self-realization/knowledge (*atmagyan*). It may be noted that humans do not always pursue happiness; rather, on many occasions (for example, marriage of daughter), we willingly give up some amount of happiness to get our life narratives moving in the right direction, improving in general.

It is believed that the end of one marks the beginning for the other. As it is reported in *Mahabharata*, 'Days end with the sun's setting and night with the sun's rise. The end of pleasure is always pain and the end of sorrow is always pleasure.' It is accepted that all the pleasures, even the highest joys of life, do not continue forever. They pass away, leaving pain in their wake. The great Indian poet Kalidas in his *Meghdoot* noted that happiness and unhappiness do not remain forever. It is like a rotating wheel where sometimes happiness and sometimes unhappiness takes the front side. Thus, happiness and unhappiness are complementary and follow each other. According to *Adhyatma Ramayana*, happiness lies within misery and vice versa. It is similar to mud containing to water and soil together.

It should not be assumed that unhappiness is always to be avoided. It also gives meaning to life in certain ways. First, happiness following misery is joyful. It is similar to the experience of reaching under the shadow of a tree after a long walk under the sun. If there is no misery, there would not be happiness at all. Second, the legendary poet Rahim believed that short-lived misery is beneficial as it provides an opportunity to discriminate friends from foes.

Equanimity in Opposites

The disposition of equanimity is considered important for cultivating stable state of happiness. Equanimity reflects the attitude of the person who is neither affected by the joy or sorrow, good or evil, pleasure or pain and gain or loss. Such a person is called a person with steady intelligence (*sthitapragya*). He/she is said to maintain his composure in spite of life's circumstances.

He/she treats others as if they were the person himself and has no desire or expectation from them. His/her senses remain under control, the person is free from love and hatred and gives equal treatment to joy and sorrow. According to *Bhagavadgita*, as a happy person, the person who acts does not concentrate on the results. Hence, the result does not alter his/her state of mind by presenting either an elating or a depressing mood. The converse of this proposition is that an agent who tries to be happy in his/her own self receives the results of his/her work equanimously. His/her intention remains focused on the goal and his/her attention on the process of activating towards this goal (Menon, 1998). Thus, a happy person is neither elated in happiness nor depressed in unhappiness. Surveying the research literature on poverty, Misra and Mohanty (2000) observed that the Indian view of happiness comes quite close to being equidistant or even tangential to both affluence and poverty.

Happiness and Education

In the Indian context, education is considered a key to success as it empowers human beings by facilitating realization of human potentials and bringing in excellence in action (*yastu kriyawan purushah sa vidwan*). It is through education and learning—*sadhana* of *vidya*—that one may attain liberation and realize true self (*Sa vidya ya vimuktaye, vidyamritmashnute*). As narrated in one of the famous Sanskrit verses, education imparts intellectual culture; intellectual culture secures capacity and stability; capacity and stability enable to secure wealth; wealth so secured enables to perform *dharma*, which in turn secures happiness (*Vidya dadati vinayam, vinayam yati patratam, patratwad dhan mapnoti, danaddhamam tatag sukham*). Happy people typically feel empowered and remain in control of situations. Those who feel empowered rather than helpless typically would do better in school, cope better with stress and live more happily. When people are deprived of control over one's life, they suffer lower morale and worse health (Srivastava and Misra, 2003). Therefore, the ultimate pursuit of education should be to make people happy.

In conclusion, it can be said that the model of man in the Indian tradition articulates life goals that are different from that of the Western world. The self in the Indian context is more relational and interdependent. As a consequence, the experience of happiness is not restricted to personal accomplishments; rather, happiness is seen in terms of fulfilling familial and social obligations and maintaining harmony with the inner and outer world. Pleasure and pain are considered two aspects of the same coin.

On many occasions, people welcome suffering, which becomes a cause for happiness. Moderation in behaviour is the key element of happiness in the Indian context.

REFERENCES

Ahrens, A. H. (1991). Dysphoria and social comparison: Combining information regarding others' performances. *Journal of Social and Clinical Psychology*, 10, 190–205.

Allardt, E. (1976). *Dimensions of welfare in a comparative Scandanavian study*. Finland: Research Group for Comparative Sociology, report 9, University of Helsinki.

Andrews, F. M. and Withey, S. B. (1976). *Social indicators of well being: America's perception of life quality*. New York: Plenum Press.

Argyle, M. (1987). *The psychology of happiness*. London: Methuen.

———. (1999). Causes and correlates of happiness. In D. Kahneman, E. Diener and N. Schwarz (Eds), *Well being: The foundations of hedonic psychology* (pp. 353–73). New York: Russell Sage Foundation.

Armor, D. A. and Taylor, S. E. (1998). Situated optimism: Specific outcome expectations and self-regulations. In M. P. Zanna (Ed.), *Advances in experimental social psychology*, Vol. 30 (pp. 309–79). New York: Academic Press.

Bond, M. (2003, October 4). The pursuit of happiness. *New Scientist*, pp. 40–43.

Broadburn, N. M. (1969). *The structure of psychological well-being*. Chicago: Aldine Publishing.

Bruner, J. (1986). *Actual minds, possible world*. Cambridge: Harvard University Press.

Campbell, A. (1981). *The sense of well-being in America*. New York: McGraw-Hill.

Campbell, A., Converse, P. E. and Rodgers, W. L. (1976). *The quality of American Life: Perceptions, evaluations, and satisfactions*. New York: Russell Sage Foundation.

Cantor, N. and Sanderson, C. A. (1999). Life task participation and well-being: The importance of taking part in daily life. In D. Kahneman, E. Diener and N. Schwartz (Eds), *Well-being: The foundation of hedonic psychology* (pp. 230–43). New York: Russell Sage Foundation.

Cantril, H. (1965). *The pattern of human concern*. New Brunswick, NJ: Rutgers University Press.

Carver, C. S. and Scheier, M. F. (1998). *On the self regulation of behavior*. New York: Cambridge University Press.

Chang, C. M. (1996). *Kuai le de ze xue: Zhong guo ren shen ze xue shi* (The philosophy of happiness: A history of Chinese life philosophy). Taipei, Taiwan: Hong Yie.

Chaturvedi, V. (2001). Causality of Karmic justice. *Journal of Indian Council of Philosophical Research*, 18, 129–56.

Cowen, E. L. (1991). In pursuit of wellness. *American Psychologist*, 46, 404–8.

Csikszentmihalyi, C. (1990). *Flow: The psychology of optimal experience*. New York: Harper & Row.

DeNeve, K. M. and Cooper, H. (1998). The happy personality: A meta-analysis of 137 personality traits and subjective well-being. *Psychological Bulletin*, 124, 197-229.

Diener, E. (1984). Subjective well-being. *Psychological Bulletin*, 95, 542-75

——. (2000). Subjective well-being: The science of happiness and a proposal for a national index. *American Psychologist*, 55, 33-43.

Diener, E. and Diener, C. (1995). The wealth of nations revisited: Income and quality of life. *Social Indicators Research*, 36, 275-86.

Diener, E., Diener, M. and Diener, C. (1995). Factors predicting the subjective well-being of nations. *Journal of Personality and Social Psychology*, 69, 851-64.

Diener, E. and Fujita, F. (1995). Resources, personal strivings, and subjective well-being: A nomothetic and idiographic approach. *Journal of Personality and Social Psychology*, 68, 926-35.

——. (1997). Social comparisons and subjective well-being. In Buunk and R. Gibsons (Eds), *Health, coping, and social comparisons* (pp. 329-57). Mahwah, NJ: Erlbaum.

Diener, E. and Oishi, S. (2000). Money and happiness: Income and subjective well-being across nations. In E. Diener and E. M. Suh (Eds), *Culture and subjective well-being* (pp. 185-218). Cambridge, MA: MIT Press.

Diener, E., Suh, E. M., Lucas, R. E. and Smith, H. L. (1999). Subjective well-being: Three decades of progress. *Psychological Bulletin*, 125, 276-302.

Diener, M. L. and Lucas, R. E. (2004). Adults' desires for children's emotions across 48 countries: Associations with individual and national characteristics. *Journal of Cross-Cultural Psychology*, 35, 525-47.

Durant, W. (1932). *On the meaning of life*. New York: Ray Long & Richard R. Smith.

Easterlin, R. A. (2004). The economics of happiness. *Doedalus*, 133, 26-33.

Elliot, E. J. and Sheldon, K. M. (1997). Avoidance achievement motivation: A personal goal analysis. *Journal of Personality and Social Psychology*, 73, 171-85.

Emmons, R.A. (1996). Striving and feeling: Personal goals and subjective well-being. In J. Bargh and P. Gollwitzer (Eds), *The psychology of action: Linking motivation and cognition to behavior* (pp. 314-37). New York: Guilford.

Eysenck, M. W. (1990). *Happiness: Facts and myths*. East Sussex. England: Erlbaum.

Folkman, S. (1997). Positive psychological states and coping with stress. *Social Science and Medicine*, 45, 1207-21.

Fordyce, M. (1987). *PSYCHAP inventory*. Cypress Lake, FL: Cypress Lake Media.

Glatzer, W. and Zapf, W. (Eds). (1984). *Lebensqualitat in der Bundersrepublik*. (Quality of life in West Germany). Frankfurt: Campus Verlag.

Goodwin, N. R. (1997). Interdisciplinary perspectives on well-being. In F. Ackermann, D. Kiron, N. R. Goodwin, J. M. Harris and K. Gallaghar (Eds), *Human well-being and economic goals* (pp. 1-14). Washington: Island Press.

Gurin, G., Veroff, J. and Feld, S. (1960). *American's view their mental health: A nation wide interview survey*. New York: Basic Books.

Halbfass, W. (1997). Happiness: A Nyaya-Vaisesika perspective. In P. Bitmoria and J. N. Mohanty (Eds), *Relativism, suffering, and beyond: Essays in memory of B.K. Matilal* (pp. 150-63). Delhi: Oxford University Press.

Headey, B. and Wearing, A. (1992). *Understanding happiness: A theory of subjective well-being*. Melbourne: Longman Cheshire.

Inglehart, R. (1990). *Culture shift in advanced industrial society*. Princeton, NJ: Princeton University Press.

Inglehart, R. and Klingemann, H. (2000). Genes, culture, democracy, and happiness. In E. Diener and E. M. Suh (Eds), *Culture and subjective well-being* (pp. 165–83). Cambridge, MA: MIT Press.

Jolly, J. and Schmidt, R. (1923). *Arthasastra* (new edition, vol. 1). Lahore: Motilal Banarasi Das.

Kakar, S. (1978). *The inner world: A psychoanalytic study of childhood and society in India*. Delhi: Oxford University Press.

Kamat, J. (2003). *Indian culture: Swastika in Indian culture*. Retrieved from http://www.kamat.com/indica/culture/sub-cultures/swastika.htm on 15 July 2009.

Kammann, R. (1983). Objective circumstances, life satisfactions, and sense of well-being: Consistencies across time and place. *New Zealand Journal of Psychology*, 12, 14–22.

Kasser, T. and Ryan, R. M. (1993). A dark side of the American dream: Correlates of financial success as a central life aspiration. *Journal of Personality and Social Psychology*, 65, 410–22.

———. (1996). Further examining the American dream: Differential correlates of intrinsic and extrinsic goals. *Personality and Social Psychology Bulletin*, 22, 280–87.

Kinnier, R. T., Kernes, J., Tribbensee, N. C. and Van Puymbroeck, C. M. (2003). What eminent people have said about the meaning of life. *Journal of Humanistic Psychology*, 48, 105–18.

Kitayama, S. and Markus, H. R. (1994). *Emotion and culture: Empirical investigations of mutual influence*. Washington, DC: American Psychological Association.

———. (2000). The pursuit of happiness and the realization of sympathy: Cultural patterns of self, social relations, and well-being. In E. Diener and E. M. Suh (Eds), *Culture and subjective well-being* (pp. 113–61). Cambridge: The MIT Press.

Kitayama, S., Markus, H. R. and Kurokawa, M. (2000). Culture, emotion, and well-being: Good feelings in Japan and the United States. *Cognition and Emotion*, 14, 93–124.

Krugman, P. (1998, August 23). Viagra and the wealth of nations. *New York Times Magazine*.

Lane, R. E. (1991). *The market experience*. New York: Cambridge University Press.

———. (1996). 'The joyless market economy', paper delivered to the Conference on Economics, Values, and Organization, Yale University, New Haven, CT, April 19–21.

Lee, G. R. and Ishii-Kuntz, M. (1987). Social interaction, loneliness, and emotional well-being among the elderly. *Research on Aging*, 9, 459–82.

Lu, L., Gilmour, R. and Kao, S. (2001). Cultural values and happiness: An east-west dialogue. *The Journal of Social Psychology*, 141, 477–93.

Lu, L. and Shih, J. B. (1997). Sources of happiness: A qualitative approach. *The Journal of Social Psychology*, 137, 181–87.

Lyubomirsky, S. (2001). Why are some people happier than others? The role of cognitive and motivational processes in well-being. *American Psychologist*, 56, 239-49.

Lyubomirsky, S. and Lepper, H. S. (1999). A measure of subjective happiness: Preliminary reliability and construct validation. *Social Indicators Research*, 46, 137-55.

Lyubomirsky, S. and Ross, L. (1997), Hedonic consequences of social comparison: A contrast of happy and unhappy people. *Journal of Personality and Social Psychology*, 73, 1141-57.

Lyubomirsky, S. and Tucker, K. L. (1998). Implications of individual differences in subjective happiness for perceiving, interpreting, and thinking about life events. *Motivation and Emotion*, 22, 155-86.

Lyubomirsky, S., Tucker, K. L., Caldwell, N. D. and Berg, K. (1999). Why ruminators are poor problem solvers? Clues from the phenomenology of dysphoric rumination. *Journal of Personality and Social Psychology*, 77, 1041-60.

Marriott, M. (1976). Hindu transactions: Diversity without dualism. In B. Kapferer (Ed.), *Transaction and meaning* (pp. 109-42). Philadelphia: Institute for Study of Human Issues.

Martin, R. A. and Lefcourt, H. M. (1983). Sense of humor as a moderator of the relation between stressors and moods. *Journal of Personality and Social Psychology*, 45, 1313-24.

McFarland, C. and Miller, D. T. (1994). The framing of relative performance feedback: Seeing the glass as half empty or half full. *Journal of Personality and Social Psychology*, 66, 1061-73.

Menon, S. (1998). The ontological pragmaticity of Karma in Bhagavadgita. *Journal of Indian Psychology*, 16, 44-52.

Miller, J. G., Bersoff, D. M. and Harwood, R. L. (1990). Perceptions of social responsibilities in India and in the United States: Moral imperatives or personal decisions. *Journal of Personality and Social Psychology*, 58, 33-47.

Misra, G. (2010). The cultural construction of self and emotion: Implications for well-being. In R. Schwarzer and Peter A. Frensch (Eds), *Personality, human development, and culture: International perspectives on psychological science*, volume 2 (pp. 95-111). New York: Psychology Press.

Misra, G. and Mohanty, A. K. (2000). Poverty and disadvantage: Issues in retrospect. In A. K. Mohanty and G. Misra (Eds), *Psychology of poverty and disadvantage* (pp. 261-84). New Delhi: Concept.

Myers, D. G. (1992). *The pursuit of happiness: Who is happy and why.* New York: William Morrow.

——. (1993). *The pursuit of happiness.* New York: William Morrow.

——. (2000). The funds, friends, and faith of happy people. *American Psychologist*, 55, 56-67.

——. (2001). *The American paradox: Spiritual hunger in an age of plenty.* New Haven, CT: Yale University Press.

Myers, D. G. and Diener, E. (1995). Who is happy? *Psychological Science*, 6, 10–19.
———. (1996, May). The pursuit of happiness. *Scientific American*, 274, 54–56.
Nezu, A. M., Nezu, C. M. and Blisett, S. E. (1988). Sense of humor as a moderator of the relation between stressful events and psychological distess: A prospective analysis. *Journal of Personality and Social Psychology*, 54, 520–25.
Nolen-Hoeksema, S. and Morrow, J. (1991). A prospective study of distress and posttraumatic stress symptoms after a natural disaster: The 1989 Loma Prieta earthquake. *Journal of Personality and Social Psychology*, 61, 115–21.
Outlook. (2005, January 10). *Kya hai khusi ka khazana* (What is the secret of happiness), pp. 24–25.
Paranjpe, A. C. (2009). In defence of an Indian approach to the psychology of emotion. *Psychological Studies*, 54, 3–10.
Rice, T. W. and Steele, B. J. (2004). Subjective well-being and culture across time and space. *Journal of Cross-Cultural Psychology*, 35, 633–47.
Roland, A. (1984). The self in India and America: Toward a psychoanalysis of social and cultural contexts. In V. Kovolis (Ed.), *Designs of selfhood* (pp. 123–30). New Jersey: Associated University Press.
Ross, L. (1990). Recognizing the role of construal processes. In L. Rock (Ed.), *The legacy of Solomon Asch: Essays in cognition and social psychology* (pp. 77–96). Hillsdale, NJ: Erlbaum.
Ryff, C.D. and Keyes, C. L. (1995). The structure of psychological wellbeing revisited. *Journal of Personality and Social Psychology*, 69, 719–27.
Salve, V. T. (2000, February 15). Bliss as the state beyond happiness. *The Times of India* (New Delhi), p. 14.
Scarr, S. (1988). How genotypes and environments combine: Development and individual differences. In L. Bolger, A. Caspi, G. Downey and M. Moorehouse (Eds), *Persons in context: Developmental processes* (pp. 217–44). New York: Cambridge University Press.
Scheier, M. F. and Carver, C. S. (1993). On the power of positive thinking: The benefits of being optimistic. *Current Directions in Psychological Science*, 2, 26–30.
Schyns, P. (1998). Crossnational differences in happiness: Economic and cultural factors explored. *Social Indicators Research*, 43, 3–26.
Seidlitz, L. and Diener, E. (1993). Memory for positive versus negative life events: Theories for the differences between happy and unhappy persons. *Journal of Personality and Social Psychology*, 64, 654–64.
Seligman, M. E. P. (1991). *Learned optimism*. New York: Knopf.
Shashin (2004, November 22). Life is celebration, be happy. *The Times of India* (New Delhi), p. 18.
Sheldon, K. M. and Elliot, A. J. (1999). Goal striving, need satisfaction, and longitudinal well-being: The self-concordance model. *Journal of Personality and Social Psychology*, 76, 482–97.
Sirgy, M. J. (2002). *The psychology of quality of life*. Dordrecht: Kluwer Academic Publishers.

Srivastava, A. K. and Misra, G. (2003). Going beyond the model of economic man: An indigenous perspective on happiness. *Journal of Indian Psychology*, 21, 12-29.

Suh, E. M. (2000). Self, the hyphen between culture and subjective well-being. In E. Diener and E. M. Suh (Eds), *Culture and subjective well-being* (pp. 63-86). Cambridge, MA: MIT Press.

Triandis, H. C. (1994). *Culture and social behavior*. New York: McGraw Hill.

Tversky, A. and Griffin, D. (1991). Endowment and contrast in judgments of wellbeing. In F. Strack and M. Argyle (Eds), *Subjective well-being: An interdisciplinary perspective* (pp. 101-18). Oxford, England: Pergamon Press.

Veenhoven, R. (1984). *Conditions of happiness*. Dordrecht: Kluwer Academic.

———. (1997). Quality-of-life in individualistic society, a comparison of 43 nations in the early 1990s. In H. Vanderbraak, M. J. Delong and A. C. Zijderveld (Eds), *The gift of society: Social capital and institutions in a (post)modern world* (pp. 157-86). Amersfoort, Holland: Enzo Press.

———. (2000). *World database of happiness*. Retrieved from http://www.eur.nl/fsw/research/happiness on 17 July 2009.

Wilson, W. (1967). Correlates of avowed happiness. *Psychological Bulletin*, 67, 294-306.

Wolfensohn, J. D. (2004, November 18). Tryst with destiny: Globalisation can be India's hour of glory. *The Times of India* (New Delhi), p. 14.

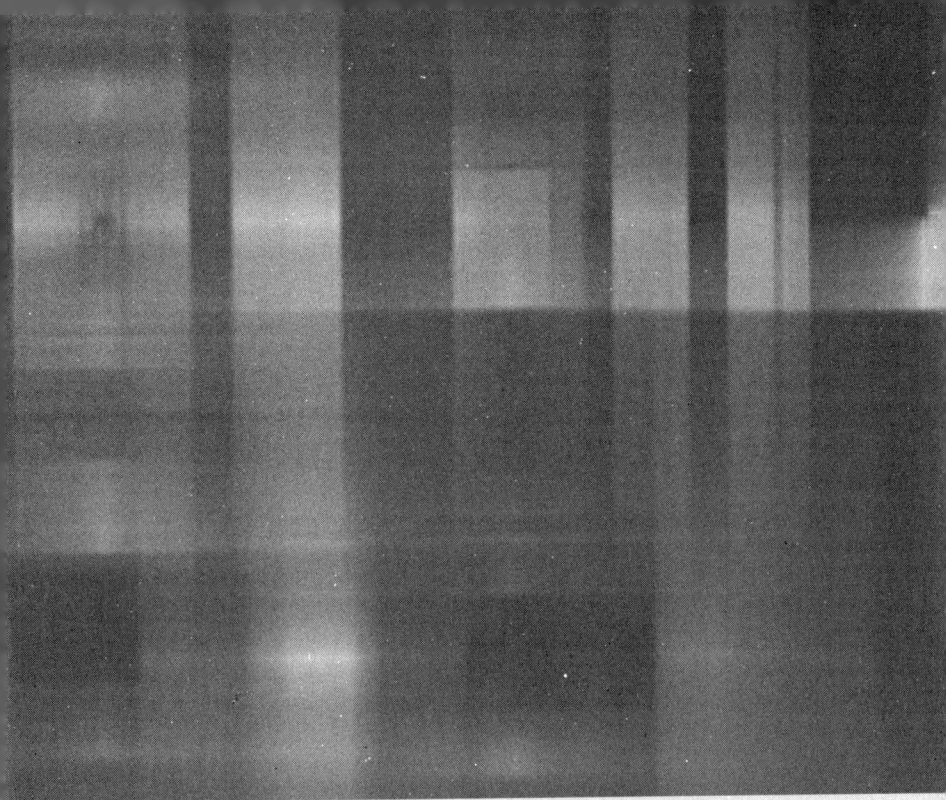

Part II

SOCIAL AND DEVELOPMENTAL CONTEXT OF HEALTH

Introduction

The domain of health is located in the societal context and the challenges for ensuring health for all can be meaningfully understood and addressed only in the context of the socio-cultural configuration of the groups and communities under consideration. In the Indian setting, the contextual dimension assumes greater degree of complexity as Indian society has to deal with cultural diversity being shaped by the forces of continuity and change. The Indian people simultaneously live with many of the age-old traditions and beliefs as well as modern ideas side by side. They have assimilated many modern influences during the last two centuries, particularly under the colonial rule. During the period spanning a little more than a half century after gaining political independence in 1947, the forces of Westernization, urbanization and industrialization have introduced many new elements in the social and economic order. More recently the forces of globalization, privatization and liberalization have added new dimensions to this context. The newer conditions require more complex skills for adaptation. The economy, ecology and the mindset of the people are seized by many new challenges in the wake of these developments.

This section tries to bring into focus some of the psychologically significant developmental and social aspects that have bearing on health. By placing health in the developmental and social context, we recognize the fact that during our life course our health is shaped by a variety of factors (Resnick and Rozensky, 1996). For instance, the roles and responsibilities vary with age, and age is correlated with diverse types of vulnerabilities. Thus, while chronic diseases are more likely to affect the health of middle aged and elderly, the younger population is more vulnerable to accidents and unintentional injuries, and have distinctive health-related issues (Kapur, 1995). We think that socio-cultural factors immensely contribute to the states of health and disease. Also, we must recognize that there are gender-bound health problems and gender barriers to health care. The gender bias in treatment and health care has been pointed out by many researchers (Davar, 2001; Ussher, 1997). In addition to gender, our belongingness to a particular type of family, social support, poverty and community and the kind of identity that we hold also play important role in determining our health (Dalal, 1995; Patel, Ricardo, Mauricio and Ana, 1999).

In particular, the stages of life to which we belong become a crucial determiner of the nature of health-related issues and priorities. It is well-known that human lifespan is organized in certain major developmental stages, which have specific developmental tasks. As Erikson states, the stages are characterized by specific conflicts and virtues and smooth transition occurs only when the conflicts are properly resolved. The preconditions of optimal development are met in certain groups, but in many, the developmental ecology is impoverished and functions at below that level. In fact, certain disadvantaged and marginalized groups are put under unhealthy circumstances (Misra and Tripathi, 1980).

Coming to the developmental context, we are reminded of the view that according to the Indian tradition, the human lifespan is organized in four life stages, i.e., *brahmcharya*, *grihastha*, *vanprastha* and *sanyas*. These stages are sequentially arranged in such a manner that they are linked with preparation, acceptance of the adult societal role, development of detachment and providing space and opportunity to the younger generation and finally withdrawing from the various worldly responsibilities and concentrating on spiritual development. Following the metaphor of seed and tree, this scheme maintains the continuity of life across different births. The traditional Indian view posits that one has to grow and equip to meet the life challenges, play the designated and chosen roles and learn to happily withdraw from the scene. One is required to live a life to realize all the four goals (*purusharthas*), i.e., *dharma*, *artha*, *kama* and *moksha*. The life in contemporary conditions has changed but it still shows certain parallels with the traditional view (Kakar, 1978).

It has been noted that certain stages of development, like childhood and old age, are intrinsically more vulnerable. Within the health sector, there is a trend to attend more to the health problems of adults. Similarly womenfolk, due to the patriarchal and hierarchical nature of society, lack of education and opportunities, do remain largely unattended. The people with handicap or some kind of disability are also put to specific health problems. Keeping these variations in view, this section tries to sensitize the readers to the problems of these neglected groups. Also, journey in one's life is often a personal story written by the circumstances peculiar to that person. The study of individual lives is often very instructive and helps one to learn and reflect on one's own conditions. This idiographic orientation is often missed in the quantitative research that looks for the generalization. Keeping this in mind, the selections included in this section present a cross section of work that involves review of a problem domain, study of a group as well as the life story of a person. The purpose is to show the readers the diversity of perspectives or vantage points from which health can be viewed and understood.

The younger children grow and move towards adolescence, which has often been termed as a period of increased stress. The physiological and psychological changes taking place during this period transform the lives of adolescents. The first chapter of this section addresses some of these issues through a qualitative inquiry. Namita Rangnathan has provided a qualitative account of the experiences of stress during the transformative period of adolescence among girls. Puberty and sexuality are closely related. However, their representation and analysis is oftentimes obscured by myths, fallacies, fantasies and apprehensions. Rangnathan draws attention to the kind of change in ethos that is taking place due to media and advertisements. The study shows an innovative way to address a very sensitive topic. Using samples from a public school and a government school, an effort was made to develop an experiential account of the perceptions of puberty, concomitant changes in body and related feelings and physiological changes like breast development and menstruation. The method adopted was focused on group discussion that allowed sharing and exploring the different perspectives of adolescent girls. The approach had an added advantage of avoiding socially desirable responses. The analysis offers insights into girls' perception and experience of sexuality and working with related stresses. Rangnathan observes that while girls were dealing about sexuality, they resorted to vicarious and sublimated methods of dealing with it. This was largely due to training received from cultural and social institutions. It is clear that puberty in adolescence do have elements of discontinuities and incongruities. The author draws attention to the gendered socialization practices that accentuate the feminine identity, thereby facilitating, accepting puberty and sexual development as 'natural'.

While the preceding chapter shared the life story of one person, the problems of health and well-being have a societal angle also. Vindhya, Kiranmayi and Vijayalakshmi have analysed the problems of women in psychological distress using hospital setting. The data are used to argue that a biomedical perspective undermines and ignores the role of sociocultural factors. The psychological disorders are often distributed in the population by gender. This denies the pattern in community samples that show that female patients outnumber the male counterparts. There is gross gender-based inequity of access to health care in India. Also, it seems that the various methods used by doctors are not adequate for dealing with the illnesses of women. In the absence of alternate approaches to health care, the women remain deprived of health care facilities.

The chapter also explores the biases and difficulties in the academic discourse of psychological disorders among women. It is indicated that changes in life course, particularly in the case of menopause, are not intrinsically related to psychological trauma. A number of social factors like occupation, education, mental life, etc., are related to it. The chapter strongly makes the case that health cannot be understood in isolation from the social context, which in the case of women, owing to unequal social status, leads to mental health problems.

In the preceding chapters, the aspects of health relevant to the common man or the general population were taken into account. The problems often multiply in groups, which live in special circumstances or have additional disadvantages. Leena Kashyap has looked at the problems faced by females with people suffering from disability as any limitation experienced by the impaired or challenged person with reference to physical function or affecting any specific organ (see Ghai, 2002). The nature and type of the disability has been described. Disability has been distinguished from other terms like handicap. The analysis based on various studies tries to analyse the effects on the family. The inter-relationships, expectations and everyday functioning and present problems are highlighted. This area is less researched and many domains have not been covered. Within the family, a number of factors like parental attitude play important role. The family's coping strategies and the need of professional intervention have been examined. Counselling, facilitating parent child interaction, parent education, need further research. It is concluded that the ultimate goal is to reach the physically challenged through their family. Role of professional social worker is important in this context.

In general, the chapters included in this section underscore the need to address the problems of health at the level of multiplex reality and the order of society. It may, however, be noted that it would be wrong to emphasize on the social or developmental context alone. Health status behaviour is determined by a complex interaction of biological, social and psychological factors. These factors mutually influence each other and operate in a systemic manner (Dalal and Ray, 2005).

REFERENCES

Dalal, A. K. (1995). Family support and coping with chronic diseases. *Indian Journal of Social Work*, 15 (1), 44–52.

Dalal, A. K. and Ray, S. (2005). Social dimensions of health and well-being: An overview of research trends. In A. K. Dalal and S. Ray (Eds), *Social dimensions of health* (pp. 1-33). Jaipur: Rawat Publications.

Davar, B. V. (Ed.). (2001). *Mental health from a gender perspective*. New Delhi: Sage.

Ghai, Anita. (2002). Disability in the Indian context: Post colonial perspectives. In M. Corker and T. Shakespeare (Eds), *Disability and postmodernity: Embodying disability theory* (pp. 112-26). London and New York: Continuum.

Kakar, S. (1978). *The inner world*. New Delhi: Oxford University Press.

Kapur, M. (1995). *Mental health of Indian children*. New Delhi: Sage.

Misra, G. and Tripathi, L.B. (1980). *Psychological consequences of prolonged deprivation*. Agra: National Psychological Corporation.

Patel, V., Ricardo, de Lima, Mauricio, L. and Ana, T. C. (1999). Women, poverty and common mental disorders in four restructuring societies. *Social Science and Medicine*, 49, 1461-71.

Resnick, R. K. and Rozensky, R. H. (Eds). (1996). *Health psychology through the life span*. Washington DC: American Psychological Association.

Ussher, J. M. (1997). Gender issues and women's health. In A. Baum, S. Newman, J. Weinman, R. West and C. McManus (Eds), *Cambridge handbook of psychology, health, and medicine* (pp. 110-12). Cambridge, UK: Cambridge University Press.

6

Puberty, Sexuality and Coping: An Analysis of the Experiences of Urban Adolescent Girls

NAMITA RANGANATHAN

With acceleration and preponement in the age of puberty, adolescence no longer remains a transitional stage which can be dismissed as a brief experience in the life of a growing girl. With the shortening of childhood, puberty and adolescence have got elongated and, therefore, warrant recognition as legitimate phases in the human life span, especially in the urban context. It thus is important to document and understand how girls feel about this phase in their lives because psychological impact of pubertal events is a product of both biological and social forces (see Berk, 1996; Rice, 1993)

Puberty is no longer interpreted as a biological phenomenon with adolescence being its consequential social construction. This study is embedded in this interactionist framework, but goes a step further, in that it lays greater emphasis on the inner voices and experiences of the growing girls as their bodies change and their sexual desires take shape.

Dealing with puberty and sexuality often remains a matter for individuals to make independent sense of, using their own resources and abilities. As a consequence, many myths, fallacies, sexual fantasies, fears, apprehensions and worries often emerge.

Further, given that adolescence has been redefined by contemporary theorists as an age of 'challenge and potential' as opposed to the traditional notions of viewing it as a period of 'storm and stress', there is an urgent need to know and understand the experiences of adolescents from a different perspective. The expansion in media, especially women's magazines, help-line columns and television programmes which strive to either directly or indirectly address issues concerning girls' and women's changing bodies and sexuality have also enhanced the awareness levels of girls in general. The boom in beauty pageants and extensive advertising of women's beauty products have also contributed towards focusing girls' attention on their bodies. All these factors gave impetus to the present study. The specific objectives were as follows:

1. To know how girls perceive and describe the experience of puberty.
2. To identify the changes which they observe in their bodies and how they feel about them.
3. To know their reactions and feelings towards breast development and menstruation, in particular.
4. To locate their sources of knowledge and information about issues concerning puberty and sexuality.
5. To document and evaluate their experiences at home, school and with friends during this phase of their lives.
6. To understand how they feel about their emerging sexuality and the methods of coping which they use.

Method

The Setting

Each of the above listed objectives were studied with a view to identifying general adolescent trends and take cognizance of class differences wherever they occurred. The rationale for including social class as a factor was that society and culture place different standards of behaviour and expect-ations on different socio-economic strata. It was thus deemed worthwhile to study class as a factor mediating pubertal experiences and sexuality. This has already been studied in a Western context wherein some interesting trends have emerged (Dornbusch et al., 1987; Martin, 1987; Simmons and Blyth, 1987). Accordingly, a sample of 120 girls drawn from three different types of schools—an elite public school with a very high fees structure, a Kendriya Vidyalaya and a government girls' school run by Delhi Administration were identified. The schools were located within a radius of three kilometres from each other. It was felt that since schools reflect the class structure in society by virtue of the fees charged by them determining access, the public school would typify the upper class, the Kendriya Vidyalaya which charges a relatively low fees and is largely patronized by the government and quasi government children would represent the middle class, and the state government school which charges a very nominal fee and consists mainly of children from the lower strata and lower middle class would typify the lower class. The total sample of 120 girls was equally distributed across each of the three types of schools to ensure adequate representation of adolescent girls from different social and cultural backgrounds and also to report class differences wherever they existed, with more conviction. The girls were selected at random depending upon their willingness to participate in the research. They were all studying in class XI and XII, with their age ranging between 16-18 years. The rationale for focusing on this age group was that having experienced puberty over a span of a couple of years, they would be in a better position to articulate and discuss their experiences, including their feelings of sexuality and the methods of coping which they use. Furthermore, it was expected that by the stage of late adolescence, the psychological concomitants of puberty would be well inscribed in their personalities, thereby facilitating a more relevant and meaningful understanding of them. It must be pointed out here that since the study dealt with a relatively unusual theme especially in the Indian cultural context, considerable time and effort had to be given to building up rapport with the girls, before any data collection could be done. The concerned school principals and teachers also had to be convinced about the necessity and significance of this kind of a study.

Methodological Strategy

The study used 'focused group discussions' which were held in groups of 10 girls each. These were done in each of the three schools. In these discussion groups, the themes which were probed and explored, centred around issues encompassed within the objectives. The focused group discussions which were transformed into sharing occasions were held over several sessions with each group, ranging from at least 6-8 sessions of 60-90 minutes duration each over a span of 3-5 weeks. The discussions were recorded and later transcribed. The focused group sharing sessions were used since they helped many girls to shed their inhibitions and share their perceptions and feelings more freely. In the rapport formation stage itself, the self consciousness and discomfort level of the girls in addressing issues allied to their pubertal experiences and sexuality had been diagnosed by the researcher. It was thus felt that using a group approach in a sharing mode would be more worthwhile than administering individual questionnaires or interviews, where girls were likely to be awkward or felt compelled to give socially desirable answers. The data were recorded and later transcribed. The transcribed data were analyzed with reference to the focus of each of the objectives.

Results and Discussion

Analysis of the data was done at two levels—the first attempting to delineate trends for adolescent girls in general, and the other relating to identification of class differences, wherever they surfaced. The findings, however, are being presented holistically.

The Experience of Puberty

With respect to the perceptions and descriptions about the experience of puberty, majority of the girls had negative associations and memories. These included:

1. 'It is horrid.'
2. 'I wish I was a boy and could escape it all.'
3. 'It's a curse to be born a girl.'
4. 'I dread every month as the time comes closer because I get cramps and stomachaches.'
5. 'Why should girls suffer like this?'
6. 'Changing sanitary napkins is just so difficult.'
7. 'I'm always worried that my school uniform which is white will stain.'
8. 'Could God have not thought of other ways for girls to grow up?'
9. 'When I first started, I thought I had cut a vein, or had cancer or AIDS.'

From these descriptions it is clear that the girls had interpreted puberty very narrowly, as almost being synonymous and inter-changeable with menstruation. They seemed oblivious of the fact that puberty was actually a long process which began with breast budding, followed by a number of secondary sex changes and culminated with menarche. There were hardly 10 or 12 girls who knew these facts and they had also either been told by their mothers or elder sisters or had read about them. Secondly, most of the girls had no scientific awareness or understanding of what puberty actually entailed, even though four to five years had elapsed since they had entered this phase. They complained that they had not been given any prior preparation for breast development or menstruation before they had themselves started the cycle. The few who knew about menstruation had discovered these phenomena either through friends or television programmes, or the magnanimity of some empathetic women in their families whom they were close to. They expressed a great deal of surprise when they were told that boys also undergo pubertal processes and should thus not be objects of girls' envy. They were, however, not convinced and felt that 'at least boys don't suffer month after month'. It was clear that the strongest association in girls' minds with puberty was menstruation. Further, in comparison with boys, there was an element of self-pity at being girls and a distinct feeling of gender inequality.

There were no discernible class differences with respect to the experience of puberty, excepting for the fact that the girls from the public school were much more articulate and vociferous in stating their views and opinions.

Breast Development and Menstruation: Feelings and Reactions

In the context of reactions towards breast development, most girls recalled feeling very awkward and self-conscious at the time of initial breast development and also at the time when they first began to wear bras. Some of them said that they had begun 'to stoop their shoulders', others used 'to cover their chest with a book or with their hands folded across.' Some girls said that 'they kept their plaits in front to cover the chest region'. They felt that breast development had reduced their running and jumping activities since they had felt uncomfortable until they started wearing bras, to give their breasts support. After this however, their worries changed to the adequacy of their breast-size and having a good bust-line consonant with socially upheld norms and standards of what constituted a good figure. This was very much their current concern. Breast size was seen as a determinant of the ability or inability to dress fashionably.

There were noticeable class differences with respect to the experience of breast development. While the reactions of self consciousness and awkwardness at the initial stages were found to be similar among all the adolescent girls, the persistent pre-occupation with bust-lines and breast size thereafter was seen much more prominently in the public school girls. Girls from the Kendriya Vidyalaya and government school seemed to have accepted breast size as a natural acquisition and were more concerned about body proportion in the context of the total figure, rather than breast size alone.

In their reactions towards menstruation too, apart from the consensus in the physical discomfort and the nuisance of a recurrent monthly cycle, there was found to be considerable variation in the myths and fallacies associated with menstruation. Girls from the Kendriya Vidyalaya and government school, for instance, had been led to believe by their mothers that 'menstrual blood was impure thereby warranting that they avoid going to temples or performing puja on those days'. Many of the Kendriya Vidyalaya girls said that they had questioned these notions and practices on scientific principles and often resisted following them, but found themselves getting into many conflicts with their mothers as a consequence. However, they all seemed to think that 'having one's period was to be a top secret never to be divulged to their fathers or brothers'. They thus attributed a strong hush-hush orientation to menstruation. This was also the case with many of the public school girls who also admitted 'to not being free enough with their fathers or brothers to talk about menstruation'. They also seemed to believe that 'menstrual problems and difficulties were to be shared with their mothers'. Some of them expressed 'acute self-consciousness at having to buy sanitary napkins from male sales persons who they claimed felt equally awkward at having to sell them'. Some of them also admitted to being victims of strictures based on religious considerations imposed on them by their mothers, but the number in comparison to Kendriya Vidyalaya and government school girls was much lower. For the girls of the government school there was a meek acceptance of all the strictures which menstruation imposed on them. They, however, admitted to feeling angry about the restrictions on entering the puja room, the kitchen, touching the pickle jars of the household and being asked to eat food in separate vessels, but felt helpless and unable to do anything about them in their present life situations. They unanimously said that 'they would never subject their own daughters to these practices'. Thus, while on the one hand there was reconciliation to being female, there was a sense of optimism and hope that they could mediate change when in a position of power and control, on the other.

Bodily Changes and Allied Feelings

Most of the girls focused on height and weight gain, development of adult-like figures, broadening of their hips, and breast development. While height gain did not bewilder them, weight gain and broadening of the pelvis, they said, was a source of great worry to them. They often 'wondered why their arms and thighs were becoming fat and their hips expanding'. This was a concern expressed by most girls, excepting those with thin, skeletal figures, and cut across all the three classes.

Another prominent source of tension and anxiety for many of the girls was their skin colour, texture and the emergence of acne and pimples. They said that, 'they were perplexed at the change in their skins and their sudden proneness for pimples'. They also admitted to becoming more self-conscious about their appearance. Many girls expressed discomfiture with too much facial hair around the eye-brows, side-burns and upper lip regions. Most girls admitted to spending much more time looking at themselves in the mirror and examining their facial features in detail. Many girls of the public school had very noticeably shaped their eye brows, removed their unwanted facial hair and waxed their arms and legs. In fact, the public school girls seemed to be very concerned about the shape of their legs and were seen to always wear ankle length socks in their quest to display their legs. Body-image had undoubtedly become a very important component of the life of the adolescent girls. The role models for most girls varied, but were all derived from the glamour industries of fashion, television or films. Within body-image, the two major sub-concerns were firstly, the overall figure determined by body contours, and the second was the general appearance in terms of how they looked, dressed, wore their hair and used accessories to highlight their features.

While body-image, especially mediated through personal appearance was a very important component of the adolescent girls' 'psyche' in general, once again it surfaced much more prominently for the public school girls. Almost all of them went to beauty parlours for grooming, routinely. In fact, the public school girls had begun to evaluate their sex-appeal and rate their attractiveness on various critical dimensions such as glossiness of hair, skin quality, facial features, shape of the legs, overall figure, etc. These dimensions in turn were derived from the points of emphasis in beauty pageants and international design and fashion magazines. For the Kendriya Vidyalaya and government school girls, while being 'too short, too tall, too fat, too thin or too dark' were issues of concern, they did not seem obsessed with their body-image and the culture of beauty parlours was still alien to most of them. However, there was a general desire to 'look nice'.

Home, School and Peer-related Experiences

With respect to the factors of home, school and peer-related experiences, almost all the girls reported major changes. They all felt that the naturalness and spontaneity with which they used to previously interact with members of their family, especially males had disappeared. They now had a more formal and distant relationship with their fathers, uncles and elder brothers. The public school girls felt that their fathers had distanced themselves from their daughters, in that they very seldom kissed them, fondled them or hugged them, which had not been so when they were younger. The government school girls in fact reported, 'having very little verbal communication with their fathers after coming of age'. Girls from the Kendriya Vidyalaya said that 'while personal issues and difficulties were discussed with their mothers, fathers were consulted for educational or career related guidance, although this had not been so when they were younger'. Many of them recalled 'having being scrubbed and bathed by their fathers when they were much younger'.

The mother–daughter relationship also seemed to have undergone a transformation. Mothers were perceived by most girls to be 'like regulatory control authorities' who kept reminding their daughters that they had grown up and must thus behave in a more mature and controlled manner. For the government school girls, growing up meant 'having to shoulder the responsibilities of domestic chores, especially cooking, cleaning and washing and looking after younger siblings'. They also felt that

> ... their freedom to play and interact in the neighbourhood had been curtailed. They were discouraged by their parents to go out to the market or spend the evening walking with friends—both being activities they had engaged in when younger. They were encouraged to remain indoors instead.

The girls of the Kendriya Vidyalaya also felt that their mothers were constantly monitoring them and questioning them on 'whom they were talking to on the telephone, or whom they were playing badminton with, or why they wanted to go out with their friends every evening'. Also, strict deadlines were imposed on them in terms of having to return home by 7.00 p.m. or before it became dark. They also reported feeling very unhappy at having to leave the telephone number and address of their friends at home whenever they went over to their houses. Some girls reported serious conflicts with their mothers on matters of dress. All of them unanimously said that 'their mothers' encouraged them to be friends with girls and not with boys and if any boy came over or rang up, it became a matter of great storm in the house. In fact, 'it was carried to the extreme with reference to the neighbour's son whom they had played with all along, becoming an object of their mothers' suspicion', as some girls said.

In the case of the public school girls, mother–daughter conflicts were found to be high on matters of 'dress, fashion, use of cosmetics, wanting to be with friends, wanting to go to parties, having long telephone chats with friends and returning home late'. Most girls reported that their mothers were like 'detectives who kept a continuous vigil on them'. They reported that 'their mothers were constantly warning them, about undesirable men and girls being at risk' unless they were careful. Their mothers also disapproved of male friends, unless it was in a large group.

With regard to school life, the girls of the government school said that since they were in a single-sex school, life at school continued in the same way for them, excepting that sometimes they felt that their teachers were very critical of them and demanded very adult-like, mature and controlled behaviour from them. They were also very strict about the girls' adherence to the school uniform, especially the length of the skirt and socks. They made the girls tie their hair in two plaits with ribbons and any digression from this was punished. Their teachers often spoke about the need for girls to 'be virtuous, modest, simple and more focused towards their studies'. All the girls complained that there was not a single teacher whom they could approach for personal problems related to matters of body-image, puberty or sexuality, as these were seen as extraneous to the school curriculum.

The experiences of the girls in the Kendriya Vidyalaya were also similar with the additional burden of their behaviour being under constant scrutiny from their teachers, especially in their interaction with boys. They felt that although their school was co-educational, this was only notional since in spirit it operated more like 'an all boys school' and 'an all girls school', with intermingling of the sexes being discouraged. While this was not the case in the public school, girls felt that 'their teachers, especially the female teachers were always gauging the length of their skirts, asking them to pull up their socks to knee length and observing their interaction and friendship patterns with the boys of their class'. They, however, mentioned that there were some 'empathetic teachers who could be approached for personal counselling'.

As far as friends were concerned, all the girls felt that friends were their biggest support system. Friends were persons

> ... whom one could freely talk to, discuss even the most confidential matters with, seek advice on personal difficulties from, discuss matters of fashion, body-size, dressing up, cosmetics, etc. They felt non-threatened and completely at ease with their friends and relished the fact that they could be themselves without fear of being watched or analyzed.

From the above cited experiences of the adolescent girls, it is evident that during puberty and adolescence they are looking for empathy and uncritical and unconditional acceptance which seems to be forthcoming only from their friends, which is why friendship assumes such strength and significance. Also, since their friends themselves are undergoing similar changes and transformations, the element of peer solidarity is very high.

Sexuality and Coping

When the girls were asked to describe their sexuality, they initially drew a blank, not knowing how to respond. They kept saying that they had not thought about it. The researcher began to realize that the term 'sexuality' was evoking reactions of alarm and resistance since the girls were probably interpreting it in terms of heterosexual relationships and physical intimacy, both of which carried social and moral taboos which had evidently been internalized by them. It was only after being prodded about their feelings towards the opposite sex and their concern about their appearance that they began to share their feelings and experiences. All of them admitted to 'having strong personal desires to look attractive'. While some girls were more vocal in stating this fact, all the others seemed to nod in agreement. They also said that they felt 'attracted towards boys and enjoyed being in their company'. Some government school girls who usually walked to school said that while they felt angry at men staring at them or making passes at them on the road, they also felt glad at having been noticed by these men. They also admitted to harbouring secret dreams about marriage, sex and family life. The Kendriya Vidyalaya girls and public school girls described some of the very enjoyable moments which they had in class, especially with the boys. Some girls also spoke about crushes which they had on some boys and how glad they felt when they were noticed by those boys. It is thus quite evident that all girls experience sexual feelings during the phase of puberty and adolescence, but because of the 'guilt and shame orientation' which culture and society socialize them into on matters of sexuality, they are apprehensive about discussing these issues or even thinking about them. At best they derive satisfaction from vicarious or disguised, often sublimated, sources. For instance, reading romantic fiction, watching Hindi films and television serials, especially those based on themes of love and romance, enjoying music centred on these themes, glancing through magazines dealing with fashion, glamour and dressing-up, having detailed debates and discussions on film and television heroes and heroines, anchors and video and disc jockeys—are all activities the girls engage in, which constitute their forms of 'coping with sexuality'. Their conversations with their friends focus mainly on boys, marriage, sex, romance, love, honeymoons, boy-girl relationships in their school and neighbourhood, latest fashions and any sex-related scandals which they come across. For the public school girls, there was an additional dimension of going out in groups with their friends and mixed parties. Very few girls admitted being involved in a heterosexual relationship and almost all of them rejected the ideas of sexual experimentation, dating, going steady and pre-marital sex. They felt that there 'was an appropriate time and place for everything and thus relationships and sex could also wait'—an idea which culture had evidently socialized them to internalize. Marriage was seen as the legitimate institution for this.

It was thus quite clear that while girls were aware about their sexuality, they resorted to vicarious and sublimated methods of dealing with it, resulting from the training given to them by culture and society. Also, the associative bonds which they had formed with the term 'sexuality' were largely moralistic in tone and flavour 'which good girls did not think about or engage in' and in their quest to be 'good girls' they felt the need to conform.

It would be meaningful to point out at this juncture that studies on puberty and sexuality experiences in the West have also obtained similar findings. The travails of menstruation, breast development, heightened mother-daughter conflict emanating from the controls exercised by the mother, fears of unwanted pregnancy, importance given to chastity and virginity and sublimated approaches to dealing with sexuality during the stage of adolescence have all been identified by researchers (Brooks-Gunn, 1987; Brooks-Gunn and Ruble, 1983; Brooks-Gunn and Zahaykevich, 1989; Crockett and Peterson, 1987; Delaney, Lupton and Toth, 1988; Koff, 1983; Martin, 1987).

Conclusions

The findings of this study have raised some very fundamental but potent issues about 'growing up female'. It is quite evident that puberty and adolescence are fraught with internal conflicts, discontinuities and incongruities for growing girls brought about by the basic mismatch between biological forces on the one hand and societal interpretations of them on the other. While there are class-related variations in the intensity of these conflicts and discontinuities, there are many issues in growing up female which merit attention.

For instance, a major incongruity exists between the developmental needs of adolescent girls such as freedom, autonomy, self expression, identity and sexuality and the sensitivity shown towards these needs by significant others around them, which is reflected in the rigorous moral codes, advanced social expectations and 'you have grown up; girls don't do this' syndromes used by parents, teachers and other adults.

Yet another basic discontinuity exists between the stage of childhood on the one hand and adolescence on the other, which prevails in the popularly held and practised perception that childhood and adolescence represent two mutually exclusive categories, with advent into adolescence symbolizing the magical and dramatic end of childhood and, therefore, the emergence of a completely new set of expectations from the growing girls. Actually, adolescence should be perceived as the stage of transition which allows for overlap and continuity with childhood. This will then safeguard against the development of a discontinuity in socially approved roles, expected behaviour and levels of indulgence experienced by the girl child and the adolescent girl.

It has also to be recognized that vesting sexuality, which is a natural process, with moral overtones leads girls to develop a guilt and shame orientation and considerable unfulfilled curiosity about their sexuality, which in turn causes high levels of anxiety, conflict and dilemma.

Further, during puberty and adolescence, the internalization of a feminine personality characterized by traits like being virtuous, obedient, conforming, adaptable and submissive brought about by gendered socialization leads to the development of learned helplessness, feelings of dependence, inferiority and acceptance of male supremacy in the growing girls. This gendered socialization constantly reminds the girls that the three most important aspects of feminine identity are 'being good daughters, wives and mothers'. Sexuality is also expected to be synthesized with these roles. These then become the primary goals in many girls' lives, leading them often to sacrifice their competence in other spheres which may later generate feelings of bitterness, resentment, etc. This gets further impetus from the fact that social rewards are usually given to girls who conform to the 'good girl' image. As a consequence, many girls have to deny what their inner subjective world and experience tell them and replace this with what is desirable as objective external reality. Even their sense of self and identity is defined in relation to others.

It is thus important that puberty and adolescence be given the due importance and attention which they warrant and growing girls be suitably prepared for and facilitated to make their 'growing up' experiences more worthwhile and memorable. This can be achieved by harmonizing the girls' inner subjective experiences and their wishes and desires with the objective reality of their life situations. A beginning can be made by accepting puberty and sexual development as natural developmental processes which are as integral to a human being as are cognitive, social, emotional and moral development. This will help to facilitate the required attitudinal and experiential transformation of society. A major onus for this can be undertaken by schools in this regard by making Sexuality Education a core component of the school curriculum.

REFERENCES

Berk, E. (1996). *Child development.* New Delhi: Prentice Hall of India.
Brooks-Gunn, J. (1987). Pubertal processes and girls psychological adaptation. In R. M. Lerner and T. T. Foch (Eds), *Biological-psychosocial interactions in early adolescence* (pp. 123-53). Hillsdale, NJ: Erlbaum.
Brooks-Gunn, J. and Ruble D. N. (1983). Dysmenorrhea in adolescence. In S. Golub (Ed.), *Menarche: The transition from girl to woman* (pp. 251-61). Lexington: Lexington Books.
Brooks-Gunn, J. and Zahaykevich. (1989). Parent-daughter relationships in early adolescence: A developmental perspective. In K. Kreppner and R. Lerner (Eds), *Family systems and life-span development.* Hillsdale, NJ: Erlbaum.
Crockett, L. J. and Peterson, A. C. (1987). Pubertal status and psychosocial development: Findings from the Early Adolescence study. In R. M. Lerner and T. T. Foch (Eds), *Biological psychosocial interactions in early adolescence: A life span perspective.* Hillsdale, NJ: Erlbaum.
Delaney, J., Lupton, M. J. and Toth, E. (1988). *The curse: A cultural history of menstruation.* Urbana, IL: University of Illinois.
Dornbusch, S. M., Ritter, P. L., Leiderman, P. H., Roberts, D. F. and Fraleigh, M. J. (1987). The relation of parenting style to adolescent school performance. *Child Development,* 58, 1244-57.

Koff, E. (1983). Through the looking glass of menarche: What the adolescent girl sees. In S. Golub (Ed.), *Menarche: The transition from girl to woman* (pp. 77-86). Lexington, MA: Lexington books.

Martin, E. (1987). *The woman in the body*. Boston: Beacon Press.

Rice, P. F. (1993). *The adolescent: Development, relationships and culture*. Boston: Allyn and Bacon.

Simmons, R. G. and Blyth, D. A. (1987). *Moving into adolescence: The impact of pubertal change and school context*. New York: De Gruyter.

7

Mental Disorders in Women: Evidence from a Hospital-based Study[1]

U. VINDHYA, A. KIRANMAYI
AND V. VIJAYALAKSHMI

INTRODUCTION

In the past few decades, significant changes in mental health research have come from epidemiological findings and in particular from the recognition that mental illness had social as well as biological and psychological causes. In recent years, it is being increasingly demonstrated that mental illness has an identifiable social distribution and that elements of each kind of mental disorder and socio-cultural structures are inexorably dependent with regard to causation, labelling, classification and response (Prior, 1993).

Mental health problems currently are said to constitute about 8 per cent of the global burden of disease and more than 15 per cent of adults in developing societies are estimated to suffer from mental illness (World Health Organization, 2001). According to the new concept of measuring disability called Disability Adjusted Life Years (DALY), mental

---

[1] This chapter is partly based on the doctoral dissertations of the second and third authors, supervised by the first author. An earlier version was presented at the Regional Seminar on Women and Regional Histories, organized by the Indian Association for Women's Studies and University of Hyderabad, 30 August–1 September, 1999, at Hyderabad.

disorders constitute a significant part of total disability adjusted life years (8.1 per cent) more than the disability caused by several well-recognized disorders such as cancer (5.8 per cent) and heart diseases (4.4 per cent) (World Health Organization, 2001). In our country, it was estimated that more than 3 crores of individuals suffer from mental illnesses every year and that 1.75 lakh new cases are added every year (Prabhu and Raghuram, 1987), indicating the magnitude of the problem of mental illness. The overall prevalence rate estimated from psychiatric surveys has been found to be about 11 per cent, with men averaging 10 per cent and women 15 per cent (reviewed in Davar, 1999).

It was commonly believed that the prevalence of mental illness in India was much less than in the Western countries, citing the 'oriental philosophy of life', the limited urbanization and industrialization, the strong family ties as factors responsible for this 'low prevalence' of mental illness (Prabhu and Raghuram, 1987). Representative surveys of mental morbidity were also not taken up till the 1960s. Since then, however, the accumulated evidence, based either on hospital data or community samples, points out that the prevalence rate of mental illness is not significantly less than it is in the west (Prabhu and Raghuram, 1987). However, much of the work in the area of mental health continues to be directed at treatment of illness rather than towards preventive or promotion efforts.

More women than men the world over are said to suffer from mental disorders. And yet, psychological distress of women has not been articulated as a distinct agenda by the mainstream psychological approaches. Viewing mental illness from the biomedical model, these approaches usually consider somatic and psychological factors in their diagnostic efforts, ignoring the impact of socio-cultural and socio-demographic factors (Haslam, 2000). Opponents of the biomedical model point to evidence of the substantial roles of exogenous life circumstances and social influences on psychopathology, and to the inadequacies of reductionist analyses of psychological processes (for example, Meehl, 1995). Challenging both biomedical and intrapsychic approaches to mental illness, feminist psychological research has pointed out that consideration of women's mental health needs requires recognition of the impact of the social context on mental health (Carmen, Russo and Miller, 1981). The unique aspects of women's health are those which are affected by women's social roles, and not purely by their biology. The feminist psychological viewpoint has been at pains to present mental illness of women in an expanded explanatory context of life circumstances and stresses, social influences and stereotyping, vulnerabilities and developmental pathways, rather than locating cause in any specific abnormality (Nicolson and Ussher, 1992). The feminist conception of women's health and illness is in fact in line with the recent biopsychosocial perspective that examines the interaction of biological, psychological and social factors rather than focusing on aberrant somatic processes to identify the cause of an illness as in the traditional biomedical model (Stroebe and Stroebe, 1995).

Mental disorders are not randomly distributed throughout a population but rather subgroups differ in the frequency of various disorders. Knowledge of this uneven distribution can be used to investigate causative factors and to lay the groundwork for programmes of prevention and control. Epidemiological studies attempt to relate the distribution of mental disorders to population characteristics. When a high rate of disorder is found to be associated with a particular population characteristic, a possible implication is that this characteristic contributes to producing the disorder.

The demographic, social and ecological factors that are believed to be associated with psychological disorders are age, gender, marital status, economic conditions, educational level, occupation, social class, social mobility, density of habitat, family structure, opportunities for work and recreation, trauma, injury, addictions, etc. By themselves, these factors may not be the only causative factors but they interact with others such as genetic and psychological to give rise to disorders in predisposed individuals.

Although epidemiological investigations of mental health in our county have been conducted since the 1960s, albeit in a scattered manner, studies on mental health of women are meagre. It was only recently that a gender-sensitive analysis, perhaps the first of its kind in the country, of the data gathered in these epidemiological studies was made, questioning the gender-biased assumptions of this research and highlighting the psychosocial stressors associated with women's position and roles in society (Davar, 1999).

There is a dearth of region-specific studies also and, to the best of our knowledge, no research attempting to determine the vulnerable groups in the population in terms of socio-demographic correlates has been done in the state of Andhra Pradesh so far.

With these considerations in view, it was felt that a growing urbanized and industrialized city like Visakhapatnam and its surrounding villages and smaller towns in Visakhapatnam district in north coastal Andhra Pradesh would constitute an appropriate locale to ascertain not only the extent of mental disorders in the population, but also to explore the factors in the socio-demographic environment, which may be causally linked with these disorders. Although Visakhapatnam has the oldest hospital for mental care in the state (established in 1863, as some records indicate) an epidemiological study of this kind, drawing upon a psychosocial model and with a focus on gender-specific distribution of mental disorders, has not been conducted so far.

The aim of the present chapter is to delineate the mental illness profile of women seeking psychiatric help and the construction of a sociodemographic profile of these women. The larger project was concerned with obtaining a global picture of the distribution of various psychological disorders and their relationship with socio-demographic variables such as age, educational and income levels, occupation, marital status, number of children and place of residence. For reasons of space, only a few major findings that serve to illustrate the theoretical underpinnings of the present research will be highlighted here. While qualitative in-depth studies can reveal much about social processes that women experience and perhaps hold the key to discovering the quality of women's mental health problems, empirical data as from the present study lay the preliminary groundwork for intensive research on women in psychological distress. While representation of numbers may appear rather gross, they are an obvious measure of the magnitude of the problem and are essential for an understanding of some of the social factors that relate to mental illness.

WOMEN AND MENTAL ILLNESS

Considerable research in the West has been devoted to interrogation of the scientific and social underpinnings of the mental health discourse that determine the health status of women. Since the 1970s, due to the influence of feminist theory and the women's movement, research studies began to document the complex ways in which gender bias, gender role stereotyping and devaluation of women affect the nature, diagnosis and treatment of mental health problems (Zuckerman, 1979). The feminist critique of psychology's construction of women's mental illness has been cited widely enough to need further elaboration here (for example, Chesler, 1972). It is being increasingly recognized that gender inequalities and the stresses that differentially affect women by virtue of their unequal social status have led to pervasive mental health problems for women. There is accumulating evidence that links mental disorders with alienation, powerlessness and poverty, conditions most frequently experienced by women (Dennerstein, Astbury and Morse, 1993). In fact, three of the five priority areas outlined in the National Institute of Mental Health document in the USA, namely, violence against women, multiple roles and poverty focus specifically on the ways in which women's actual experience and their subordinate position in society contribute to problems in their mental health (Russo, 1990). All these issues are as of much relevance and concern to the conditions of women's lives in India as well.

Both community surveys and hospital-based studies indicate that women are disproportionately affected by mental health problems and that their vulnerability is closely associated with their marital status, work and roles in society (Russo, 1990). Examination of women's position in society reveals that there are sufficient causes in current social arrangements to account for the depression, anxiety and distress experienced by women. Recent research has demonstrated the ways in which social inequities and social assumptions about womanhood influence different aspects of women's lives, and thereby their physical and emotional health (Lee, 1998). Whether it is poorer nutrition, health care and education; limited access to material resources; or less compensation for a disproportionate share of socially necessary labour or sexual and other forms of physical and mental abuse across the lifespan; research evidence globally points to women being at the greatest risk (Dennerstein, Astbury and Morse, 1993). These issues not only fall within the rubric of human rights but also are those that understandably affect mental health. Furthermore, women's reproductive role of bearer and nurturer of children produces unique potential for stress-related effects. Thus, the well-documented higher morbidity in women's health across the lifespan has clear biosocial underlying causes (Dennerstein, Astbury and Morse, 1993).

Consideration of women's mental health requires, therefore, recognition of the impact of social factors on mental health, a position that challenges traditional intrapsychic, biomedical approaches to mental illness. Central to the socio-cultural perspective is the idea that there are two main routes through which women's position in society might contribute to poor mental health outcomes; one more indirect and insidious and the other more direct and extreme. The first is concerned with role-related stressors including multiple role strain, role overload and role conflict. The second route which is more direct and extreme has just begun to capture substantial research interest, although these experiences of women have long been identified as crucial forms of oppression by the women's movement. These include actual sexual victimization whether through brutal stressors like rape, battering, incest or other forms of violence against women (Russo and Green, 1993). While experiences of gender oppression—ranging from employment discrimination and sexual violence to the trivialization of women's work—occur, to quote Rubin (1975, cited in Frederickson and Roberts, 1997) with both 'endless variety and monotonous similarity', the variety of intra-individual psychological consequences leading to poor mental health outcomes in women are just about beginning to be identified. Accumulation of such experiences help account for mental health risks that disproportionately affect women: unipolar depression, anxiety and somatization disorders, eating disorders and some phobic disorders (Russo, 1990).

Frequencies and patterns of mental disorder have also been found to be different for men and women. In the Western context, the widely acknowledged and cited National Institute of Mental Health (NIMH), USA, Epidemiological Catchment Area Programme, which sampled the non-institutionalized population, found that for the 15 diagnostic categories studied, there were substantial gender differences in prevalence rates of lifetime diagnoses: (*a*) women predominated in diagnoses of major depressive episodes, whereas men predominated in antisocial personality and alcohol abuse/dependence; (*b*) women were more likely than men to have received a diagnosis of dysthymia, obsessive-compulsive disorder, schizophrenia, somatization and panic disorders; and (*c*) no gender differences were apparent in manic episode or cognitive impairment (Eaton and Kessler, 1985).

Patterns of gender differences for six-month prevalence rates also indicated that major depression, phobias, dysthymia and obsessive-compulsive disorder were the most common diagnoses for women. Men, on the other hand, predominated in alcohol abuse/dependence (Myers et al., 1984). This pattern of gender differences in diagnoses has also been found to vary by marital status and class. While single and widowed/separated men have been found to have higher overall admission rates than women in the same marital status categories, married women have higher admission rates than married men. This has been the pattern in the Western context, despite variations across samples of different ethnic categories (Russo, Amaro and Winter, 1987). In India, however, in addition to the higher frequency of illness in married women, a higher frequency has been found in single women as well when compared to single men (Chakraborti, 1990). The difference between the findings of the Western and Indian studies can perhaps be attributed to cultural differences in the centrality of the institution of marriage. While the potential stressors associated with marriage are reported to be applicable to women, the social stigma and related tensions attached to single status have more adverse effects on women once again.

The findings underscore the importance of understanding complex relationships among gender, ethnicity, sex roles and mental health if effective mental health policies and programmes are to be developed. Furthermore, the psychosocial nature of these variables points to the need to go beyond narrow biomedical approaches in building the research knowledge base.

In the Indian context, there have scarcely been any focused studies on gender differences in the prevalence of disorders or access and utilization of mental health services, or on the specific vulnerabilities of women in various age, occupational, socio-economic groups. Drawing on the data gathered by epidemiological studies conducted in our country since the 1960s, Davar (1999) in her critique of these studies pointed out that despite their methodological shortcomings and politically misleading inferences, the data converged qualitatively on some significant dimensions of being a woman in psychological distress in India. Women were found to be at least twice as frequently ill as men in the case of *common* mental disorders or the erstwhile neuroses, while no gender difference was seen in the prevalence of *severe* mental disorders (see Table 7.1 for classification of severe and common mental disorders).

These epidemiological surveys have indicated that around 1 per cent of men and 1.3 per cent of women received a diagnosis of *severe* mental disorder, whereas 6.7 per cent of men and 10–11 per cent of women were diagnosed with *common* mental disorder (Davar, 1999). In other words, where mental illness has a biological basis, as in the case of *severe* mental disorders, frequency of illness is the same across gender. On the other hand, where mental illness has a psychosocial basis, women are more mentally ill than men. Therefore, a biomedical approach to women's mental health is inadequate since a larger part of mental disorder epidemiology in women is constituted by the *common* mental disorders which have a psychosocial etiology. This underscores the necessity of adopting a different and exclusive approach to women's mental health concerns.

The National Mental Health Programme (NMHP, introduced in 1982), however, does not have a women's mental health agenda, despite its stated objective of 'ensuring availability of minimum mental health care for all ... particularly to the most vulnerable and under-privileged sections of the population' (GOI, 1982). Furthermore, adverse implications for women follow from the focus of the NMHP on the mental illness categories that it has chosen for intervention, namely, epilepsy, mental retardation

TABLE 7.1: Diagnostic Categories of Mental Illness

Severe Mental Disorders	*Common Disorders*
Schizophrenia	**Stress and Adjustment Disorders**
Paranoid schizophrenia	Brief depressive reaction
Schizophrenia unspecified	Mixed anxiety and depression
Prolonged depressive reaction	
Acute transient psychoses (with symptoms of schizophrenia)	
Puerperium	
Schizoaffective disorders	
Other categories in schizophrenia (catatonic, hebephrenic, delusional and residual)	
Mood (affective) Disorders	**Behavioural and Emotional Disorders**
Manic Episode	Hyperkinetic disorder
Depressive Episode	Conduct disorder
Bipolar Disorder	
Dysthymia	
Mental Disorders Due to Brain Damage	**Neurotic Disorders**
Organic brain syndrome	Somatoform disorder
	Panic disorder
Dementia (presenile, senile, Alzheimer's, Parkinson's)	Anxiety disorder
	Obsessive-compulsive disorder
Seizures	**Psychoactive Substance Use**
Epilepsy	Substance abuse and dependence
General tonic clonic seizures	Substance psychosis
Temporal lobe epilepsy	

Source: Goldberg and Huxley (1992).

and the psychoses, which are *severe* disorders. Although these disorders are marked by severe impairment of functioning in all three areas of psychological life—cognitive, emotional and relational—their symptoms are stable and the epileptic and psychotic disorders, in particular, respond swiftly to chemotherapy and electrotherapy, which are the dominant modes of treatment in most psychiatric institutions. The NMHP prioritizes the *severe* mental disorders for intervention because of the exclusive reliance on the biomedical approach. Such a prioritization is especially problematic for women since more women than men have been found to suffer from *common* mental disorders, whose clinical picture and treatment vary considerably from that of *severe* disorders. Such a prioritization in effect therefore, denies delivery of appropriate mental health services to women.

This is not to suggest that there is a conspiracy on the part of the NMHP to keep women out of the ambit of mental health care services. However, the point to be noted here is that the ways in which care and treatment of psychiatric disorders are organized serve to reflect the socio-political organization of institutionalized psychiatry in India. The NMHP was and remains basically a psychiatric preserve; its illness-driven approach to mental health care and mental health financing does not respond adequately to mental health needs of women.

METHOD

Sample

Data collected from hospital case records of 11,726 patients registered in two major psychiatric facilities over a five-year period, i.e., 1991–95, were analyzed, for the purpose of the present chapter, to construct socio-demographic and mental illness profiles of women who have sought psychiatric help. The first admission cases in the two mental health facilities, i.e., the cases who were attending the hospitals as inpatients or outpatients for the first time constituted the sample.

Locale of the Study

The two institutions from which the data were taken were the Government Hospital for Mental Care (GHMC) and a private psychiatric facility named Shantiniketan Hospital (SNH), both located in Visakhapatnam city in the north coastal region of Andhra Pradesh.

The GHMC, located in Visakhapatnam, is one of the two government hospitals in Andhra Pradesh and caters to not only the people of the city but also to those in Visakhapatnam district and in the adjoining districts in the north coastal region. Established in 1863, it has a bed strength of 300 (225 for males and 75 for females). Shantiniketan, started in 1984, is the only private clinic in the city rendering both inpatient and outpatient services and has a bed strength of 12. There is understandably a variation in the socio-economic profile of patients who seek the facilities of the government hospital and those of the private clinic.

The catchment area of these facilities is not only the city of Visakhapatnam but the entire north coastal region, which is characterized predominantly by economic backwardness. The city itself has grown from a small fishermen's village in the beginning of the century to a bustling city with a heavy concentration of both public and private sector industries and ancillary units. The city has one of the fastest growth rates in Asia; large-scale migration of people from rural areas and smaller towns in the region has contributed to the striking growth of the city and has been a significant feature of economic and demographic transformation. Most of the industries, however, are capital-intensive, utilizing high technology, and the high growth rate of population poses a problem of labour absorption. As a result, problems like unemployment and underemployment, pressure on civic facilities, congestion, pollution, etc., which can affect the psychological well-being of people have increased in recent times. A recent study also documented a high rate of domestic violence against women in the city, with Visakhapatnam showing the highest incidence of deaths due to such violence (per lakh of population) when compared to the other major city, Hyderabad, and representative districts of the three distinct regions (coastal Andhra, Telengana and Rayalseema) of the state (Vindhya, 2000).

These aspects of structural and socio-demographic change have been elaborated because they serve as a backdrop to our understanding of mental health problems in this region.

Procedure

Information about the socio-demographic variables and the psychiatric diagnoses was taken from the hospital case records of the patients. The diagnoses, made by the psychiatrist on duty, were as per the Tenth Revision of the *International Classification of Disorders* [ICD-10] of the WHO. It needs to be mentioned here that in view of the ICD-10 coming into use from 1993, the case records of earlier years (i.e., 1991 and 1992) were recorded according to the latest revision of the ICD. Also, since seizures are not included in ICD-10, the third revision of the Diagnostic and Statistical Manual (DSM III) of the American Psychiatric Association (APA) had been used by the psychiatrists in the two hospitals for diagnosing seizures.

Results and Discussion

Socio-demographic Profile of Mentally Ill Women

Prevalence of mental disorder has been studied through different parameters such as age, literacy levels, marital status and occupation in order to construct a socio-demographic profile of women affected by mental illness (Table 7.2). Evidence from our data identified the following groups to be the most affected: (a) women in their reproductive years (16-40 years); (b) those who were married; (c) those who are principally housewives; (d) those who were employed as agricultural or daily wage unskilled labourers; and (e) those with no or little formal education.

Table 7.2: Socio-demographic Profile of Women Patients

(n = 4,458)

Age	
Childhood and Adolescence (1-17 yrs)	6.1 %
Reproductive Years (18-45 yrs)	80.5 %
Menopausal and Elderly (46 yrs and above)	13.4 %
Education	
No Formal Education	55.3 %
Primary	15.4 %
Secondary	22.7 %
College and Above	6.6 %
Marital Status	
Married	69.3 %
Unmarried	22.1 %
Single (separated, widowed, divorced)	8.6 %
Occupation	
Daily Wage/Agricultural Labourer	20.0 %
Cultivator	10.1 %
Housewife/Unemployed	67.0 %*

Sources: Kiranmayi (1999); Vijayalakshmi (2000).
Note: *Rest of the sample was found scattered across occupation categories such as clerical, business, services, etc.

Traditional and socio-biological theories have suggested that women's well-being declines once their biological usefulness has passed, after about 40 years of age (Gergen, 1990). Feminist researchers, however, have not only questioned the view that menopause translates to psychological trauma (for example, Ussher, 1989), but have also argued that midlife may in fact be women's prime of life related to increased autonomy and self-determination (Mitchell and Helson, 1990). Certain features such as *identity certainty* or the subjective sense of having a strong and clear identity; a sense of *generativity* or an enlarged vision of one's role in the social world and a sense of responsibility and commitment; feelings of *confident power or efficacy* and finally a conscious and direct *awareness of aging* itself have been shown to be experienced as central by women in middle age (Stewart and Ostrove, 1998). These findings, admittedly, pertain to currently middle-aged, college-educated middle class white women. Although there is scarcely any research that has focused on the impact of different aspects of social location such as class, caste and historical circumstances might make to the experience of middle age in India, we could perhaps speculate that a realistic sense of aging and an enhanced sense of personal identity would be shared by several sections of currently middle-aged women in our country.

Furthermore, in contrast to the menopausal theory, widely held both by mental health practitioners and the lay public, the reproductive years have in fact been identified as the most vulnerable years of women's lives in terms of psychological distress. The reasons for such vulnerability are not far to seek and can be located in the psychosocial context of women's lives.

It is not surprising that marriage and reproduction related events like pregnancy and motherhood are implicated among the social stressors impinging on mental illness in view of the cultural imperatives associated with the centrality attributed to the institution of marriage. Much has been written about the socialization of Indian women, and the social stressors acting on women relating to marriage, family and ageing. Current research in the West has indicated that it is not just women who figure more prominently in psychological disorders, but rather that it is married women who experience more emotional distress than married men, while within each of the single statuses (unmarried, divorced or widowed), men were found to have higher rates of mental illness when compared to their female counterparts (Gove and Geerken, 1977). In short, this means that marriage is more advantageous for men because their emotional worries are laundered and processed by their wives while the same cannot be said for women who seem to be left with their own dependency needs unfulfilled. Studies focusing on interaction of marital status and employment have revealed that from the point of view of mental illness, the unemployed housewife is the most vulnerable. While such findings have by now been documented widely enough (Gove and Geerken, 1977; Brown and Harris, 1978), what is of interest to note is that our data showed marriage to be stressful for both men and women. Admittedly, the proportion of married people in the population may be sizeable compared to those who are single; even so, the high frequency of mental illness among men who are married points to the psychological costs of marital life for men as well and implicates the lack of fulfilling marital relationships as a contributory factor to mental distress. By and large, in our context, marital relationships are so closely bound within kinship structures of family life that intimate interaction between the spouses is minimized, with a harmonious and egalitarian relationship often being discouraged. Marriage, viewed more in terms of responsibilities and duties rather than in terms of companionship, may perhaps thus act as an inhibiting factor in forging an equitable and mutually satisfying relationship.

Among the occupational categories, those most affected by mental illness were found to be housewives and daily wage labourers. It is not as if the feminine role identity of the housewife is especially related to psychological distress. Rather, factors like lack of paid employment, unrelieved child care (in fact, correlation of number of children with mental illness showed women with three or four children to be the single largest group), responsibility for care-giving functions in the family and a poor non-confiding marital relationship associated with mental illness among housewives could mean lack of instrumentality, i.e., the perceived freedom to be active and instrumentally effective in directing one's life. In the case of daily wage labourers, this lack of instrumentality is born out of the deficits, obstacles and threats to health inherent in poverty and the chronic life conditions imposed by lack of basic amenities, disproportionate exposure to dangerous environments and crime, violence and discrimination, isolation from information and the like.

Finally, lack of education was found to be correlated with mental illness. Given the low literacy levels in our country and the lesser than the national average in Visakhapatnam district (48.6 per cent for men and 29.8 per cent for women), it is not surprising that a large proportion of those with little or no education are represented among the mentally ill. Research has indicated that education seems to have a positive effect on psychological well-being, the impact being more on women than men, with education being associated not only with an increase in knowledge but also with skills that can enhance one's coping potential and one's sense of competence, mastery and life control, thereby alleviating psychological distress (Radloff, 1975).

Overrepresentation of Male Patients

The two hospital samples showed a predominance of male patients with 61.9 per cent of the total sample being men, while only 38 per cent were women patients (Table 7.3). The gender gap was slightly narrowed in the case of the private hospital sample where the proportion of male and female patients was 56.2 per cent and 43.7 per cent, respectively; in the case of the government hospital, it was 63.1 and 36.8 per cent, respectively. This preponderance of male patients in psychological disorders is in line with several earlier hospital-based studies (reviewed in Davar, 1999) done in our country but is at variance with community samples (for example, Chakraborty, 1990) and with trends reported in the West where asylum statistics from 1850s onwards have confirmed that female patients outnumber their male counterparts (Kromm, 1994).

Table 7.3: Distribution of Male and Female Patients

Men	Women	Total	
7,268 (61.9 %)	4,458 (38.0 %)	11,726	
Hospital	**Men**	**Women**	**Total**
GHMC	6,139 (63.1 %)	3,579 (36.8 %)	9,718
SNH	1,129 (56.2 %)	879 (43.7 %)	2,008

Sources: Kiranmayi (1999); Vijayalakshmi (2000).

Most epidemiological studies employ either data obtained from hospital records or from field surveys in the community. While the advantage with field data is that the prevalence rate of psychological disorders (even untreated) in the community can be known, the present study had to suffice with hospital data. Studies based on hospital data as the present one, therefore, indicate the prevalence rate of only treated disorders and the utilization and access to hospital care and facilities. Such studies provide information about the socio-demography of those receiving mental health care, since who has access to what kind of mental health services in our country depends to a considerable extent on the user's social location, including social and economic status and gender.

The hospital-based studies conducted in India have recorded a predominance of male patients from which researchers have concluded that there is a greater frequency of mental illness among men. The explanation offered by some of these researchers (for example, Sethi and Manchanda, 1978, cited in Davar, 1999) is that it is men who carry the onerous burden of responsibility and stress while women have a relatively stress-free time. In her critique of epidemiological studies in the country, Davar (1999) points out that such explanations are too facile and 'methodologically questionable and politically misleading' (p. 287). She argues that first, these studies have been based on hospital samples using data on utilization of hospital facilities and services as if they were prevalence data. While doing so, these researchers, according to Davar, have glossed over the fact that there is gross gender-based inequity of access to health care in this country. Second, to say that it is only the male role that is stressful is to overlook the compelling and crucial issues that the women's movement over the past several years has been drawing our attention: the potentially stressful factors affecting women's psychological health such as the unequal work distribution, unequal decision-making power, unpaid labour and rigid role functions and stereotyping. To ignore these issues therefore and to conclude that the supposedly greater prevalence of mental illness among men is due to greater stress reveals a gender-blind approach.

Community surveys, on the other hand, from the 1970s to the 1990s, have recorded a greater female morbidity (Chakraborty, 1990). Patterns of mental disorder too vary markedly for men and women, whether data from community surveys or from hospital studies are used. Most of the studies show that women report significantly more frequent symptoms of common mental disorders. The overall gender-based difference in prevalence of severe disorders, on the other hand, is negligible compared to the overall difference in the prevalence of common disorders.

From a gender perspective, this divergence between the data obtained from hospital samples and community surveys, and between patterns of mental disorder in men and women has important implications for the mental health programme in the country. Two inferences can be drawn from these findings:

1. The pattern of predominance of male patients in hospital statistics indicates restricted access of women to health care services. The fact that in community surveys across the country more 'unidentified cases' of women have been reported indicates that women's mental distress is either untreated or they may be seeking help from

alternate settings (Primary Health Centres [PHCs] and General Practitioners [GPs]) or from native healers.
2. The approach of hospital services and treatment programmes, characterized chiefly by electrotherapy and chemotherapy and geared for severe mental disorders, is inadequate for dealing with the illnesses of women, which differ in nature and etiology and the kind of treatment required.

Since there is a paucity of traditional psychiatric services such as counselling and psychotherapeutic centres in the country, what this means, in effect, is that women, for whom a biomedical approach is inadequate to deal with the symptoms of common mental disorders, do not have recourse to appropriate psychological help. These inferences have been borne out in our study too.

The two hospital samples showed a predominance of male patients with 62 per cent of the total sample being men, while only 38 per cent were women patients. The gender gap was slightly narrowed in the case of the private hospital sample. The implications drawn from research findings mentioned in the section above seem to hold good for this study too. Hospital statistics confirm an overall overrepresentation of male patients, although this might not correlate with prevalence rates of distress in the community. The deduction then is that women are underserved by hospital services.

The patient profile of the government and private hospitals showed further differences, which are again in accordance with earlier research findings in psychiatric epidemiology. While patients from rural areas and lower socio-economic groups formed the bulk of persons seeking help in the government hospital, the private hospital had a relatively higher urban, better educated and economically advantaged clientele. It is women from the urban, educated and comparatively higher socio-economic groups that had access to the facilities of the private hospital. Therefore, despite the higher frequency of male patients in both the samples, the related findings mentioned above point to the relatively better access of women from the upper socio-economic strata to the private facilities and the poorer access of women from disadvantaged sections to state hospitals. In fact, it has been recognized in recent years that mental health services are not evenly distributed in the country. Access and quality of such care services has been found to be the best for economically advantaged men in the cities, with women from city slums and rural areas receiving the least satisfactory services in the country (Raghavan, Murty and Lakshminarayana, 1995). Once again, these findings underscore the importance of making available mental health services to sections like economically disadvantaged women from rural areas and poorer settlements in the cities.

Mental Illness Profile of Women

The multiple ways of being female in a society impact women's subjective experiences in negative ways, which can accumulate and contribute to a subset of mental health risks. The disorders commonly affecting women, as revealed in our study, were found to be *stress and adjustment disorders and neurotic disorders* (Table 7.4). Both these categories are common mental disorders whose origins are closely associated with women's work and roles in society. In these categories, it was *prolonged depressive reaction* in the category of *stress and adjustment disorders* and *somatoform and dissociative disorders* in the category of *neurotic disorders* that were found to be the most frequent diagnoses.

Table 7.4: Prevalence of Common Mental Disorders in Male and Female Patients

Type of Disorder	Men	Women
Stress and Adjustment Disorders	30.7 %	53.9 %
Behavioural and Emotional Disorders	3.8 %	2.3 %
Neurotic Disorders	19.9 %	40.6 %
Substance Abuse	45.5 %	3.2 %

Sources: Kiranmayi (1999); Vijayalakshmi (2000).

Certainly, not all women experience and respond to potential stressors in the same way. Unique combinations of class, caste, age, physical and personal resources undoubtedly create unique sets of experiences across women, as well as by experiences shared by particular subgroups. Yet, amid the heterogeneity evident among women, being female in a culture that devalues women may create a shared social experience, which, in turn, may create a shared set of psychological experiences and of mental health risks and outcomes. It is significant to note here that despite the diversity in socio-economic status of patients seeking consultation in the government hospital and private clinic, a commonality in the type of disorders was evident across the sample of women patients in the two hospitals.

Depression

Stress and adjustment disorders, in the ICD-10 classification, have been further subdivided into brief depressive reaction, prolonged depressive reaction and mixed anxiety and depression; women from both the hospital samples in our study predominated in the category of prolonged depressive reaction. This finding is in line with community-based studies and studies of treatment-seekers in many Western countries and in community studies in India which have indicated depression to be the most frequently encountered women's mental health problem (Chakraborty, 1990; Dennerstein, Astbury and Morse, 1993; Goldberg and Huxley, 1992; Russo and Green, 1993).

Depressive reactions, characterized by prolonged depressed mood, loss of pleasure in most activities are common in both men and women; even so, women are about twice as likely as men to become depressed (Nolen-Hoeksema, 1990). A related finding of our study was that even in a category such as mood (affective) disorders, the two binary extremes—mania and depression—were represented by a predominance of men and women, respectively, confirming the stereotype of the manic male externalizing mental disorder as an aggressive and potentially combative figure with constant physical agitation, elation of mood and activity, and of the depressive female on the other hand, as primarily a self-abusing figure who internalizes mental disorder.

Multiple theories have been advanced to explain the consistent gender difference in risk for depression. These theories can be distilled into three classes of explanations. The fist, focusing on female biology, attributes gender differences in depression to women's hormonal fluctuations and periodically low levels of estrogen. Puberty, premenstrual phases, the postpartum period and menopause are thus identified as times when women should be highly susceptible to depression. Empirical investigations of these life phases, however, offer only mixed evidence, suggesting that the direct relationship between hormonal changes and depression is weak, at best temporary and far from universal (Nolen-Hoeksema, 1990).

A second category of explanations for women's greater depression focuses on women's inferior social status and relative lack of power. Enumerating the social conditions that are stressful in women's lives and precipitate illness is an elaborate task that is beyond the scope of the present chapter. However, among the correlates of depression identified in community studies, high levels of depressive symptoms have been associated with long-term social adversity, including poverty, homelessness and economic dependence, role strain and an overload of role-related functions, a poor non-confiding marriage and lack of intimacy with the spouse, particularly the lack of spousal approval for employment and violence and victimization (Brown and Harris, 1978; Pearlin and Johnson, 1977). While environmental adversity including poverty, joblessness, inadequate housing, etc., has been associated with psychiatric morbidity in men as well, it is important for the mental health disciplines to take into consideration of the low social status of women and the particular stresses associated with such status in their evaluations of mental distress.

Learned helplessness theory (Seligman, 1975) and other cognitive models of depression have been used to explain how powerlessness that women experience in relationships and in the workplace can lead to reduced motivation and depression. The critical component of these models is the learning that one's actions have little or no effect upon the environment. This lack of consistency between behaviour and consequences becomes internalized, producing the expectation that nothing matters; this contributes to passivity and fatalism and has been termed learned helplessness. The theory also helps to explain why women who are low-income, single parents are particularly likely to become depressed (Russo, 1990). Given the multiple sources of oppression faced by women of colour, a power-status explanation would predict that ethnic minority women ought to experience depression at higher rates than white women. This, however, does not appear to be the case (Frederickson and Roberts, 1997). The lack of a neatly consistent relationship between depression and low social status points to the complex and nuanced factors affecting the susceptibility of people to psychological illnesses such as depression.

In our country, we do not have research that specifically addresses the question of depression in women (or men) in lower socioe-conomic classes, although there is some evidence of psychiatric morbidity being high in the most deprived sections and unclassified categories of the workforce such as beggars, prostitutes and domestic maids (Davar, 1995) and in low-income, slum-dwelling and uneducated women (Blue et al., 1995).

A third class of explanations describe how certain personality characteristics, more typical of women than men, can increase risk for depression. Women are often characterized as nurturant, emotional, non-assertive, self-sacrificing and relationship-oriented. Even if we consider these traits to pertain more to the 'private domain' (where such characteristics are manifested in the context of women's relationships with their family) rather than to the 'public sphere', a range of theories has been offered to explain how women develop these characteristics and how they can compromise mental health. Carol Gilligan's theory, for instance, is illustrative of such theories which suggest that women's strivings for interpersonal intimacy, combined with cultural prescriptions for being a 'good woman', combine to create an experience that has been described as 'loss of self' (Gilligan, 1989; Jack, 1991). According to these theorists, loss of self can result when, in efforts to smooth and protect valued relationships, women develop habits of censoring their own expression and restricting their own initiatives (Gilligan and Brown, 1992; Jack, 1991). Over time, habitual self-censorship can lead to a duplicity of experience in which outer compliance is paired with inner confusion and frustration, often with ensuing depression (Jack, 1991).

Despite the lack of consensus across explanations for the gender difference in depression, strands of each of these classes of explanations can be drawn together. Building on a view advanced by researchers in the biopsychosocial tradition (for example, Goldberg and Huxley, 1992), an integrated explanation can be posited which suggests that biochemical stressors (like hormonal fluctuations) and psychosocial stressors (from the external social environment) work through the person's own cognitive appraisal mechanisms, i.e., the person's interpretation or meaning given to the event, or one's schema for organizing reality resulting in experience of distress. As Davar (1999) has pointed out: 'In the end, the comparative importance that one justifiably gives to the physical, the cognitive and the social components of mental distress would be determined by negotiating a pool of facts within an integrated research domain' (p. 304).

Somatoform and dissociative disorders

Among the neurotic disorders, women patients in our study were found to predominate in somatoform and dissociative disorders. Both these classes of disorders essentially focus on the body. Somatoform disorders involve a pattern of recurring multiple, clinically significant bodily complaints without any diagnosable general medical condition to account for the physical symptoms. The essential feature of dissociative disorders is a disruption in the usually integrated functions of consciousness, memory, identity or perception of the environment. While dissociative amnesia belonging to this category is perhaps a frequently seen condition in popular films, a more frequently diagnosed condition in hospital data is depersonalization disorder, characterized by a persistent or recurrent feeling of being detached from one's mental processes or body, precipitated by severe stress and subsequent to life-threatening traumatic situations.

It is not surprising that women's mental ill-being is predominantly manifested through disorders such as somatoform and dissociation.

Medically unexplained symptoms, preoccupation with physical illness, trance-like experiences characteristic of these disorders may constitute culturally shaped 'idioms of distress' that are employed to express concerns about a broad range of personal and social problems. Although the forms of these symptoms may reflect cultural ideas about acceptable and credible ways to express distress, what is important to note is that women's idioms of distress are expressed through the body.

In the traditional debate between biological and environmental determinants of psychological gender differences, the body has most often been explored in terms of its anatomical, genetic or hormonal influences on personality, experience and behaviour. Feminist psychologists have been understandably suspicious of such perspectives because of their deterministic flavour and essentialist stance, and have done a great deal to illuminate the multiple ways that the body conveys social meaning and how these meanings shape gendered experience (for example, Kaschak, 1992; Ussher, 1989). According to these theorists, accumulation of experiences in cultures that objectify the female body may help account for mental health risks that centre around the 'normative discontent' women feel towards their bodies and that disproportionately affect women: somatoform, dissociative and eating disorders.

Conclusion

Issues related to women's mental health in our country have not received much attention from mainstream psychological approaches. Viewing mental illness from the biomedical model, these approaches have, by and large, ignored the impact of socio-cultural factors. However, in an area such as women's mental health, it is all the more necessary to consider the socio-cultural context of their health since it is being increasingly recognized that the stresses that differentially affect women by virtue of their unequal social status have led to pervasive mental health problems for them. This chapter has attempted to map the mental illness profile of women seeking psychiatric help and construct a socio-demographic profile of these women. Data from hospital case records of 11,726 patients in two major psychiatric facilities in the city of Visakhapatnam in South India formed the empirical basis for the study. The disorders that women were found to be affected most were common mental disorders such as depression, dissociation and somatoform disorders, whose origins are closely associated with women's position, work and roles in society.

The socio-demographic profile of the mentally ill women indicated that women in their reproductive years, those who were married, those employed as agricultural labourers or as housewives and those with little education were the most affected groups. It is not surprising to recognize these socio-cultural barriers that diminish women's psychological wellbeing and limit their potential; what is surprising but heartening is that despite the enormity of these stressors, women continue to be resilient and negotiate for spaces and a position for themselves.

REFERENCES

Blue, I., Ducci, M., Jaswal, J., Ludumir, A. and Harpham, T. (1995). The mental health of low-income urban women: Case studies from Bombay, India; Olinda, Brazil; and Santiago, Chile. In T. Harpham and I. Blue (Eds), *Urbanization and mental health in developing countries* (pp. 75-102). Brookfield, VT: Ashgate.

Brown, G. W. and Harris, T. (1978). *Social origins of depression*. London: Tavistock.

Carmen, E. H., Russo, N. E. and Miller, J. B. (1981). Inequality and women's mental health: An overview. *American Journal of Psychiatry*, 138(10), 1319-30.

Chakraborty, A. (1990). *Social stress and mental health: A social-psychiatric field study of Calcutta*. New Delhi: Sage.

Chesler, P. (1972). *Women and madness*. New York: Doubleday.

Davar, B. V. (1995). Mental illness among Indian women. *Economic and Political Weekly*, 30(45), 2879-886.

———. (1999). *Mental illness in Indian women*. New Delhi: Sage.

Dennerstein, L., Astbury, J. and Morse, C. (1993). *Psychosocial and mental health aspects of women's health*. Geneva: WHO.

Eaton, W. W. and Kessler, L. G. (1985). *Epidemiologic field methods in psychiatry: The NIMH Epidemiologic Catchment Area Program*. Orlando, FL: Academic Press.

Frederickson, B. L. and Roberts, T. (1997). Objectification theory: Towards understanding women's lived experiences and mental health risks. *Psychology of Women Quarterly*, 21(2), 173-206.

Gergen, M. M. (1990). Finished at 40: Women's development with the patriarchy. *Psychology of Women Quarterly*, 14(4), 471-93.

Gilligan, C. (1989). *Mapping the moral domain: A contribution of women's thinking to psychological theory and education*. Cambridge, MA: Harvard University Press.

Gilligan, C. and Brown, L. (1992). Meeting at the crossroads: Women's psychology and girls' development. Cambridge, MA: Harvard University Press.

Goldberg, D. P. and Huxley, P. (1992). *Common mental disorders: A bio-social model*. London: Routledge.

GOI. (1982). *National Mental Health Programme for India*. New Delhi: Directorate General of Health Services.

Gove, W. R. and Geerken, M. D. (1977). The effects of children and employment on the mental health of married men and women. *Social Forces*, 56(1), 66–76.
Haslam, N. (2000). Psychiatric categories as natural kinds: Essentialist thinking about mental disorder. *Social Research*, 67(4), 1031–58.
Jack, D. C. (1991). *Silencing the self: Women and depression.* New York: Harper.
Kaschak, E. (1992). *Engendered lives: A new psychology of women's experience.* New York: Basic Books.
Kiranmayi, A. (1999). Socio-demographic correlates of psychological disorders: A hospital-based study in Visakhapatnam district. Unpublished doctoral dissertation, Andhra University.
Kromm, E. (1994). Feminization of madness in visual representation. *Feminist Studies*, 20(3), 507–20.
Lee, C. (1998). *Women's health: Psychological and social perspectives.* London: Sage.
Meehl, P. E. (1995). Bootstraps taxometrics: Solving the classification problem in psychopathology. *American Psychologist*, 50(4), 266–75.
Mitchell, V. and Helson, R. (1990). Women's prime of life: Is it the 50s? *Psychology of Women Quarterly*, 14(4), 451–70.
Myers, J. K., Weissman, M. M., Tischler, G. L., Holzer, C. E., Leaf, P. J., Orpaschel, H., Anthony, J. C., Boyd, J. H., Burkey, J. D., Kramer, M. and Stoltzman, R. (1984). Six-month prevalence of psychiatric disorders in three communities. *Archives of General Psychiatry*, 41(10), 959–67.
Nicolson, P. and Ussher, J. (1992). *The psychology of women's health and health care.* Basingstoke, UK: Macmillan.
Nolen-Hoeksema, S. (1990). *Sex differences in depression.* Stanford, CA: Stanford University Press.
Pearlin, L. and Johnson, M. (1977). Marital status, life strains and depression. *American Sociological Review*, 42(October), 704–15.
Prabhu, G. G. and Raghuram, A. (1987). Mental health in India. In *Encyclopaedia of Social Work in India*, 2 (pp. 188–89). New Delhi: Ministry of Welfare.
Prior, L. (1993). *The social organization of mental illness.* London: Sage.
Radloff, L. (1975). Sex differences in depression: The effects of occupation and marital status. *Sex Roles*, 1, 249–65.
Raghavan, K. S., Murty, R. S. and Lakshminarayana, R. (1995). *Symposium on women and mental health: Report and recommendations.* Bangalore: NIMHANS.
Rubin, G. (1975). The traffic in women: Notes on the 'political economy' of sex. In Rayna Reiter (Ed.), *Toward an anthropology of women.* New York: Monthly Review Press.
Russo, N. F. (1990). Overview: Forging research priorities for women's mental health. *American Psychologist*, 45(3), 368–73.
Russo, N. F. and Green, B. L. (1993). Women and mental health. In F. L. Denmark and M. A. Paludi (Eds), *Psychology of women: A handbook of issues and theories* (pp. 379–436). Westport: Greenwood.
Russo, N. F., Amaro, H. and Winter, M. (1987). The use of inpatient mental health services by Hispanic women. *Psychology of Women Quarterly*, 11(3), 427–42.

Seligman, M. E. P. (1975). *Helplessness: On depression, development and death.* San Francisco: Freeman.

Sethi, B. B. and Manchanda, R. (1978). Family structure and psychiatric disorders. *Indian Journal of Psychiatry,* 20, 283–88.

Stewart, A. J. and Ostrove, J. M. (1998). Women's personality in middle age: Gender, history and midcourse corrections. *American Psychologist,* 53(11), 1185–94.

Stroebe, W. and Stroebe, M. S. (1995). *Social psychology and health.* Milton Keynes, Buckingham: Open University Press.

Ussher, J. M. (1989). *The psychology of the female body.* London: Routledge.

Vijayalakshmi, V. (2000). Mood Disorders and their socio-demographic correlates: A hospital based study. Unpublished doctoral dissertation, Andhra University.

Vindhya, U. (2000). 'Dowry deaths' in Andhra Pradesh, India: Response of the criminal justice system. *Violence against women: An international and interdisciplinary journal,* 6(10), October: 1085–1108.

World Health Organization. (2001). *The World Health Report–Mental health: New understanding, new hope.* Geneva: World Health Organization.

Zuckerman, E. (1979). Changing directions in the treatment of women. *Mental Health Bibliography* (pp. 494–505). Washington: DHEW Publication.

8

Research on Families with Disabled Individuals: Review and Implications

LINA KASHYAP

A paradox of the phenomenal advances in medical and engineering sciences, in technology and research, is the increasing number of disabled individuals. There has been a gradual increase in the incidence of these conditions as a result of improved methods for early detection, diagnosis and treatment and intensive public education. The control achieved over contagious diseases has also led to an increase in life expectancy.

However, the concern today is not just to save life; the quality of survival is now regarded as of equal, if not of greater significance. Hence, the realization that physical restoration is only one aspect of total rehabilitation; inseparable from it are psychological and social adjustments. A vast number of disabled individuals are being cared for by their families generally throughout their lifetime. Yet, until the early twentieth century, very little was known about their social non-medical needs or about the needs of their family members who cared for them or about the manner in which the perceptions and attitudes of the family influenced their overall rehabilitation.

The past few decades have seen tremendous changes in the philosophy and provision of services for such individuals. There has been a definite movement away from the concepts of custody, care and treatment to the concepts of prevention, education and rehabilitation. Institutional services, till recently, were the major forms of specialized care provided to such individuals. In recent years, there has been a growing movement towards de-institutionalization and the development of community-based rehabilitation services. This trend has received impetus from an emphasis on the 'normalization' principle, which seeks to promote conditions which would allow such individuals to develop their full potential and live as ordinary a life as possible. Another major change has been the growing emphasis on a multi-disciplinary team approach, in which each specialist contributes his or her knowledge and skills towards providing comprehensive rehabilitation services. There has been a growing recognition among specialists that these individuals cannot be viewed as isolated entities, but need to be seen within their familial and societal contexts because of the reciprocal and interdependent relationships between such individuals and their families, and the influence that the family exerts on their overall rehabilitation. Since the family can play a vital role in supporting such members, its direct involvement in the rehabilitation process, as an active partner in the multi-disciplinary team, is increasingly considered necessary.

At the same time, it is being accepted that the presence of a disabled family member disrupts family equilibrium. The reactions of the family to this member are as crucial as the actual impact of the presence of such a member on the family's daily life. Therefore, families need guidance, training and comprehensive counselling in order to meet their own needs, as well as to adjust to their member's condition, and to function effectively as a member of the rehabilitation team. Thus the disabled individual needs to be seen in his or her familial and societal context, and professional intervention needs to be focused not on him or her alone, but on his and her family also taken together as a unit.

DEFINITION OF KEY CONCEPTS

In the literature on the disabled, the terms 'impairment', 'disability' and 'handicap' are often used synonymously and interchangeably. They are not synonymous. Impairment refers to any loss or abnormality of psychological or anatomical structure or function (WHO, 1980). Disability refers to any restriction on, or lack of ability (resulting from impairment) to perform the activity within the manner or within the range considered normal for a human being (WHO, 1980). Disability, therefore, refers to any limitation experienced by the impaired person with reference to his physical function, whether locomotor or sensory, or affecting any specific organs. The effects of the disability generally extend beyond a particular pathological condition and embraces the psychological, educational and vocational aspects as well. The term handicap refers to a disadvantage for an individual with an impairment or disability, which limits or prevents the fulfilment of a role that is normal, depending upon sex, age and social or cultural factors (WHO, 1980). A disabled person feels handicapped or is made to feel handicapped. Thus, more than the disability, it is the psycho-social handicap that adversely affects the life of the disabled, as it has its root in the stigma attached to disability or impairment.

The primary goal of intervention programme is to prevent or reduce the occurrence of an impairment, prevent an impairment from developing into a disability, and prevent the deterioration of a disability into a handicap. Thus, rehabilitation refers to the restoration and development of disabled persons to their fullest physical, mental, social, vocational and economic potential and the prevention of their disability from turning into a lasting handicap, or at least reducing its handicapping effects to its minimum.

Four categories of disabilities have been considered in this paper, namely, blindness, deafness, orthopaedic handicap and mental handicap.

When a person has visual acuity of 20/200 or even less, he is considered legally blind (Government of India, 1978). If the visual acuity in the better eye is 20/70 or less, he is considered to have impaired vision, and visual ability is substantially reduced. Visual impairment also includes loss of peripheral or central vision.

The deaf are those in whom the sense of hearing is non-functional for the ordinary purpose of life (Brill, 1974). These are people for whom the sense of hearing is so impaired as to have precluded normal acquisition of language hearing. The hard of hearing are those in whom the sense of hearing, though defective, is functional with or without a hearing aid.

The orthopaedically handicapped are those who have a physical defect or deformity which causes interference with the normal functioning of the bones, joints and muscles (Government of India, 1978). There are a variety of orthopaedic handicaps, such as those caused by congenital anomaly such as club foot, absence of limbs, etc., impairments caused by diseases such as poliomyelitis, bone tuberculosis, etc. and impairments from other causes such as cerebral palsy, amputation, etc.

A mentally handicapped person is one who has sub-average general intellectual potential and slow intellectual development, which may be the result of genetic factors, trauma, organ damage or social deprivation (Barker, 1987). The retardation may be of different degrees ranging from a mild form of mental retardation or dullness to severe retardation.

Scope

This paper attempts to examine the type of research studies done in India on families having disabled individuals, indicate significant trends in this field and point out gaps in research.[1]

For the review, only those studies have been selected which are wholly or partly concerned with some aspect of the effect on the family of the disability of a member, and/or the influencing factors within the society and the family, leading to problems in coping with such members and/or the family's coping strategies and/or the professional intervention for helping the family to cope. Although there are quite a few studies which have focused on surgical and technological research and innovations in the educational and vocational training of this special group, as well as on demographic or socio-economic, or personality characteristics of such individuals, they have been excluded from the review, unless these characteristics have been looked at by the researchers in their studies as precipitating factors within the family or as influencing the family's coping strategies. By and large, master's level research has not been considered, but doctoral dissertations have been reviewed. The review has been limited to the more general aspects of the research studies and only main findings have been included.

The disabled, their needs and problems have drawn more attention from researchers in the present decade, as is evident from the fact that of the 36 studies reviewed for this paper, as many as 25 of them have been undertaken in this decade.

Of the four categories of the disabled, the mentally handicapped and their families have received the maximum attention, as 21 studies deal with some aspect relating to such individuals and their families. Only four studies could be found on the visually handicapped and their families and four on the orthopaedically handicapped and their families. In four more studies, the sample consisted of an equal number of individuals from the four categories. Only three studies could be located on the hearing handicapped and their families.

Nine studies have been conducted by multi-disciplinary teams and these were hospital or clinic based. One team was from the National Institute of Visual Handicap. All the remaining studies have been conducted by

---

[1] The research methods of the studies are not reviewed here as they are reviewed in detail by J. C. Sharma later on.

researchers from single disciplines, foremost among them being psychologists, followed by psychiatrists. Other disciplines which are beginning to show interest in research in this field are professional social workers, child development and home science specialists, occupational therapists and medical teams.

Overview of Research Findings

Research on families having disabled members has been reviewed with reference to the following aspects:

1. The effect on the family of the presence of a disabled individual.
2. The influencing factors within the family.
3. The family's coping strategies.
4. Professional invervention for helping the family to cope.

It may be noted that some studies have been cited in more than one area, depending upon the number of aspects examined by them.

Effect on the Family of the Presence of a Disabled Individual

No family is prepared for the presence of a disabled person. Therefore, the occurrence of a disabling condition in a family member shakes the family to its foundations. The perceived condition of the disabled person affects not only every member of the family, but the reactions of each of these will, in turn, have their effect on each of the others including the disabled person. It, thus, affects family inter-relationships and may call for an adjustment of certain family functions. It will affect the family's expectations from their disabled family member. It will also affect the practical aspects of the family's daily life.

Seven studies have focused on the effect on the family of the presence of a disabled member. Of these, four are on families of mentally handicapped children (Gera, Wellington and Purohit, 1978; Seshadri, Verma, Verma and Pershad, 1983; Behere and Sinha, 1985 and Rastogi, 1984); two on families of deaf children (Kashyap, 1983, 1986); one on families of adults suffering from head injury (Sabhesan, Arumugham, Andal and Natarajan, 1988); and one on families of different categories of disabled children (Gandotra, 1984).

Family inter-relationships

As the family is a system of inter-dependent relationships, it follows that the presence of a disabled person in it affects the relationship between all its members.

Gera et al. (1978) studied the social interaction between 15 pairs of mother–mentally retarded child in a simulated game situation. It was observed that the mother's perception of dependency in the retarded child seemed to have a positive correlation with her verbal interaction with the child in a game situation. The mother's verbal interaction had a negative association with the child's verbal interaction. But her non-verbal interaction was positively associated with the child's non-verbal interaction.

One medium of interpersonal interaction is communication. Kashyap's study (1983) on 100 deaf children in the age group of 5 to 14 years, studying in special schools in Bombay, has brought out the nature and extent of communication between mother–child, father–child and child–sibling dyads. It was found that there was a greater amount of communication between mother and child than between father and child. Of the three family members, the deaf child expressed himself to the greatest extent to the mother, next to the sibling and least to the father. On the whole, the overall extent of communication within the family was at a medium level. It was low while communicating in situations related to eliciting action from the child and in situations related to helping the child understand self. It was medium in situations related to information exchange, explaining cause-and-effect relationships and for eliciting emotional expression. There was also a high degree of reciprocity between mother–child and between father–child dyads. A high degree of such reciprocity coupled with just low or medium levels of communication from either person in the two dyads led to a low level of responsive communication from the other. The conclusion arrived by the researcher was that the initiative in raising these levels must obviously rest with the parents.

Kashyap has also talked about the relationship between other family members. The mothers of 30 per cent of the children studied expressed their concern over the fact that there was a decrease in their interactions with their other children. Sibling relationship was also affected. The mothers of more than half the children in the study reported that they had to cope with sibling rivalry between their deaf child and their other children. The study by Sabhesan et al. (1988) of 75 male agriculturists who had suffered head injury and who were followed up for one and a half years has brought out that psychological sequelae, particularly cognitive disturbances and disturbed interpersonal relations, were some difficulties prevalent among the patients and they affected their occupational resettlement.

The first two studies have depicted that there is a reciprocity in the level of interaction between members of the family and the disabled individual. Seshadri et al. (1983) studied 30 families having a mentally retarded child. They observed that the children's degree of mental retardation had not affected the marital adjustment between the parents, as there was no significant marital disharmony in the sample. Kashyap (1986) has brought out similar findings in her study of 100 school-going deaf children. In her study, too, a majority of the parents felt that the presence of the deaf child had not affected their marital relationship. However, of significance were seven mothers and four fathers who confided that they had come closer to their spouse in their common concern over the deaf child, and an equal number of parents stated that their marital relationship had deteriorated. It can, therefore, be surmised that the presence of a disabled member will not create marital disharmony in a stable marriage, but it may precipitate conflict between marital partners when their personalities and interactions have already predisposed them to conflict.

Expectations from disabled persons

Most families have some expectations from each of their members. The occurrence of disability in a family member, however, calls for considerable adjustment on the part of the family regarding its hopes and plans for that individual's future.

Behere and Sinha (1985), who studied the expectations of 38 parents of mentally retarded children, have stated that a majority of the respondents were illiterate and had unrealistic expectations from their child as well as the clinic. Most of these unrealistic expectations were that their mentally retarded child would be able to take education on a par with other normal children, and be able to share the financial burden of the family. Parents also expected a miracle cure following the administration of 'brain tonic' demanded by them from the clinic.

There is a variation in parental expectations from their deaf children, according to Kashyap's data (1986). While 39 per cent and 36 per cent of the mothers and the fathers, respectively, had positive expectations from their deaf child, the remaining parents had low or unrealistic or no expectations at all. In this sample, the mother's expectations were significantly related to the child's age group, but not the father's. Moreover, the parent's age and educational level did not affect their expectations from the deaf child.

The effect on the practical aspects of daily life

The presence of a disabled person can have an effect for better or worse on some of the practical aspects of daily life, such as social life, leisure-time activities, household responsibilities, work life, etc.

Gandotra's study (1984) has made an analysis of the problems faced by 25 home-makers having disabled children. The sample consisted of five families from each of the groups: orthopaedically handicapped, blind, deaf-mute, mentally retarded and cerebral palsy affected. Deaf-mute children were perceived as the least dependent on others for carrying out day to day activities and the cerebral palsy children, the most dependent. So according to this study, the nature and extent of the disability affected the problems faced by the family members. The main problems identified were in the areas of direct care, social contacts, inadequacy of day-care facilities for the disabled family member, lack of funds, time and expense of treatment and physical health of the home-maker.

In Kashyap's study (1986), mothers of almost half the deaf children reported an increase in household responsibilities. A few complained of deterioration in their social life and leisure-time activities. Three mothers stated that they had to give up their careers because of the deaf child. Half the mothers and a quarter of the fathers felt an adverse effect on their health.

Rastogi's study (1984) of the personality patterns of parents of 50 mentally retarded children reports that both the parents of mildly retarded children obtained high scores on scales of anxiety, phobia and depression. A higher degree of neurotic traits were found in the mothers of retarded children rather than in the fathers.

Gaps in research

From the above review it is clear that very little and very limited research has been done on disabled people and their families. Not all categories of the disabled have been included in the research either.

Though there is some research on the inter-relationship patterns between disabled children and their families, specifically the parents, research is also needed to understand the inter-relationship patterns among other members of the family, for example, between the disabled child and its siblings, as this will have implications for professional intervention.

Moreover, the inter-relationships between a disabled adult or a disabled parent and his or her spouse, children and other members of the extended family are still unexplored empirically, in spite of the growing number of adults disabled due to accidents, which create a family crisis, needing professional intervention. Also, many disabled persons are now marrying either similarly disabled partners or able-bodied persons. Interpersonal relationships in both groups need research for more effective intervention.

The expectations of family members with reference to all the disabled groups need study. It would be of relevance to determine the nature of basic family functions which such families are able to perform, the degree to which they perform certain functions and the factors influencing their performance, as it will have implications for professional intervention as well as for social policy. For example, the economic function is basic to all families. During his or her early years, a disabled child usually makes greater demands on the family's financial resources by way of medical care, prosthetic aids and appliances, special educational services, transport costs, etc. The ability to provide these facilities would depend upon the economic and employment status of its members, and the number of children it has. Not only does the disabled child increase demands on the family's financial resources, he may also decrease its productive power when members have to give up lucrative jobs or promotions to take care of the needs of the disabled person.

The effect of the presence of a disabled individual on the practical aspects of daily life also needs deeper research for all the disabled groups. Such studies would indicate the type of support services needed by the family. It would also give some indication of the family's reactions to the disabled person and its capacity to cope with the situation.

Influencing Factors within the Family

A number of factors within the family influence its perception and coping strategies vis-à-vis the disabled individual. It is obvious that certain factors influence the type of problems faced by a family having a disabled person and the coping strategies used by it. These factors could be related to the family's characteristics, such as composition, mobility, socio-economic status, stage of the family life cycle, role expectations and role behaviour, reactions to the disabled person, etc.

Fourteen studies have dealt with the influencing factors within the family. Eight studies are on parents of mentally handicapped children, two are on parents of deaf children, one each on blind women and on families with adults recovering from head injury. In two more studies, the sample consists of groups of children having different types of disabilities.

One major influencing factor is the attitude of the family towards the disabled individual. It is interesting to note that 12 out of the 14 studies in this area have examined only this factor. Only two studies, Gandotra (1984) and Kashyap (1983), have discussed other influencing factors.

Parental attitudes towards mentally retarded children were reported as negative by Chaturvedi and Malhotra (1983), Rastogi (1981) and Prabhu (1968). Rastogi also observed that mothers had more negative attitudes than fathers. According to Jehan and Ansari (1981) and De Sousa and Iyer (1968–69), a majority of the parents had a rejecting attitude, though a few parents did have an accepting attitude towards their mentally retarded child. In complete contradiction to these studies, Seshadri et al. (1983) report that most mothers of the 30 mentally retarded children in their study had favourable attitudes towards their mentally retarded child. It is of interest to note that only Seshadri et al. used the Parental Attitude Scale (Bhatti and Narayanan, 1980), for investigating this aspect, whereas, all the other researchers used either the interview schedule or a structured questionnaire. Seshadri's findings also showed that the higher the education, the more favourable the attitudes. Also, the child's degree of retardation was not correlated to parental attitudes. A study by Mudgil, Singh and Srivastava (1982), of 100 mentally retarded children from a child guidance clinic, has related child's behaviour to parental attitudes. The authors in this study have surmised that psychological symptoms, such as hyperactivity, bed-wetting, temper tantrums, aggressiveness and anti-social behaviour could be a reaction to the disease and are partly caused by parental attitudes of rejection and indifference.

Ishtiaq and Kamal (1981), in a comparative study of mentally retarded and blind children, found that the former faced more negative attitudes from their families than the latter. This study used the case-history method to analyze the social climate of the respondents. In a study of attitudes of parents of deaf and hard-of-hearing children towards total rehabilitation of their children, Nigam and Kakar (1981) found that the parents were more interested in 'medical and surgical treatment' than in 'educational treatment', although most of them reported satisfaction about the overall treatment. Forty out of 45 blind women employed in a sheltered workshop and contributing to the family income, when interviewed by Sethuraman (1979), felt that their employment had not changed the negative attitude of their parents and relatives towards them.

Sabhesan et al. (1988) reported that among the male agriculturists who had recovered from head injury, those who were overprotected by the family took a longer time to go back to work, and that this protective attitude was often derived from certain culture-sanctioned concepts about the nature of head injury.

Gandotra's (1984) analysis of the managerial behaviour of 25 home-makers, who had a major role in the care of a disabled family member, indicated that the extent of the problem faced by home-makers in caring for their disabled child, was related to the economic status of the family, family structure, extent of help received by her from other members of the family and lack of awareness about facilities available in the city. Her follow-up study showed that families could tackle the problem of rehabilitation of the disabled person better when they became aware of the available facilities.

Gandotra's study also considered the age of the disabled persons and the nature and extent of the disability as other influencing factors. Thus, in her sample, the deaf–mute group had the lowest disability score and the cerebral palsy group, the highest. In contrast to this data, a study by Channabasavanna, Bhatti and Prabhu (1985) on attitudes of parents towards their mentally retarded children showed that the degree of retardation did not affect the attitudes, and neither did the socio-demographic variables of these families. The authors have surmised that in their sample, the attitudes were dependent on the parents' level of knowledge of the handicap and, therefore, removal of misconceptions brought about a positive change in them.

In her study of deaf children, Kashyap (1983) observed that among 55 per cent of the families, both parents had poor knowledge of the disability, and only one mother had a good knowledge of the disability. The rest had only average knowledge. Of the parents who had poor knowledge, the majority did not see this lack of knowledge affecting their ability to cope with the disabled child. However, among those who had average knowledge, the majority felt that this lack of information adversely affected their coping ability. This implies that only when parents have some knowledge of the disability, do they realize that the lack of full knowledge affects their communication and interaction with the disabled child.

Most of the studies reviewed have focused on the attitudes of parents and family as an influencing factor and only two studies have indicated other influencing factors. More studies for all categories of the disabled and their families are required, which will comprehensively study this area, as only thorough knowledge of the factors influencing the family's coping strategies will enable professional intervention and service provision to be more need-based and, thus, more effective. The family's perception of the availability of and extent of usefulness of supportive and educational services also needs to be explored empirically.

Family's Coping Strategies

Disability in a family member is a major crisis in the family and all families go through a reactive period of mourning, but eventually most of them evolve strategies for coping with this situation. Knowledge of the family's manner of and the extent of ability to do so will throw light on the type of professional intervention needed by it in this endeavour. In spite of the importance of this topic, there is an absolute paucity of research in this area, which is evidenced by the fact that only one research study has examined this topic.

Only Gandotra (1984) has studied the ways and means used by 25 home-makers to cope with the problems arising from the presence of a disabled person in the family. Her case studies on these families show that the high-priority goals of the families studied were to make the disabled person self-reliant with respect to daily needs and to find employment for him. Towards this end, families secured the necessary aids for their disabled family members and made relevant changes in certain household facilities. A lot of time and expense were spent on their treatment and members of the family did overtime jobs in order to meet financial needs. Gandotra reports that in some families, home-makers were relieved of some of their household chores, so that they could have more time to meet the needs of the disabled family member. Other family members also helped in the disabled child's care. Education and vocational training were provided by most families for their blind, deaf–mute and orthopaedically handicapped members, but only a few families did so for their mentally retarded and cerebral palsy members. They made efforts to help the disabled person to be self-employed or to get a job outside, although not all families succeeded in this endeavour. Finally, all families made efforts to provide for the future financial security of the disabled person.

The important area of coping strategies has been almost totally unexplored empirically. Research in this area is important because it is necessary to know in some depth the family's actual coping strategies in dealing with the presence of a disabled member. Such data would help in arriving at a typology of families, based on the extent of their coping abilities. For example, there will be some families who will be able to cope with the situation with their own resources, while others will be able to cope only with the help of professional intervention and other available services. There will be still others who will not be able to cope with the situation at all and will require services on a more permanent basis. The characteristics, ability to cope and manner of coping of all three types of families will differ and will have implications for the type of professional intervention and supportive services needed.

Professional Intervention for Helping Families to Cope

Many families seem willing to assume total responsibility for their disabled member, despite considerable financial, physical and emotional burdens. However, since most families need some guidance to assume such a role, it is desirable that they get to know about the rehabilitation facilities available. Comparatively speaking, the family experiences little difficulty in obtaining a diagnosis. The major problems encountered are in the area of availability of therapeutic services. Families need help in coping with a painful situation in a way most constructive to their disabled member as well as to the family as a unit. They need help in understanding their disabled member, guidance in the use of resources, encouragement for active participation in remedial programmes and support and acknowledgement for the care provided in the home.

From a review of research on professional interventions, one thing that stands out is that in this aspect too, the mentally handicapped group has received maximum attention from professionals. Of the seven studies reviewed, five are on mentally handicapped persons. Except for one study which assesses an intervention programme for mentally retarded children, all the other studies have assessed parent-training programmes.

Mehta and Ochaney (1984), Singh and Kaushik (1982) and Kaushik (1984) have evaluated training programmes in which parents of mentally retarded children were trained in behaviour-modification techniques. Kaushik (1984) felt that the critical factor in the programme was the method of training. Singh and Kaushik (1982) observed that the demonstration procedure was very important for teaching behavioural skills. Mehta and Ochaney were of the opinion that the involvement of one or both parents, as co-therapists, contributed to the success of the programme.

The parent-training programmes assessed by Embar (1979), Parikh (1981) and Siddiqui, Sultana and Ahmad (1984) for parents of mentally retarded children had a more broad-based approach. Though the techniques used in different programmes differed, as did the assessment tools, all the studies reported an improvement in social behaviour of the mentally retarded children and the parents' ability to cope with them as a result of the training. There was positive acceptance of the programmes from the parents. Siddiqui et al. (1984) found that the younger the child, the better were the effects of behavioural training given by the parents on the advice of professionals.

Deshmukh and Rawat (1977) had experimented with teaching simple passive exercises to rural illiterate mothers to work on at home with their polio-affected children. They found that these mothers were able to follow the exercises so well that they were able to prevent complications in their children, such as deformity or contractures. They concluded that rural people can be taught simple physiotherapy methods that achieve the same results at home as in a modern hospital. Mathur, Chokshi and Singh (1986) have focused on a community-based rehabilitation programme for rural blind individuals and have surmised that community-based programmes are definitely effective in terms of cost-benefit and rehabilitation measures in the home environment.

The maximum attention of professionals has been on the mentally handicapped and their families. Here also, the emphasis has been on educational programmes for training parents in behaviour modification techniques. The outcome of different kinds of professional interventions with all the categories of the disabled and their families, such as individual, group and family counselling programmes, vocational rehabilitation programmes, community-based rehabilitation programmes, programmes enhancing parent–child relationships, parent-education and community-education programmes, etc., need to be assessed in terms of their usefulness and effectiveness. A variety of research methods such as need survey, monitoring programmes, documentation of services provided, implementation, evaluation, process analysis of the delivery system, research on utilization of services, cost-benefit analysis, follow-up research, etc., could be used, depending upon the type of intervention to be assessed.

IMPLICATIONS FOR SOCIAL WORK PRACTICE, TEACHING AND SOCIAL POLICY

One of the basic needs of the disabled people and their families is to receive comprehensive, instructional and therapeutic counselling to enable them to meet their own needs and to achieve a wholesome adjustment to the disabling condition of their family member.

The social work professional trained in working with individuals and families is well equipped to provide family-counselling services to families having disabled individuals. Family-centred programmes are viable means of reaching the disabled person because although the primary thrust of therapeutic attention is directed towards the family, its ultimate goal is to reach the disabled individual through the family. As the approach of most of the other specialities in the field is client- or patient-centred, the social work professional can be a vital link between different professionals and the family and the disabled individual on the one hand, and between the family and its disabled member on the other. In addition, professional social workers also have the necessary skills to participate actively at the community level in developing local services, advocating on behalf of the rights of the disabled and working to prevent the occurrence of the chronic problems through programmes of community education.

The social worker's role as a team member is gradually being recognized as a significant one in the rehabilitation process by social workers themselves, as well as by the other members of the rehabilitation team.

From the review of research on the effects on the family of the presence of a disabled person, it is quite clear that the presence of a disabled person affects family relationships. The entire inter-relationship pattern in the family needs to be strengthened, specially parent–child, sibling and marital inter-relationships. It is seen from the studies that family expectations, especially parental expectations, are mostly negative or unrealistic, except in a few rare cases. Therefore, many parents will need guidance in setting up realistic expectations about their child's performance and accomplishment. They often need encouragement to believe in the possible achievements of their handicapped child. They need guidance in understanding the limitations imposed by the child's handicap on certain aspects or the child's development, as well as his or her capacities for full growth in most areas. Therefore, a major task of the social worker would be to help parents resolve feelings about their child's handicap, in terms of its effect on the practical aspects of daily life and parental expectations.

The fact that the practical aspects of daily life are negatively affected has implications for social policy in terms of the need to provide support systems such as day-care services, respite care, etc. This could also suggest the need for a scheme to give aid to families having severely disabled individuals. Counselling services would also be required to look after the mental health of the caregivers.

The review on precipitating factors within the system has pointed to the adverse attitudes of society towards the disabled. This has implications for social policy in terms of the use of mass media for community education. For social workers, it shows the need for organizing community-education programmes for specific groups of people in whom attitudinal changes are sought.

The findings have pointed out that families do not have much knowledge of the disability of their family member and its consequences on his or her development and prospects. This shows the need for family-education programmes, to give the whole family a better understanding of the ramifications of the disability. This will, in turn, inculcate more positive attitudes.

As the essence of professional social work is to help families to help themselves, the study on the family's coping strategies has clearly pointed to the type of help that families require, both from the support services and from the professionals. This should give clear indications for social work intervention.

The review of research on professional intervention for helping families to cope had some interesting findings, which have implications for social work intervention. Firstly, it has shown chat parents are ready to accept professional intervention. Secondly, the fact that programmes directly involving parents were more effective than those where parents were mere passive receivers shows the need for professional intervention to be experiential. One study has also brought out the need for treating parents as active partners in the rehabilitation process and not just as care-takers or go-betweens. Thirdly, parent-education/training programmes helped parents to cope better with their child, but did not change attitudes. Social work professionals need to keep all these points in mind while designing intervention strategies.

One of the main reasons why fewer professional social workers have ventured into this field, as compared to other fields such as child or women welfare, is that social work practice with this special group has not received adequate back-up from professional social work training programmes. According to the University Grants Commission's Curriculum Development Centre for Social Work Education at the Tata Institute of Social Sciences, there arc barely two schools of social work in India, which offer practice-based courses on social work intervention with the disabled and their families. Social workers desiring to work with the specific problems experienced by disabled children, adults and their families would require, in addition to generic social work knowledge and skills, some specialized knowledge and skills, which would equip them to provide appropriate and useful information, counselling and support to this special group.

The social work tasks that have been drawn up based on the review of research in this area have provided clues regarding training that will be required to prepare social workers for working with the disabled and their families. Broadly speaking, the training inputs will have to be in the areas of knowledge, attitudes and skills. Knowledge covers the needs and problems of families having disabled individuals, factors influencing their coping strategies and information on available resources. Skill training will be required for selection and use of appropriate intervention strategies. Attitudes essential for being sensitive, emphatic and positive towards families of the disabled and for effective social work intervention will need to be inculcated first in social workers themselves, before these professionals can attempt to change family and societal attitudes towards this special group of people.

Since independence, there has been a marked development in the national concern for the disabled in India. However, the trend in the planning and administration of services for the disabled is more towards a centralized approach to the problem. At present, different types of national schemes, programmes and concessions have been formulated for education, training and employment of the disabled. Four national institutes for each of the four categories of disabled have been established to serve as apex bodies to develop manpower and suitable service models, and to serve as premier information and documentation centres. Serious attempts to formulate a national policy for the disabled during the International Year of the Disabled in 1981 failed to produce anything tangible. Also, though some of the national schemes and programmes for disabled persons indirectly benefit their families, there are no family-based schemes or programmes in spite of the pressing need for such services as studies in this area have shown.

CONCLUSIONS

The purpose of this review has been primarily to summarize the findings of available Indian research studies on families having disabled individuals. What has emerged is a clear picture of the areas studied and the gaps in research in this field.

From among the four categories of the disabled, the mentally handicapped and their families have received maximum attention from researchers. The effects on the family of the presence of a disabled family member have been studied with reference to inter-relationships between different members of the family, the expectations of parents from their disabled children and the effects on practical aspects of daily life. Areas that have remained unexplored are sibling relationships and those between the disabled adult and his/her spouse, children and other members of the extended family. The effect on family functions also needs to be examined empirically. The attitudes of society as well as the family have been researched to some extent, but not other influencing factors. The family's coping strategies is one area which, though very important, has been almost left unexplored. Research on professional intervention on helping families to cope has been very limited, considering the variety of interventions made by professionals from different disciplines. Finally, the review has given good indication for the direction that social work practice and teaching should take. The implications drawn for social policy and intervention need further prompting and action on the part of all the professionals involved in the rehabilitation of the disabled and their families.

REFERENCES

Akhtar, S. and Verma, V. K. (1972). Guidelines for the parents of mentally retarded children. *Indian Journal of Mental Retardation*, 5, 75-88.

All India Institute of Medical Sciences. (1979). *The Implications of mentally handicapped to the family*. New Delhi: All India Institute of Medical Sciences.

Anand, J. S. and Patel, S. C. (1983). Prevalence and patterns of handicaps in urban children. *Indian Paediatrics*, 20(6), 434-38.

Arya, S. C. (1970). Parents may reduce retardation. *The Retarded*, 2(1), 5-10.

Barker, R. L. (1987). *The Social work dictionary*. Silver Spring: National Association of Social Workers.

Basu, S. N. (1981). The handicapped child and his problems. *Archives of Child Health*, 23(1), 11-13.

Behere, P. B. and Sinha, A. K. (1985). Expectations of the parents from their mentally retarded children. *Indian Medical Gazette*, 69(5), 173-74.

Bhalerao, U. (1983). *Educated blind of urban Madhya Pradesh*. New Delhi: Sterling Pub.

Bhat, K. N. (1981). Law and the handicapped. *Swasth Hind*, 25(7), 179-81.

Bhatia, B. D. (1964). Education and guidance of parents of the mentally retarded. *The Journal of Rehabilitation in Asia*, 5(2), 14-16.

Bhatt, U. (1963). *The physically handicapped in India*. Poona: Oriental Watchman Publishing House.

Bhatti, R. S. and Narayanan, H. S. (1980). Parental Attitude Questionnaire. Unpublished manuscript, NIMHANS, Bangalore.

Bhatti, R. S., Channabasavanna, S. M. and Prabhu, L. R. (1985). A tool to study the attitudes of parents towards the management of mentally retarded children. *Child Psychiatry Quarterly*, 18(2), 35-43.

Brill, R. G. (1974). *Education of the deaf: Administrative and professional developments*. Washington: Gallandet College Press.

Chakraborty, B. (1981). The handicapped and their attitude towards society: Some observations. *Journal of Social Research*, 24(1), 131-38.

Channabasavanna, S. M., Bhatti, R. S. and Prabhu, L. R. (1985). A study of attitudes of parents towards the management of mentally retarded children. *Child Psychiatry Quarterly*, 18(2), 44-47.

Chaturvedi, S. K. and Malhotra, S. (1983). Parental attitudes towards mental retardation. *Child Psychiatry Quarterly*, 16(3), 135-42.

———. (1984). A follow up study of mental retardation focusing on parental attitudes. *Indian Journal of Psychiatry*, 26(4), 370-76.

De Sousa, A. and Iyer, D. S. (1968-69). Mental deficiency—An analysis of 100 cases. *Child Psychiatry Quarterly*, 1(2), 56-72.

Deshmukh, Y. N. and Rawat, M. S. (1977). Domestic management of acute poliomyelitis in a rural set up. *The Journal of Rehabilitation in Asia*, 18(2), 18-20.

Dharitri, R. and Murthy, V. N. (1987). Handicapped children—Their abilities and behaviour. *Indian Journal of Clinical Psychology*, 14(1), 13-18.

Dhillion, P. K. and Chaudhari, S. (1988). A scale to measure attitude towards the mentally retarded. In D. M. Pestonjee (Ed.), *Second handbook of psychological and social instruments* (p. 391). New Delhi: Concept Publishing Co.

Embar, P. (1979). Workshop for parents of the mentally retarded. *Indian Journal of Mental Retardation*, 12(1 and 2), 31-42.

Fueller, S., Sen, A. K. and Chedha, N. K. (1989). Mother's attitude towards her mentally retarded child: An exploratory study. In A. K. Sen and N. K. Chedha (Ed.), *Research in psycho-social issues* (pp. 175-206). Delhi: Akshet Publications.

Gandotra, V. S. (1984). Management problems and practices of home-makers with a disabled member in the family. *The Indian Journal of Social Work*, 45(4), 485-90.

Gera, K., Wellington, M. and Purohit, S. (1978). An exploratory study of retardate's interaction with mother in game situation. *Indian Journal of Mental Retardation*, 11, 1-11.

Ghai, A. and Sen, A. (1985). Work adjustment and job anxiety of the handicapped in open employment: An empirical study. *Indian Journal of Industrial Relations*, 20(4), 439-50.

Ghatak, R. and Inderesan, J. (1983). Family dynamism and performance on educable mentally retarded children. *Journal of Psychological Research*, 27(2), 66-79.

Government of India. (1978). *National employment service manual*. New Delhi: Ministry of Labour.

Harisara, M. (1981). A developmentally handicapped child in the family: Parent's perception, attitude and their participation in the programme. *Mental Health Review*, 1(2), 55-60.

Huque, H. (1980). Primary health care approach to care of mentally disadvantaged children. In M. V. Singh (Ed.), *Disadvantaged child* (pp. 57-61). New Delhi: Delhi Association of Clinical Psychologists.

Ishtiaq, K. (1976). Sociological aspects of mental retardation. *Indian Journal of Menial Retardation*, 9, 77-82.

Ishtiaq, K. and Kamal, S. (1981). A comparative study of the mentally retarded and the blind. *Indian Journal of Mental Retardation*, 14(1), 13-18.

Jayashankarappa, B. S. and Puri, R. K. (1984). Parental counselling of the mentally retarded children. *Child Psychiatry Quarterly*, 17(3), 109-12.

Jehan, Q. and Ansari, Z. (1981). A study of certain psycho-social characteristics of mentally retarded children. *Indian Journal of Clinical Psychology*, 8(1), 47-48.

Kashyap, L. D. (1983). *Communication between the deaf child and his family*. Unpublished Doctoral Thesis, Tata Institute of Social Sciences, Bombay.

——. (1986). The family's adjustment to their hearing impaired child. *The Indian Journal of Social Work*, 47(1), 49-53.

——. (1989). Family's role in providing support to disabled persons in India's changing times. *International Journal of the Advancement of Counselling*, 12(4), 261-71.

Kaushik, S. S. (1984). Behaviour modification workshop for parents and teachers of mentally retarded: Programme evaluation. *Journal of Rehabilitation in Asia*, 25(2), 47.

Krishna Iyer, V. R. (1979). Legislation for the mentally handicapped. In S. Sinclair (Ed.), *National planning for the mentally handicapped: Report of the Expert Group on National Planning for the Mentally Handicapped in India*. New Delhi: Mehta Offset Work.

Krishnamurthy, K., Reddy, P. R., Bageerathy, G. M. and Rama Rao. (1985). The model programme for rural mentally handicapped children—the Naraspur experience. *Child Psychiatry Quarterly*, 18, 124-29.

Krishnaswamy, S. (1987). The demography of the disabled and the handicapped in India. *The Indian Journal of Social Work*, 48(1), 85-94.

Mallick, P. K., Bannerji, D., Bowmik, P., Bhadra, B. K. and Sen, S. (1983). Biosocial characteristics of the orthopaedically handicapped: A pilot study. *Journal of Rehabilitation in Asia*, 2, 44-51.

Mani, D. R. (1988). *Physically handicapped in India*. New Delhi: Ashish Publishing House.

Mathur, M. L. Chokshi, Y. J. and Singh, T. B. (1986). Appropriate strategy for rehabilitating the rural blind: Education of parents and counselling of visually handicapped persons in Bhagwanpur Block. *International Journal of Rehabilitation Research*, 9(3), 251-83.

Mathur, S. and Nalwa, V. (1987). Misconceptions about mental retardation, *Indian Journal of Clinical Psychology*, 14(1), 19-21.

Mazumdar, B. N. and Prabhu, G. G. (1972). Mental retardation: Parent's perception of the problem. *Child Psychiatry Quarterly*, 5(1), 13-18.

Mehta, D. S. (1983). *Handbook of disabled in India*. New Delhi: Allied Publishers.

Mehta, M. and Ochaney, M. (1984). Training mental retardates: Involving mothers in operant conditioning programme. *Indian Journal of Clinical Psychology*, 11(2), 45-50.

Mohsini, S. R. and Gandhi, R. R. (1982). *The physically handicapped and the Government*. Delhi: Seema Publication.

Moudgil, A. C., Kumar, H. and Sharma, S. (1985). Buffering effect of socioemotional support on the patterns of mentally retarded children. *Indian Journal of Clinical Psychology*, 12(2), 63-70.

Moudgil, A. C., Sharma, S. and Kumar, H. (1985). Hospitalization facilities for mentally retarded children. *Indian Journal of Clinical Psychology*, 12(2), 79.

Mudgil, A., Singh, S. B. and Srivastava, J. R. (1982). An etiological and psychological study of mentally retarded children. *Indian Paediatrics*, 19(8), 689-93.

Nigam, J. C. and Kakar, S. K. (1981). Attitude of parents of deaf and hard of hearing children towards their rehabilitation. *Hearing Aid Journal*, 2(4), 9-10.

Nimbkar, K. V. (1980). *A new life for the handicapped*. Bombay: Nimbkar Rehabilitation Trust.

Ojha, K. N., Verma, S. K. and Sinha, A. K. (1977). Psychological evaluation of change and progress in the mentally retarded: Implications for teachers and parents. *The Journal of Rehabilitation in Asia*, 18(1), 23-25.

Parikh, J. and Yadav, R. (1979), Developing and evaluating a programme for the parents of developmentally handicapped children. *Indian Journal of Mental Retardation*, 12(1 and 2), 63-70.

Parikh, J. K. (1981). An experiment with helping parents of developmentally handicapped children. *Child Psychiatry Quarterly*, 14(3), 79-84.

Patil, N. M. (1964). Home care for the chronically ill-hemiplogies. *The Journal of Rehabilitation in Asia*, 5(1), 47-48.

Prabhu, G. (1968). The participation of parents in the services for the retarded. *Indian Journal of Mental Retardation*, 1(1), 4-11.

Prabhu, G. G. (Ed.). (1977). *Report of the Third Asian Conference on Mental Retardation*. New Delhi: Federation of the Welfare of the Mentally Retarded.

Punani, B. (1981). Home bound programme for economic rehabilitation. *NASEOH News*, 11(2), 17-19.

Punani, B. and Rawal, N. (1987). *In the fold of the family: A report on awareness creation, training and counselling the parents of disabled children*. Ahmedabad: Blind Men's Association.

Purwar, A. K. (1983). Facilities available for the speech and hearing handicapped in hospitals in India. *Journal of Rehabilitation in Asia*, 24(3), 33-44.

Ramachandran, P. (1971). *Visually handicapped persons as physiotherapists: A feasibility study*. Bombay: TISS (Mimeo).

Ramadwar, D. K. and Oza, B. (1960). Prevalence and patterns of handicapped at Kelod. In The Report of Central Advisory Council for Education of the Handicapped (pp. 28-31). New Delhi: Government of India.

Rastogi, C. K. (1981). Attitude of parents towards their mentally retarded children. *Indian Journal of Psychiatry*, 23(3), 206-09.

Rastogi, C. K. (1984). Personality pattern of parents of mentally retarded children. *Indian Journal of Psychiatry*, 26(1), 46-50.

Sabhesan, S., Arumugham, R., Andal, G. and Natarajan, M. (1988). Vocational restitution after head injury. *The Indian Journal of Social Psychiatry*, 3, 104-12.

Sabhesan, S., Ramasamy, P., Andal, G. and Natarajan, M. (1987). Determinants of burden experienced by the families of head injured patients. *Indian Journal of Social Psychiatry*, 3, 104-12.

Sabhesan, S., Ramasamy, P., Ramaniah, T.B.B.S.V. and Natarajan, M. (1986). Marital interaction following head injury. Paper presented at the Annual Conference of ISPS W, Cochin.

Sahasrabhdha, B. G. and Sancheti, K. H. (1980). Survey of handicapped. *Journal of Rehabilitation in Asia*, 21(4), 30-35.

Seetharam, M. (1986). Evaluation of integrated education system. *International Journal of Rehabilitation Research*, 9(4), 389-90.

Sen, A. (1981). Education and care of mentally retarded. *Indian Journal of Public Administration*, 27, 700-712.

———. (1988). *Psycho-social integration of the handicapped.* Delhi: Mittal Publishers.

Sen, A. K. (1982). *Mental retardation.* Varanasi: Rupa Psychological Corporation.

Seshadri, M., Verma, V. K., Verma, S. K. and Pershad, D. (1983). Impact of a mentally handicapped child on the family. *Indian Journal of Clinical Psychology*, 10(2), 475-78.

Sethuraman, S. (1979). A study of blind women in a sheltered workshop. *Journal of Rehabilitation in Asia*, 20, 11-13.

Sharma, U. and Gupta, S. (1985). Mental health status of parents of physically handicapped children. *Indian Paediatrics*, 22(3), 185-90.

Siddiqui, A. Q., Sultana, M. and Ahmad, P. (1984). Social class, parental attitudes and acceptance of parental counselling in mentally retarded subjects. *Indian Journal of Clinical Psychology*, 11(2), 22-28.

Sinclair, S. (Ed.). (1979). National planning for the mentally handicapped. *Report of Expert Group on National Planning for the Mentally Retarded in India.* New Delhi: Mehta Offset Work.

Singh, M. V. (1972). Counselling needs of parents of mentally retarded children. *Indian Journal of Pediatrics*, 39, 361-63.

Singh, P. (1987). Mainstreaming of exceptional children. *New Frontier Education*, 17(2), 28-33.

Singh, R. and Kaushik, S. S. (1982). Parent training techniques in acquisition and generalization of behaviour modification skills to train the retardate. *Indian Journal of Clinical Psychology*, 9, 193-201.

Singh, T. B. (1988). Temperament of pre-school age visually handicapped children. *Insight* (NIVH Newsletter), 3(3), 7-8.

Singh, V. K. (1979). Problem children—handicapped, maladjusted and mentally retarded. *Indian Psychological Review*, 18(14), 122-28.

Somasundaram, O. and Papakumari, M. G. (1979). Down's Syndrome cases from Madras City: Their socio-economic status. *Child Psychiatry Quarterly*, 12, 43-47.

Srivastava, O. P. (1981). *Stress and coping mechanism of physically handicapped children.* Unpublished Doctoral Thesis, Psychology Dept., Allahabad University, Allahabad.

Srivastava, R. K., Saxena, V. and Saxena, N. K. (1978). Attitudes of mothers of mentally retarded children toward certain aspects of child-rearing practices. *Indian Journal of Mental Retardation*, 11(2), 62–74.

Unkovic, C. M. and Zook, L. (1969). Mental retardation: The role of the counsellor in effective application of the case history and the family interview. *Journal of Social Research*, 12(2), 79–85.

Verghese, A. (1984). Problems encountered in rehabilitating the mentally disabled. *The Journal of Rehabilitation in Asia*, 25(2), 26–30.

Verma, M. (1961). The socio-economic survey of 500 families of the physically handicapped in Kanpur. *The Indian Journal of Social Work*, 21(4), 447–50.

Verma, S. K. (1985). Cultural aspects of mental disorders: A review of recent studies in India—I: Knowledge and attitudes. *Journal of Personality and Clinical Studies*, 1(1), 1–4.

Vohra, R. (1987). Services for the mental retardates in India. *Disabilities and Impairments*, 1, 91–117.

Vohra, R. and Sen, A. K. (1989). Rehabilitation centres for the mentally retarded individuals in India: A glimpse. In A. K. Sen and N. K. Chedha (Ed.), *Research in psycho-social issues* (pp. 143–58). Delhi: Akshat Publication.

World Health Organization. (1980). *International classification of impairments, disability and handicaps: A manual of classification relating to the consequences of diseases.* Geneva: WHO.

Part III

PERSPECTIVES ON HEALING

Introduction

Healing is a concept that draws attention to a process of restoring health and well-being primarily by an internal mechanism which is self-regulatory. In common usage, we do refer to healing of a wound. In this process, we recognize some kind of malfunctioning and utilize internal and external supports to resume the state of fitness necessary to conduct ourselves in everyday affairs. Thus, thinking about 'healing' necessarily implies a state of disequilibrium or disturbance that is unwelcome to the state of being. This may emanate from physical or bodily malfunctioning or may be caused by the frustrations, losses, aspirations that may happen at the psychological plane (Kazarian and Evans, 2003). The efforts involve various strategies that get rid of incapacitating symptoms, facilitate effective functioning in social and personal lives and feelings of well-being. Healing also occurs at social and spiritual planes when we empathize and experience pain for the community or people at large and move on the path of self-realization and inner growth. In any case, healing starts from within and takes care of the problems in such a way that the person starts feeling rejuvenated and again starts investing his or her energies in the efforts aimed at personal growth. Keeping the significant role of healing in peoples' lives, societies have created various formal and non-formal systems of healing. Being a process located in the socio-cultural context, any understanding of healing has to attend to the diversity of healing systems.

In the Indian tradition, healing is a multi-faceted process and many institutions and people participate in it. For instance, the institution of guru still operates in many parts of India. The literal meaning of guru is a person who destroys darkness. People have their gurus who act as healers and help in restoring health of people by guiding, supporting and extending help in various ways. Having a spiritual guru is a common experience. In the *bhakti* tradition, devotional surrender is emphasized and a guru is treated as lord. In the *tantra* tradition, idealization of mystery and power was emphasized. Therefore, the disciple moved from the status of a man to a child and the guru moved from the status of man to God (*Guruh sakhat parabrahama*). In recent years, the role of a guru as healer of emotional suffering and various somatic manifestations is becoming increasingly prominent. Guru is being treated as the physician of world diseases. In terms of Kohut's framework, there is idealizing transference, with its strong need for the experience of merging into a good and powerful, wise and perfect self-object—the guru. When a disciple forms a relationship with a guru, the disciple is in fact forming a relationship with his own best self.

Today we find a number of *babas, swamis, sadhus, bhagwans* and *matajis* in different parts of India, to whom people of different faiths are devoted. Also, there are many sacred places where people go and worship to feel better and to get healed. In fact, there is a wide spectrum of such resources that cater to the needs of people in trouble. In *Shamans, Mystics and Doctors*, Sudhir Kakar (1982) has provided fascinating and rich accounts of the healing process in three traditions, i.e., local and folk, mystical and medical. The case studies of various healing institutions and masters included by Kakar are the Pir of Patteshah Dargah, Balaji, Oraon Shamana, Lama of Macleodganj, Radha Soami sect and Mata Nirmala Devi. Kakar also provides an analysis of healing in the Ayurveda and *tantra* systems. In all these traditions, the role of sacred is very important. As Kakar notes, it is the introduction of the sacred in the assumptive worlds of the healer and his patient's *being* that they jointly seek to make *well*. These traditions offer a glimpse of social values as well as the symbolic universe of the Indian society. As Kakar says, the Indian emphasis has been on the pursuit of an inner differentiation while keeping the outer world constant. He also thinks that the Indian society is organized around the primacy of the therapeutic. Protection and care has received more attention than performance or equality. The Indian healing traditions emphasize on the supportive-suggestive processes. Also, health is considered more in a relational term. In the medical tradition, India has a pluralistic system. In addition to the Western style biomedicine (allopathy), we have the Ayurveda, Siddha and Unani-Tibb systems. These systems employ different methods of healing.

Anthropologist R. S. Khare (1996) notes that in India, accessibility and affordability are important considerations. Because of the socio-economic considerations, we must attend to the diverse forms of health care practices. Khare discussed the health models rooted in the culturally shared assumptions, ethical values, reasoning patterns and sensibilities. Khare noted that the medical reasoning shows continuity from the Vedic period onwards, and context-sensitive reasoning runs across all the traditions in the Indian subcontinent. It leads to plurality and overlaps with the practiced medicine. Khare rightly observed that practiced medicine does have to confront the issues of cultural alienation, economic affordability and just safe and accountable availability of medical services.

Introduction • 207

This section presents contributions which relate to indigenous and contemporary perspectives on healing. In the first contribution, Kakar examines the eastern spiritual healing traditions in relation to psychoanalysis. He observes that the religio-spiritual phenomena have often been treated as antithetical to psychoanalysis. However, spiritual practices like meditation do have therapeutic value since both view mind as the centre that creates suffering and disturbance. They do share the view that life happens through us and we are responsible for our distress. The impurities of mind are treated as the causes leading to mental illness, distress and disease. A purified mind makes for a pure body and a perfected mind for the perfection of the body. Here, it is important to note that the spiritual disciplines are believed to be accompanied by alterations in the bodily system.

Kakar observes that Kohut's theory is most pertinent for understanding healing in eastern traditions. It views cure in terms of restoring to the self the empathic responsiveness of the self-object. In spiritual healing, patients often display access to archaic modes of contact in which a hallucinatory image of the guru is created to sustain a self in danger of losing its cohesion. Also, surrender is indispensable for the mutative changes in self as it is the full-flowering of the idealized transference. The idealizing transference, leading to the merging experience, is thus the core of the healing process in the guru–disciple relationship. In this context, empathy is emphasized. A complete empathic knowledge of another person is supposed to involve the activation of a normally dormant higher faculty of consciousness. Kakar thinks that the Eastern meditative discipline can become part of training. By emphasizing on the guru's empathy and in claiming that meditative practices radically reduce the noise and glare produced by the sensual self the teacher-healer's empathic capacity can be significantly enhanced.

Adulthood is a stage in which people have to share a number of responsibilities and perform diverse roles. People have to become bread-earners and relate to various social institutions. The increase in the range or scope of responsibilities also increases the possibility of challenges, problems and possibilities. However, the narratives of people are very different. Every one of us has a different story to tell. Jyoti Anand has explored the problem of handling emotional pain. Using narrative inquiry with a case of an adult woman, she has looked at her life struggles and the way healing takes place. We find that the life challenges can be taken in such a way that the adverse conditions do not continue to hamper health and well-being. The narrative shows a series of emotional episodes which challenge the whole existence of a person. The study is important in the sense that life does not move normally in a logical, rational and linear manner. Also, some sort of self-directed self-rejuvenation does occur even in the adverse conditions. People do grow out of those traumatic conditions. The process of self-transformation and healing by the use of resources within and personal strengths is exemplified in the reported case study. Working with emotions in the course of life struggles is not unusual in a country like India where patriarchy and traditions are very strong. The study throws a challenge in the sense that any given theoretical model developed in the Western world does not suit to explain the social and personal reality in the Indian context. Devotion to God (*bhakti*), working with emotions, healing and contemplation do play an important role in self transformation.

Ravi Kapur, a psychiatrist by training, has described the state of mind from the Yoga perspective. In this third contribution of this section, we find a new methodological approach which may be termed as a first person perspective. He views Yoga as a science for positive mental health. Yoga, defined as inhibition of fluctuation of mind (*yogaschittavriti nirodhah*), involves psychophysiological processes, conscious control of instinctual demands, surrender to a higher will and reordering of one's relationship with the external world. Kapur shares his own experiences of Yogic training and the concomitant changes. He received training over a period of one year under the guidance of a guru. He wrote his own observations everyday in the evening. He started with experiencing Yoga and subsequently learned the Yogic texts from a guru. He observed that the witness function of *purush* is central to the entire process. *Prakriti* consists of the three *gunas*, *sattva*, *rajas* and *tamas*, which stand for ethics, creativity and negative/destructive impulses, respectively. *Purush* is tainted by *prakriti* and its *gunas*. Mind fails to distinguish which leads to *kleshas* or sufferings. To end miseries, one engages in *karma*, *vasana* and *sanskar*. Yoga leads to actions that have no consequences. As a result, one engaged in Yoga becomes inert and sequence or chain of actions is resolved. Practice (*abhyasa*) is needed for controlling the emotional as well as cognitive fluctuations that frequently take place and work as obstacles. Therefore, one has to follow austerity, contemplation and surrender to a higher will (*ishwar*). Following the path of eightfold (*ashtang*) Yoga, one may move towards *kaivalya*—a state of non-attached being. Kapur's own journey of personal experiences showed gradual change. He experienced spontaneity, order and flexibility, self-awareness and self-examination, slowing of thoughts and feelings, willed control, reduction in anxiety and worry, perceptual sensitivity, more space in mind, control over thoughts and emotions, relaxation, strong will and joy.

In the next contribution, Alok Pandey examines psychotherapy in the Indian tradition. He begins by questioning the past- and future-oriented therapies. He notes that the attempt to discover causes in the past and preparing the person for the future has limited value. Working from a different vantage point, Pandey proposes that the point of crisis in one's life may be taken as a learning experience for growth and progress. Pandey offers a critique of the divergent worldviews of man and his goal, as developed in the Western thought and Vedant. The solutions offered by both are problematic. Pandey asserts that detachment and non-involvement in this world as a solution for health is not the only way out. In actual practice, it may lead to many problems. As an alternative, he draws attention to certain powerful and positive streams of Indian thought.

Pandey introduces the ideal of inner purification and argues in favour of moderation and balance through an enlightened reason and discrimination, *sattvashudhi*. It is a conscious and deliberate cultivation of the positive qualities of the mind and heart which help one grow into *sukham* or gladness and *prakasham* or light of wisdom. Referring to different levels of spiritual development along *tamsic*, *rajsic* and *satvik gunas*, he says that all of us are mixtures of the three but there is a predominance of one *guna* or another that leads to afflictions. The therapeutic intervention shall take place according to the level of one's development. Establishing the harmony of mind and body is the goal of Yogic, meditative practices. Referring to the *Bhagavadgita*, Pandey articulates the following key assumptions: man is essentially an imperishable soul, using an enlightened will to discover his own sublime realities; divinity dwells within the human being and it is the task of each one to bring it out rather than stifle it; and conflicts are a cry for an evolutionary change. The principle of *nishkam karma* states that our everyday actions can lead us to a glad and happy state of being if we do them in a selfless spirit. It would lead to equanimity. God will deliver us from all fear and evil if we can learn to surrender ourselves into His hand.

Pandey notes that Sri Aurobindo has made a synthesis of the great tradition of knowledge. In his synthesis, the universal self is present but it is also projected in an individual soul—*the psychic being* or the secret divinity in us. It is veiled by the surface nature and its movements. The psychological maladies spring from our inability to dwell in the psychic consciousness. It is the growth in consciousness which can be thought as the aim of human life and solution of human misery and suffering. The more we grow in consciousness, the more we become progressively free of ignorance and limitations. Illness is a barometer to discover our hidden weaknesses or points that need to be developed and perfected. As Pandey states, 'the goal of psychotherapy is not just warding off of the present symptoms but the discovery of the inner healer who can heal not only this but all other anomalies of life in all times to come'. The experience of the divine within and around us as the one single simultaneously objective and subjective experience is the path as well as the destination for well-being.

The contributions included in this section bring into focus the broad range of perspectives on healing in the socio-cultural context. The emphasis has been on the practices that are usually neglected in the mainstream discussions on healing but represent reality as found in the case of masses.

REFERENCES

Kakar, Sudhir. (1982). *Shamans, mystics and doctors*. New Delhi: Oxford.
Kazarian, S. S. and Evans, D. D. (2003). *Handbook of cultural health psychology*. San Diego: Academic Press.
Khare, R. S. (1996). *Dava, daktar and dua*: Anthropology of practiced medicine in India. *Social Science and Medicine*, 43(5), 837–48.

9

The Guru as Healer

SUDHIR KAKAR

The contemporary images of the Indian guru, the sacred centre of Hindu religious and philosophical traditions, are many. He is that stately figure in spotless white or saffron robes, with flowing locks and beard, to all appearances the younger brother of a brown Jehovah. To be approached in awe and reverence, he is someone who makes possible the disciple's fateful encounter with the mystery lying at the heart of human life. He is also the Rasputin lookalike, with piercing yet warm eyes, hypnotic and seductive at once, a promiser of secret ecstasies and radical transformations of consciousness and life. The guru is also the venerable guardian of ancient, esoteric traditions, benevolently watchful over the disciple's experiences in faith, gently facilitating his sense of identity and self. He can also be (to use the imagery of Pupul Jayakar, the biographer of the Indian sage Jiddu Krishnamurti), 'the silent, straight-backed stranger, the mendicant who stands waiting at the doorways of home and mind, holding an invitation to otherness', evoking 'passionate longings, anguish and a reaching out physically and inwardly to that which is unattainable' (Jayakar, 1987, p. 9).[1]

In the above snapshots, we find little trace of the old polarity which characterized the guru image. This polarity consisted of the worldly, orthodox teacher guru at one end representing relative, empirical knowledge, and

---

[1] Here I must add the caution contained in Brent's observation that:

> In a country where there are perhaps ten million holy men, many with their own devotees, acolytes and disciples, some of them gurus with hundreds of thousands of followers, all of them inheritors of a tradition thousands of years old, nothing that one can say about them in general will not somewhere be contradicted in particular. (see Brent, 1973)

the otherworldly, mystic guru at the other pole who was the representative of esoteric, existential knowledge. In Hindu terms, the dominant image of the guru seems to have decisively shifted towards the *moksha* (liberation) guru rather than the *dharma* (virtue) guru, towards the *bhakti* (devotional) guru rather than the *jnana* (knowledge) guru or, in *tantric* terms, towards the *diksha* (initiation) guru who initiated the novice into methods of salvation rather than the *shiksha* (teaching) guru who taught the scriptures and explained the meaning and purpose of life.[2]

This was, of course, not always the case. In Vedic times (1500-500 BC), when man's encounter with the sacred mysteries took place through ritual, the guru was more a guide to their correct performance and an instructor in religious duties. A teacher deserving respect and a measure of obedience, he was not yet a mysterious figure of awe and the venerated incarnation of divinity.

In the later Upanishadic era (800-500 BC), the polar shift begins in earnest as the person of the guru starts to replace Vedic rituals as the path to spiritual liberation. He now changes from a knower and dweller in Brahman to being the only conduit to Brahman. Yet, the Upanishadic guru is still recognizably human—a teacher of acute intellect, astute and compassionate, demanding from the disciple the exercise of his reason rather than exercises in submission and blind obedience. When, in the seventh century AD, the great Shankara, in his project of reviving the ancient Brahminical tradition, seeks to resurrect the Upanishadic guru, he sees in him a teacher who:

> ...is calm, tranquil, childlike, silent and free from distracting motivations. Although learned, he should be as a child, parading neither wisdom, nor learning, nor virtue itself ... He is a reservoir of mercy who teaches out of compassion to the multitude. He is sympathetic to the conditions of the student and is able to act with empathy towards him. (Cenker, 1983, p. 41)

In the disciple's spiritual quest, Shankara's guru places reason on par with scriptural authority and constantly exhorts the student to test and verify the teachings through his own experience. Every student needs to discover anew for himself or herself what is already known, a spiritual patrimony which has to be earned each time for it to become truly one's own. Here, the ideal of the Hindu guru was not too far removed from the Buddhist

---

[2] For a comprehensive historical discussion of the evolution of the guru institution, on which this introductory section is based, see Steinmann (1986). See further (Cenker, 1983).

master who, too, constructed experience-near situations to illustrate a teaching and who saw the master–disciple relationship as one of perfect equality in self-realization, with radical insight as its goal. The relationship between the guru and disciple was of intimacy, not of merger. Both the guru and disciple were separate individuals, and potentially equals, though striving for ever-greater closeness.

From the seventh century onwards, the swing away from the teacher image of the guru received its greatest momentum with the rise of the *bhakti* cults in both North and South India. Devotional surrender on the part of the disciple, with such lectures as ritualistic service to the guru, the worship of his feet, bodily prostration and other forms of veneration, and divine grace (*prasada*) on the part of the guru, mark the guru–disciple relationship. 'Guru and Govind [i.e., Lord Krishna] stand before me', says the fifteenth century saint-poet Kabir, and asks, 'Whose feet should I touch?' The answer is: 'The guru gets the offering. He shows the way to Govind' (cited in Gold, 1987, p. 104). The operative word is now love rather than understanding. To quote Kabir again:

> Reading book after book, the whole world died
> And none ever became learned
> He who can decipher just a syllable of 'love'
> is the true learned man (pandit)

With the spread of *tantric* cults around 1000 AD, the guru not only shows the way to the Lord, but is the Lord. 'There is no higher god than guru', *tantric* texts tell us: 'No higher truth than the guru'. 'The guru is father, the guru is mother, the guru is the God Shiva. When Shiva is angry, the guru is the Savior. But when the guru is angry, there is no one who can save you' (cited in Steinmann, 1986). The guru is now an extraordinary figure of divine mystery and power, greater than the scriptures and the gods, and all that the disciple requires to realize his own godlike nature, his extraordinary identity, as Lawrence Babb (1987) puts it, is to merge his substantial and spiritual being with that of the guru. The ambiguities of thought and the agonizings of reason can be safely sidestepped since the way is no longer through Upanishadic listening, reflection and concentration but through a complete and wilful surrender—the offering of *tana, mana* and *dhana* (body, mind and wealth) in the well-known phrase of North Indian devotionalism. The responsibility for the disciple's inner transformation is no longer that of the disciple but of the guru. 'One single word of the guru gives liberation', says a *tantric* text. 'All the sciences are masquerades. Only the knowledge flowing out of the guru's mouth is living. All other kinds of knowledge are powerless and cause of suffering' (*Kulanirvana Tantra*, cited in Steinmann, 1986, p. 103).

The combined forces of the *bhakti* and *tantra* pushed towards an ever-increasing deification of the guru, a massive idealization of his mystery and power. The thirteenth century Marathi saint Jnaneshvara writes of the guru (Abhayananda, 1989):

> As for his powers,
> He surpasses even the greatness of Shiva,
> With his help,
> The soul attains the state of Brahman;
> But if he is indifferent,
> Brahman has no more worth than a blade of grass.

Complementary to the movement of the guru from man to god is the shift in the disciple from man to child. The favoured, the ideal disciple is pure of heart, malleable of character and a natural renouncer of all adult categories, especially of rational inquiry and of the sexual gift. These images of the guru and disciple and their ideal relationship pervades the Hindu psyche to a substantial extent even today. 'Guru is Brahma, guru is Vishnu, guru is Maheshwara', is a verse not only familiar to most Hindus but one that evokes complex cultural longings, that resonates with what is felt to be the best part of their selves and of the Hindu tradition.

Let me not give the impression that the triumphant procession of the liberation/salvation guru in Hindu tradition has gone completely unchallenged. In traditional texts, there are at least two instances questioning the need for a guru, admittedly an insignificant number compared to hundreds of tales, parables and pronouncements extolling him. The first one is from the *Uddhava Gita* in the sixth century text of *Bhagvata Purana* where Dattareya, on asked to account for his self-possession and equanimity, lists elements of nature, the river, certain animals and even a prostitute (from whom he learned autonomy from the sensual world) as his 24 gurus. The parable of Dattareya ends with the exhortation,: 'Learn, above all, from the rhythms of your own body'. The second incident is an episode from the Yoga Vasistha, a text composed between the ninth and twelfth centuries in Kashmir, wherein Princess Cudala, setting out on her inner journey of self-exploration, deliberately eschews all gurus and external authorities, and reaches her goal through a seven-stage self-analysis.

In more recent times, beginning in the nineteenth century, there have been reformers who have sought to revive Vedic rituals and Upanishadic religion. They would, at the most, sanction the teacher guru, such as the socially engaged intellectual *swami* of the Ramakrishna Mission or of the nineteenth century reformist movement, Arya Samaj. There have been also reluctant gurus, such as Krishnamurti, who vehemently denied the need for a guru and in fact saw in him the chief obstacle to spiritual liberation. For him and some modern educated Indians, the guru institution as it exists today is a focus of all the anti-intellectual and authoritarian tendencies in Hindu society (Chaturvedi, 1990). Yet, for the great mass of Hindus, the mystical, charismatic, divine guru image continues to be a beacon of their inner worlds. The all-pervasiveness of this image is due to more complex reasons than the mere victory of irrationality over reason, servility over autonomy or of a contemporary dark age over an earlier golden era.

What I am suggesting here is that the shift from the teacher to the master image is inevitable given the fact that perhaps a major, if not the most significant, role of the guru is that of a healer of emotional suffering and its somatic manifestations. This psychotherapeutic function, insufficiently acknowledged, is clearly visible in well-known modern gurus whose fame depends on their reported healing capabilities rather than deriving from any mastery of traditional scriptures, philosophical knowledge, of even great spiritual attainments. Of course, in cases of international gurus, the healing is tailored to culture-specific needs. In India there will be more miracles and magical healing, while in the West there will be a greater use of psycho-religious methods and techniques which are not unfamiliar to a psychotherapeutically informed population (Steinmann, 1986).

The importance of the healing guru comes through clearly in all available accounts. Ramakrishna's disciple-biographer writes (Swami Saradanand, 1983, p. 521):

> The spiritual teacher has been described in the Guru-gita and other books as the 'physician of the world-disease.' We did not at all understand that so much hidden meaning was there in it before we had the blessing of meeting the master. We had no notion of the fact that the Guru was indeed the physician of mental diseases and could diagnose at first sight the modifications of the human mind due to influence of spiritual emotions.

Perhaps the most vivid recent account of the therapeutic encounter between a guru and a disciple is contained in Pupul Jayakar's moving description of her first one-to-one meeting with Krishnamurti. The narration could very well also have been of an initial interview with a good analyst. In her early thirties, outwardly active and successful yet with intimations of something seriously wrong with her life, Jayakar is apprehensive and tries to prepare for the meeting. She begins the interview by talking of the fullness of her life and work, her concern for the underprivileged, her interest in art, her desire to enter politics. As the first flow of words peters out, Jayakar gradually falls silent. 'I looked up and saw he was gazing at me; there was a questioning in his eyes and a deep probing.' After a pause he said, 'I have noticed you at the discussions. When you are in repose, there is a great sadness on your face.'

> I forgot what I had intended to say, forgot everything but the sorrow within me. I had refused to allow the pain to come through. So deep was it buried that it rarely impinged on my conscious mind. I was horrified of the idea that others would show me pity and sympathy, and had covered up my sorrow with layers of aggression. I had never spoken of this to anyone—not even to myself had I acknowledged my loneliness; but before this silent stranger, all masks were swept away. I looked into his eyes and it was my own face I saw reflected. Like a torrent long held in check, the words came. (Jayakar, 1987, p. 4)

Jayakar talks of her childhood, of a sensitive lonely girl, 'dark of complexion in a family where everyone was fair, unnoticed a girl when I should have been a boy'. She talks *of* her pregnancies, in one case the baby dying in the womb, in other the birth of a deformed child, a girl who dies in childhood. She tells Krishnamurti of the racking pain of her beloved father's death and the tearing, unendurable agony she feels as she talks.

> In his presence the past, hidden in the darkness of the long forgotten, found form and awakened. He was as a mirror that reflected. There was an absence of personality, of the evaluator, to weigh and distort. I kept trying to keep back something of my past but he would not let me. He said, I can see if you want me to. And so the words which for years had been destroying me were said. (Jayakar, 1987, p. 5)

Krishnamurti is one of the most 'intellectual' of modern gurus, with a following chiefly among the most modern and highly educated sections of Indian society. It is nonetheless the news of his 'miracle' cures—deafness in one instance, an acute depression in another—which spreads like wildfire through the *ashrams* all over the country. Crowds *of* potential disciples gather at his talks, striving to touch his hand, to share in his benediction. 'These incidents and the vastness *of* his silent presence impressed people tremendously', Jayakar writes somewhat ruefully. 'The teaching, though they all agreed it was grounded in a total nonduality, appeared too distant and too unattainable' (Jayakar, 1987, p. 211).

In my own work with gurus and disciples, I found that many of the latter shared a common pattern in their lives that had led them to a search for the guru and to initiation in his cult (Kakar, 1982). Almost invariably the individual had gone through one or more experiences that had severely mauled his sense of self-worth, if not shattered it completely. In contrast to the rest of us, who must also deal with the painful feelings aroused by temporary depletions in self-esteem, it seems that those who went to gurus grappled with these feelings for a much longer time, sometimes for many years, without being able to change them appreciably. Unable to rid themselves of the feelings of 'I have lost everything and the world is empty', or 'I have lost everything because I do not deserve anything', they had been on the lookout for someone, somewhere, to restore the lost sense of self-worth and to counteract their hidden image of a failing, depleted self—a search nonetheless desperate for its being mostly unconscious. This 'someone' eventually turned out to be the particular guru to whom the seekers were led by events—such as his vision—which in retrospect seemed miraculous. The conviction and the sense of a miracle having taken place, though projected to the circumstances that led to the individual's initiation into the cult, actually derived from the 'miraculous' ending of a persistent and painful internal state, the disappearance of the black depressive cloud that had seemed to be a permanent feature of the individual's life. Perhaps a vignette from a life history will illustrate this pattern more concretely.

Harnam was the youngest of four sons of a peasant family from a North Indian village who had tilled their own land for many generations. As the 'baby' of the family, Harnam had been much indulged during his childhood, especially by his mother. She had died when he was 18, and ever since her death, he said, a peculiar *udasinta* (sadness) had taken possession of his soul. Though he had all the comforts at home, enough to eat and drink, and an abundant measure of affection from his father and elder brothers, the *udasinta* had persisted. For 15 long years, he said, his soul remained restless, yearning for an unattainable peace. His thoughts often dwelt upon death, of which he developed an exaggerated fear, and he was subject to crippling headaches that confined him to the darkness of his room for long periods. Then, suddenly, he had a vision in a dream of the guru (he, had seen his photograph earlier), who told him to come to his *ashram* to take initiation into the cult. He had done so; his sadness had disappeared as did his fear and headaches, and he felt the loving omnipresence of the guru as a protection against their return.

Besides cultural encouragement and individual needs, I believe there are some shared developmental experiences of many upper caste Hindu men which contribute to the intensification of the fantasy of guru as healer. In an earlier work, I have described the male child's experience of 'second birth', a more or less sudden loss of a relationship of symbiotic intimacy with the other in late childhood and an entry into the more businesslike relationships of the world of men (Kakar, 1978). Two of the consequences of the 'second birth' in the identity development of Hindu men are first, an unconscious tendency to 'submit' to an idealized omnipotent figure, both in the inner world of fantasy and in the outside world of making a living, and second the lifelong search for someone, a charismatic leader or a guru, who will provide mentorship and a guiding worldview, thereby restoring intimacy and authority to individual life. I would interpret the same phenomena more explicitly in terms of self psychology. Since I believe some of the concepts of self psychology to be of value in illuminating the healing process in the guru–disciple relationship, these concepts may first need a brief elucidation.

The major focus of the Kohutian psychology of the self is what he called a self-object (Kohut, 1971; 1977). One exists as a person, a self, because a significant other, the self-object, has addressed one as a self and evoked the self-experience. Self-objects, strictly speaking, are not persons but the subjective aspect of a function performed by a relationship. It is thus more apt to speak of self-object experiences, intra-psychic rather than interpersonal, which evoke, maintain and give cohesion to the self (Wolf, 1989). The very emergence and maintenance of the self as a psychological structure, then, depends on the continued presence of an evoking-sustaining-responding matrix of self-object experiences. Always needed, from birth to death, the absence of these experiences leads to a sense of fragmentation of the self, including, in extreme states of narcissistic starvation, the terrors of self-dissolution.

The mode of needed self-object experiences, of course, changes with age from the simple to the more complex. In a child, the required self-object experience occurs primarily, though not exclusively (remember the importance of the glow in the mother's eye and of the affirmative timbre in her voice), through physical ministrations. In the adult, symbolic self-object experiences supplied by his culture, such as religious, aesthetic and group experiences, may replace some of the more concrete modes of infancy and childhood. In the language of self psychology, the guru is the primary cultural self-object experience for adults in Hindu tradition and society. For everyone whose self was weakened because of faulty self-object relations during crucial developmental phases or for those who have been forced into defensive postures by the self's fragility where they are cut off from all normal sustaining and healing self-object responses, the guru is the culture's irresistible offer for the redressal of injury and the provision of self-object experience needed for the strengthening of the self.

It is the immanence of the healing moment in the guru–disciple relationship which inevitably pushes the guru image towards that of a divine parent and of the disciple towards that of a small child. Western psychiatrists have tended to focus more on the pathology and the malevolent regression unleashed by the psychic shifts in the images of the self and the guru when therapeutic expectations of the disciples take firm hold (Deutsch, 1982; Lorand, 1962). They have talked of the extreme submissiveness of the disciples, of a denial of strong unconscious hostility, of the devotee's deepest desire being of oral dependence on the mother, etc.

I believe the Western psychiatric emphasis on the pathological and regressive—'bad' regressive—aspects of the guru–disciple relationship does it injustice. However, one may prefer the Enlightenment virtues of reason and ideological egalitarianism, the universal power exercised by what I would call the guru fantasy is not to be denied. By guru fantasy I mean the existence of someone, somewhere, who will heal the wounds suffered in the original parent–child relationship. It is the unconscious longing for the curer of the 'world-disease', a longing which marks all potentially healing encounters, whether they are or not officially termed as such. This fantasy invariably exerts its power in changing the self-image of the seeker and of the healing other in the directions I have described above.

My own profession, psychoanalysis, in its theories of cure has not escaped from the ubiquitous power of this fantasy. Patients, of course, have always approached analysis and analysts with a full-blown guru fantasy. Analysts, on the other hand, tended at first to believe with Freud that healing took place through knowledge and an expansion of conscious awareness. Yet, beginning with one of the most original of the first generation of analysts, Sandor Ferenzci, there has been a growing body of opinion which holds the person of the analyst and his interaction with the patient, in which the analyst counteracts the specific pathogenic deficit of the parent–child relationship, as the prime barriers of the healing moment. Franz Alexander was perhaps the most outright advocate of the analyst adopting corrective postures, but the stress on the role of the analyst as someone who makes up in some fashion or other for a deficient non-empathic parent is met with again and again in analytical literature, especially in the school of object relations. Winnicott, for instance, believed that with patients who suffered from not-good-enough early maternal environment, the analytic setting and the analyst, more than his interpretations, provided an opportunity for the development of an ego, for its integration from ego nuclei. Kohut's self psychology with its stress on the curative powers of the analyst's empathy moves further in the same direction. As Ernst Wolf states the self psychological position:

> It is not the content of the information conveyed to the patient, not the substance of the interpretations and interventions made, not the correctness of the therapist's conjectures, not even the therapist's compliance with demands to 'mirror' the patient or to be his or her ideal that is pivotal: It is decisive for the progress of the therapeutic endeavor that the patient experience an ambience in which he or she feels respected, accepted and at least a little understood ... The person who is the therapist then becomes as crucial a variable as the person who is the patient. (Wolf, 1989, p. 100)

Many years earlier, Sacha Nacht had captured this shift in the psychoanalytic view of healing when he said, 'it is of more value from the curative point of view, to have a mediocre interpretation supported by good transference than the reverse' (Nacht, 1962, p. 208). In interviews with devotees, the unconscious expectation that the guru will counteract specific parental deficits becomes manifest in the way an individual selects a particular guru. It seems to be a fact that often the *master* who is experienced as an incarnation of the Divine by his own disciples leaves other seekers cold. In the politics of gurudom, reverence and worship by your own devotees does not ensure that you are not a figure of indifference, even of derision and contempt, to other gurus and members of their cults. Let me illustrate.

Amita, a 30-year-old woman who is a lecturer in Hindi in a local college, is one of the closest disciples of a contemporary female guru, Nirmala Devi. Born into an orthodox middle-class Brahmin family, she has been engaged in the 'search' ever since childhood. 'My mother used to worship five hundred and sixty million gods every day', she says in a bitter, contemptuous voice, 'but it didn't change her a bit. She was a hot-tempered, dried-up woman with little human sympathy or kindness. So what was the use of observing all the rites and praying to the gods?' As Amita talks of her past, it is clear that she has been in a hostile clinch with her mother all her life. Amita went to see many gurus but was dissatisfied with every one of them till one day, a few years ago, she attended one of Mataji's public meetings. Her conversion was instantaneous, and she has remained a devoted disciple ever since. 'Mataji is like the cloud that gives rain to everyone', she says. I am struck by the juxtaposition of her imagery in which mother is dry while Mataji brims over with the rain of love.

For Amita, then, Mataji's parental style has elements of both the familiar and the strange. The familiarity is in Mataji's fierceness, the 'hot temper'; the difference, and this is indeed crucial, is in the preponderance of warmth and love in Mataji as compared to Amita's early experience of the indifference of her mother's 'style'. A guru like the late Maharaj Charan Singh of the Radhasoami sect, I would suggest, is too remote from Amita's central conflict, while the late Bhagwan Rajneesh, of Oregon and Pune fame, would be too threatening to the moral values of a girl brought up in an orthodox, middle-class Brahmin family. Mataji's parental style, on the other hand, dovetails with Amita's self-object needs and social experience.

That the guru–disciple relationship is in important ways an extension of the parent–child relationship, constituting a developmental second chance for obtaining the required nutrients for the cohesion, integration and vigorousness of the self, is implicit in some of the older devotional literature and is often explicitly stated by modern gurus. Basava, the twelfth century founder of the Virsaiva sect, identifies the guru god with a particular aspect of the mother (cited in Steinmann, 1986, p. 36):

> As a mother runs close behind the child
> With his hand on a cobra or a fire
> The lord of meeting rivers Stays with me
> Every step of the way And looks after me.

In his instructions to disciples, a contemporary guru, Swami Satyanand Saraswathi, tells us:

> Now in relation with guru, the disciple chooses one *bhava* (emotional state) for himself, according to his personality and needs, and develops that to its fullest potential. If he feels the need for a friend, he should regard the guru as his friend. Or, if he has been lacking parental love, the guru can be his father and mother ... It all depends on your basic needs and which area of your personality is the most powerful. Sometimes in adopting a certain *bhava* toward the guru, the disciple tends to transfer his complexes and neurosis too. If he has become insecure due to the suffering meted out to him by harsh parents, then in relationship with guru too, he feels insecure. (Saraswathi, 1983, p. 92)

Swami Satyanand's remarks also tell us of the difficulties in the path of *surrender* to the guru, an emotional experience which is indispensable for mutative changes in the disciple's self.

If there is one demand made by the guru on the disciple, it is *of* surrender, an opening up and receptivity of the latter's psyche which is sometimes sought to be conveyed through (what men imagine to be) the imagery of female sexual experience. Saraswathi writes:

> When you surrender to the guru, you become like a valley, a vacuum, an abyss, a bottomless pit. You acquire depth, not height. This surrender can be felt in many ways. The OM begins to manifest in you; his energy begins to flow into you. The guru's energy is continuously flowing, but in order to receive it, you have to become a womb, a receptacle. (Saraswathi, 1983, p. 77)

Surrender of the self is, of course, ubiquitous in the religious traditions of the world. In his *The Varieties of Religious Experience*, William James called it regeneration by relaxing and letting go, psychologically indistinguishable from Lutheran justification by faith and the Wesleyan acceptance of free grace. He characterized it as giving one's private convulsive self a rest and finding that a greater self is there. 'The results, slow or sudden, great or small, of the combined optimism and expectancy, the regenerative phenomenon which ensues on the abandonment of effort, remain firm facts of human nature.' He added:

> ... you see why self-surrender has been and always must be regarded as the vital turning point of religious life .... One may say the whole development of Christianity in inwardness has consisted in little more than greater and greater emphasis attached to this crisis of self-surrender. (James, 1902, pp. 107, 215)

In Sufism, too, surrender to the master is a necessary prerequisite for the state of *fanafil-shaykh* or annihilation of oneself in the master. Of the *iradah*, the relationship between the Sufi master and his disciple, the Sufi poet says:

> O heart, if thou wanted the Beloved to be happy with thee, then thou must do and say what he commands. If he says, 'Weep blood!' do not ask 'Why?'; if He says, 'Die!' do not say 'How is that fitting?' (Nurbaksh, 1978, p. 208)

In terms of self psychology, surrender is the full flowering of the idealizing transference, with its strong need for the experience of merging into a good and powerful, wise and perfect self-object—the guru. 'This is the secret of the guru–disciple relationship', says one guru. 'The Guru is the disciple, but perfected, complete. When he forms a relationship with the guru, the disciple is in fact forming a relationship with his own best self'. The disciple, in experiencing his or her self as part of the guru's self, hearing with the guru's ears, seeing with the guru's eyes, tasting with the guru's tongue, feeling with the guru's skin, may be said to be striving for some of the most archaic self-object experiences.

Ramakrishna, the arch example of the Indian penchant for using narrative form in construction of a coherent and integrated world, of its preference for the language of the concrete, of image and symbol over more conceptual and abstract forms, tells us the following parable.

One day while driving with Arjuna (the warrior hero of the Epic Mahabharata), Krishna (who is both God and Arjuna's guru) looked at the sky and said, 'See, friend, how beautiful is the flock of pigeons flying there!' Arjuna saw it and immediately said, 'Quite so, my friend, very beautiful pigeons indeed.' The very next moment Krishna looked up again and said, 'How strange, friend, they are by no means pigeons.' Arjuna saw the birds and said, 'Quite so, my friend, they are not pigeons at all.' 'Now try to understand the matter,' Ramakrishna exhorts us. 'Arjuna's truthfulness is unquestionable. He could have never flattered Krishna in agreeing with him both the times. But Arjuna's devotional surrender to Krishna was so very great that he actually saw with his own eyes whatever Krishna saw with his' (Swami Saradananda, 1983, p. 454).

Devotees come to the guru, as do patients to the analyst, in conflicted state. On the one hand, there is the unconscious hope of making up for missing or deficient self-object responses in interaction with the guru. On the other hand, there is the fear of invoking self-fragmenting responses through the same interaction. The omnipresence of fears of injury to the sell and of regression into early primitive states of self-dissolution is what forces the devotee to be wary of intimacy. It prevents the desired surrender to the guru however high the conscious idealization of the values of surrender and letting go might be. Gurus are of course aware of the conflict and in their various ways have sought to reassure the disciples about their fears. Swami Muktananda, for instance, writes:

> There are only two ways to live: One is with constant conflict, and the other is with surrender. Conflict leads to anguish and suffering ... But when someone Surrenders with understanding and equanimity, his house, body and heart becomes full. His former feeling of emptiness and lack disappears. (Swami Muktananda, 1983, p. 35)

And one of his disciples puts it in a language which the modern self psychologist would have no hesitation in acknowledging as his own:

> We live in countless fleeting relationships, always seeking, finding and losing again. As children and adults, we learn through these relationships. We learn by taking into ourselves our loved ones' thoughts and voices, absorbing our loved ones' very presence along with their knowledge. (Swami Muktananda, 1983, p. 35)

Gurus, gurus have always emphasized, are not human beings, not objects in the inelegant language of psychoanalysis, but functions. They are the power of grace in spiritual terms and intense self-object experiences in the language of self psychology.

The psychological term 'intense selfobject experience' of course transfers the location of the fount of 'grace' from the person of the guru to the psyche of the devotee. It is a grace we have all experienced as infants when the mother's various ministrations transformed our internal world from states of disintegration to one of feeling integrated, from dreaded intimations of fragmentation to blissful experiences of wholeness. The persistent search for this inner metamorphosis in adult life is what makes the guru in India—to use Christopher Bollas' concept—a primary 'transformational object' (Bollas, 1979). He is the culturally sanctioned addressee of a collective request for the transforming experience which goes beyond healing in its narrow sense. The guru's grace is, then, the devotee's recollection of an earlier transformed state. It is a remembrance, Bollas reminds us, which does not take place cognitively but existentially through intense affective experience, even when the latter is not on the same scale as in early life. The anticipation of being transformed by the guru inspires the reverential attitude towards his person, an attitude which in secular man, especially in the West, is more easily evoked by the transformational objects of art than those of religious faith.

The idealizing transference, leading to the merging experience, is thus the core of the healing process in the guru–disciple relationship. The healing is seen in terms of an alchemical transformation of the self: 'When iron comes in contact with the philosopher's stone, it is transmuted in gold. Sandalwood trees infuse their fragrance into the trees around them' (Swami Muktananda, 1983, p. 4). Psychoanalysts, of the object relations and self psychology schools, will have no quarrel with this formulation of the basis of healing. Their model of the healthy person, however, requires an additional step—of re-emergence; the drowning and the resurfacing are both constituents of psychological growth, at all developmental levels. In Kohut's language, healing will not only involve an ancient merger state but a further shift from this state to an experience of empathic resonance with the self-object.

Gurus are generally aware of the dangers of self-fragmentation and the disciple's defences against that dreaded inner state. Modern gurus, like Muktananda, talk explicitly about the agitation and anxiety a disciple may feel when he is close to the guru. The training required en route to surrender is hard and painful. Merger experience, they know, takes place not at once but in progressive stages as, for instance, depicted in Jnaneshvara's description of the unfolding of the guru–disciple relationship in the imagery of bridal mysticism (Steinmann, 1986). They are aware of the resistances and the negative transferences, the times when the devotee loses faith in the guru, and doubts and suspicions tend to creep in. Do not break the relationship when this is happening, is the general and analytically sound advice. The development of inimical feelings towards the guru are part of the process of heating transformation. What is important about the feelings towards the guru is their strength, not their direction. Whether devoted or hostile, as long as the disciple remains turned towards the guru, he will be met by total acceptance. Muktananda describes the ideal guru's behaviour:

> A true guru breaks your old habits of fault finding, of seeing sin, of hating yourself. He roots out the negative seeds that you have sown as well as your feelings of guilt ... You will never hear the guru criticize you. Instead, when you are in his company, you will experience your own divinity. You will never be found guilty in the guru's eyes. You will find in them only the praise of your hidden inner God. (Swami Muktananda, 1983, p. 85)

The 'ambience of affective acceptance' provided by the guru and his establishment, the *ashram*, will, the master knows, make the disciple feel increasingly safe, shifting the inner balance between need and fear towards the former. Old repressed and disavowed self-object needs will reawaken and be mobilized, making the transference more and more intense. Or, put simply, as the conflict between need and fear recedes, the guru, like the analyst, will become the focus for the freshly released, though old, capacities for love, which push strongly towards a merger with the beloved.

If there is a second word besides surrender with which the guru–disciple relationship can be captured, it is *intimacy*. As Lawrence Babb remarks of his interviews with the devotees of Sai Baba:

> What emerges as one general theme in these accounts is the same kind of visual, tactile and elimentary intimacy that is so central to devotional Hinduism in general. The devotees long to see him, to hear him, to be near

him, to have private audiences with him, to touch him (especially his feet) and to receive or consume, or use in other ways, substances and objects that have been touched by him or that originate from him. (Babb, 1987, p. 173)

This striving for intimacy not only marks the disciple's response to the devotional, but also to the knowledge of the guru. Pupul Jayakar, in talking of her response to the 'intellectual' Krishnamurti, says: 'I was driven by the urge to be with him, to be noticed by him, to probe into the mysteries that pervaded his presence. I was afraid of what would happen, but I could not keep away' (Jayakar, 1987, p. 3).

The sought-for intimacy is of an archaic nature, before the birth of language which separates and bifurcates. In the intimacy scale of the sixteenth century North Indian saint Dadu (cited in Steinmann, 1986, p. 290):

> The guru speaks first with the mind
> Then with the glance of the eye
> If the disciple fails to understand
> He instructs him at last by word of mouth
> He that understands the spoken word is a common man
> He that interprets the gesture is an initiate
> He that reads the thought of the mind Unsearchable,
> unfathomable, is a god.

In the desired preverbal intimacy with the guru, Jnaneshvara highlights the devotee's infantile quiescence (Swami Muktananda, 1983, p. 85):

> To say nothing is your praise
> To do nothing is your worship
> To be nothing is to be near you.

Analysts are, of course, familiar with the regressive movements in the patient's psyche occasioned by the growing transference towards the analyst. The regression gives the patient a double vision, both in relation to himself and to the analyst. Within the transference, he 'sees' the analyst as a parental self-object; in the real relationship as a helpful doctor. The two images, in flux over time, constantly condition each other. Because of the co-presence of the patient's adult self, the illusion of relation to the analyst, though it waxes and wanes, remains more or less moderate (Moeller, 1977).

The patient's illusion of the analyst corresponds to another illusion in relation to the self. Patients in analysis often report feeling childlike, even childish, also outside the analytic setting. They imagine themselves at times to be smaller and more awkward than their actual adult selves. The infantile and the adult in relation to the self shape each other and are often in a state of partial identity. In the guru–disciple relationship, the identity between the actual and the infantile selves of the disciple on the one hand and the real and parental representations of the master on the other overlap to a much greater extent and for longer periods of time than in psychoanalysis. The double vision in relation to both self and guru representations tends to become monocular. In other words, the guru–disciple interaction touches deeper, more regressed layers of the psyche which are generally not reached by psychoanalysis. The devotee, I believe, is better (but also more dangerously) placed than the analysand to connect with—and correct—the depressive core at the base of human life from which a self first emerged and which lies beyond words and interpretations.

The healing techniques of the guru are thus designed to foster deeper regressions than those of the analyst. Elsewhere, I have talked of the importance of looking and being looked at as a primary technique of the master–disciple intercourse (Kakar, 1985). I discussed the identity-giving power of the eyes that recognize, i.e., of their self-evoking and self-sustaining functions. Taken in through the eyes, the guru as a benign self-object opens the devotee's closed world of archaic destructive relationships to new possibilities. The technical word, used in scriptural descriptions of the initiation process, is *darshanat*, 'through the guru's look' in which, as Muktananda observes: 'You are seen in every detail as in a clear mirror' (Swami Muktananda, 1983, p. 37). To the utter *clarity* of the look, he might have added its absolute love and complete forgiveness. To adapt Dostoyevski's remark on the lover's vision, in *darshanat* the devotee is looked at, and is enabled to look at himself or herself, as God might have. Even gurus with thousands of disciples, whose devotees might conceivably doubt that a one-to-one recognition by the guru is taking place at regular intervals, are at pains to confirm the operation of *darshanat* in spite of the large numbers involved. To quote Muktananda again:

> Many people become angry with me out of love. They say 'Baba did not look at me,' or 'When Baba looked at me, he didn't smile!' People who say these things do not understand that when I sit on my chair I look at everyone once, silently and with great joy ... True love has no language. If I look at someone, silently emitting a ray of love, that is sublime. This is true and should be understood: love is a secret ray of the eyes. (Swami Muktananda, 1983, p. 109)

What about the guru's words, the discourses to which the devotees listen with such rapt attention? To someone reading such a discourse or listening to it apart from a devotee group, it may seem trite, repetitious and full of well-known homilies. The power of the guru's speech, however, lies not in its insight, but has a different source. 'I did not understand but I came away with the words alive within me' is a typical reaction (Jayakar, 1987, p. 8). The psychological impact of the words is not through their literal meaning but their symbolic power, through the sound which conveys the experience of the guru's presence within the psyche. They are a form of early human contact, much as the experience of a child who is soothed by the mother's vocalizations even when he is physically separated from her and cannot feel her arms around him. In psychoanalysis, a patient will sometimes comment on the quality of the therapist's voice when he feels it as a psychological bridge which joins the two or when he feels it as distancing and evoking a self-fragmenting response. Susan Bady has suggested that it is not only the psychological reaction to the therapist's voice but its virtual ingestion by the patient in a concrete way which is significant. Taken into one's vocal chords, the pattern and rate of breathing, the movement of the diaphragm, the relaxed and self-assured voice of the therapist or the guru will calm his agitation, infuse hope and courage into his own timid and hesitant voice.

The concrete physical and psychic manifestations of the guru's speech and sound are immeasurably enhanced by the group setting in which a disciple normally hears his words. To quote from my own experience of listening to a guru in a large crowd:

> At first there is a sense of unease as the body, the container of our individuality and the demarcator of our spatial boundaries, is sharply wrenched from its habitual mode of experiencing others. For as we grow up, the touch of others, once so deliberately courted and responded to with delight, increasingly becomes ambivalent. Coming from a loved one, touch is deliciously welcomed; with strangers, on the other hand, there is an involuntary shrinking of the body, their touch taking on the menacing air of invasion by the other. But once the fear of touch disappears in the fierce press of other bodies and the individual lets himself become a part of the crowd's density, the original apprehension is gradually transformed into an expansiveness that stretches to include the others. Distances and differences of status, age and sex disappear in an exhilarating feeling (temporary to be sure) that individual boundaries can indeed be transcended and were perhaps illusory in the first place. Of course, touch is only one of the sensual stimuli that hammers at the gate of individual identity. Other excitations, channelled

through vision, hearing and smell, are also very much involved. In addition, as Phyllis Greenacre has suggested, there are other, more subliminal exchanges of body heat, muscle tension and body rhythms taking place in a crowd. In short the crowd's assault on the sense of individual identity appears to be well-nigh irresistible; its invitation to a psychological regression—in which the image of one's body becomes fluid and increasingly blurred, controls over emotions and impulses are weakened, critical faculties and rational thought processes are abandoned—is extended in a way that is both forceful and seductive. (Kakar, 1982, pp. 129-30)

Other techniques employed in the guru–disciple interaction perform a similar function of psychic loosening and fostering deep regression—an increasing surrender to the self-object experience of the merging kind. The taking in of *prasada*, food offerings touched or tasted by the guru, drinking of the water used to wash his feet, helps in a loosening up of individual bodily and psychic boundaries, transforming the experience of the guru from that of a separate Other to one of coming in line with a self-object. Gurus and devotees have always known that meditation on the guru's face or form or the contemplative use of his photograph, as required in some cults, will contribute to and hasten the merging experience. As Muktananda observes: 'The mind that always contemplates the guru eventually becomes the guru. Meditation on the guru's form, immerses the meditator in the state of the guru' (Swami Muktananda, 1983, p. 3).

In a sense, my use of the term guru–disciple interaction has been a misnomer since it has had the disciple's rather than the guru's inner state as its focus. Perhaps this is as it should be given the fact that ostensibly the disciple is the one in search of healing, and that we know infinitely more about the inner processes of disciples than those of the gurus. Yet an analyst has to wonder how a guru deals with the massive idealizing transferences of so many disciples. Negative transferences and malignant projections are of course easier to handle since they cause severe discomfort, compelling us to reject them by discriminating inside between what belongs to us and the alien attributes that have been projected onto us. This painful motivation for repelling the invasion of the self by others does not exist when projections are narcissistically gratifying, as they invariably are in case of the adoring followers.

The problem is further complicated by the fact that for the self-sustaining and self-healing responses to be evoked in the follower (or in the patient), the guru (and the analyst) must accept being the wiser, greater and more powerful parent. To accept and yet not identify with the disciple's parental representation demands, the guru remains in touch with his own infantile self. The best of the gurus, as we saw in the case of Ramakrishna, clearly do that; their own relationship to the Divine keeps intact self-representations other than those of the omniscient parent. But for many others, I would speculate, the temptation to identify with the disciple's projected parental self is overwhelming. As the parent and the stronger figure in the parent–child relationship, it is easier to unload one's conflicts and the depressive self onto the child. In the case of the analyst's counter-transference, as Michael Moeller points out, the identification with the parental role is a source of twofold relief: one, in the transferential repetition of the relationship with the patient, the analyst is the stronger and the less incriminated parent, and two, in reality he is not parent at all (Moeller, 1977). The empirical finding on the anti-depressive effect of the psychoanalytic role also applies to the guru. His calm, cheerful, loving mien is perhaps a consequence rather than a cause of his role as the healer.

I have mentioned above that the dangers of the guru role lie in the disciples' massive parental projections, which the guru must process internally. Although the guru shares this danger with the analyst, or more generally, with any healer, the intensity of these projections, their duration and the sheer number of devotees involved are vastly greater than in the case of his secular counterparts. These idealizing projections are subversive of the guru's self-representation, constitute an insidious assault which a few gurus—again, like some therapists—are not able to successfully resist. A regression to an omnipotent grandiosity is one consequence, while in the sexual sphere a retreat into sexual perversion has been reported often enough to constitute a specific danger of the guru role. It is sad to hear or read reliable reports about 70-year-old gurus who become peeping Toms as they arrange, with all the cunning of the voyeur, to spy on their teen-aged female disciples (generally Western) undressing for the night in the *ashram*. The promiscuity of some other gurus, pathetically effortful in the case of elderly bodies with a tendency to flag, is also too well-known to merit further repetition.

The sexual aberrations, however, have not only to do with pathological regression in stray individual cases, but are perhaps also facilitated by the way the fundamentals of healing are conceptualized in the guru–devotee encounter. For instance, given the significance of a specific kind of intimacy, there is no inherent reason (except cultural disapproval) why intimacy between guru and devotee does not progress to the most intimate encounter of all and be seen as a special mark of the guru's favour; why the merger of souls does not take place through their containers, the bodies. If substances which have been in intimate contact with the guru's body are powerful agents of inner change when ingested by the devotee, then the logic of transformation dictates that the most powerful transforming substance would be the guru's 'purest' and innermost essence—his semen.

REFERENCES

Abhayananda, S. (1989). *Jnaneshvar*. Naples, FL: Atma Books.
Babb, L. (1987). *Redemptive encounters*. Delhi: Oxford University Press.
Bollas, Christopher. (1979). The transformational object. *International Journal of Psychoanalysis*, 60, 97-107.
Brent, P. (1973). *Godmen of India*. Harmondsworth: Penguin.
Cenker, W. (1983). *A tradition of teachers: Sankara and the Jagadgurus today*. Delhi: Motilal Banarsidass.
Chaturvedi, Badrinath. (1990, February 13). Sense and nonsense about the 'Guru' concept. *Times of India*, New Delhi.
Deutsch, A. (1982). Tenacity of attachment to a cult leader: A psychiatric perspective. *American Journal of Psychiatry*, 137(1), 1569-73.
Gold, D. (1987). *The lord as guru*. Delhi: Oxford University Press.
James, William. (1902). *The varieties of religious experience*. New York: Longman.
Jayakar, Pupul. (1987). *J. Krishnamurti: A biography*. Delhi: Penguin.
Kakar, S. (1978). *The inner world: A psychoanalytic study of childhood and society in India*. Delhi: Oxford University Press.
———. (1982). *Shamans, mystics and doctors*. New York: Knopf.
———. (1985). Psychoanalysis and religious healing: Siblings or strangers? *Journal of the American Academy of Religion*, 53(3), 841-53.
Kohut, H. (1971). *The analysis of the self*. New York: International Universities Press.
———. (1977). *The restoration of the self*. New York: International Universities Press.
Lorand, S. (1962). Psychoanalytic therapy of religious devotees. *International Journal of Psychoanalysis*, 43(1), 50-55.
Moeller, M. L. (1977). Self and object in countertransference. *International Journal of Psychoanalysis*, 58, 356-76.
Nacht, S. (1962). Curative factors in psychoanalysis. *International Journal of Psychoanalysis*, 43, 206-21.
Nurbaksh, D. (1978). Sufism and psychoanalysis. *International Journal of Social Psychiatry*, 24, 208.
Saraswathi, Swami Satyananda. (1983). *Light on the guru and disciple relationship*. Munger, India: Bihar School of Yoga.
Steinmann, R. M. (1986). *Guru-Sisya Samhandha: Das meinster-schuler verhaltns im tradiyionll-en und modernen Hinduismus*. Wiesbaden, Germany: Franz Steiner.
Swami Muktananda. (1983). *The glory of the guru*. New York: SYDA Foundation.
Swami Saradananda. (1983). *Sri Ramakrishna, The great master, vol. 1*. Mylapore, India: Sri Ramakrishna Math.
Wolf, Ernest. (1989). *Treatment of the self*. New York: Guilford.

10

Working through Emotional Pain: A Narrative Study of Healing Process

JYOTI ANAND

Life is beset with tragedies and traumas of varied nature, namely, bereavement, life threatening diseases, loss of material possessions and relationships, etc. People not only learn to live with their losses, but many emerge enriched and invigorated. How people handle their emotional pain is an area of research rife with many possibilities of growth and self-enhancement. The main objective of the present study was to augment our understanding of the experience of emotional pain and to trace the process of healing. The study also examined the reconfiguration of self as healing progresses. A healing narrative of a middle-aged woman was generated and analysed to illuminate how people work through their pain and gain new insights.

Emotional pain refers to a feeling of loss and vulnerability, in the face of major life crises. It is akin to an experience of losing a part of oneself. It includes in its gamut a feeling of brokenness and loss of control (Bolger, 1999). Bolger considers emotional pain as a natural consequence of living in this world that gets complicated as a result of a tendency to avoid or deny painful feelings. Clinical interventions aim at working through pain as a necessary task to induce changes in the inner self and ultimately in the ability to cope with life in healthier and more satisfying ways (Bradshaw, 1990). Taylor (1997) has called attention to a profound sense of isolation, meaninglessness, hopelessness and despair as major accompaniments of emotional pain. According to him, emotional pain tends to isolate a person from the flow of contemporary events. One may often be ridden with the feeling of being abandoned and having been left alone. Bakan (1968) has focused on intimate relationships and considers emotional pain as a loss of familial world, which evokes fear of annihilation. Jain (1994) has shown in his work how emotions are construed within the Indian cultural context. Misra (2004) has further viewed all emotional experiences within the social constructionist framework. Accordingly, the experience of emotional pain is situated in a matrix of meanings, identities and relationships specific to a particular culture. Analysing the relevant scriptures, Paranjpe (1998) and Misra (2004) have argued that in the Indian culture, the oft-used term for emotion is 'bhāva', which considers cognition and emotion as indistinguishable and has its genesis in aesthetics and the *bhakti* (devotional) movement.

Healing may be understood as the other side of emotional pain. It is an *experience of an inner sense of well-being, harmony, balance and peace*. It is a process through which the harmony between mind, body and spirit is restored. It would involve a reconstruction of one's reality, a change in emotions and broadening of one's perspective. Thus, healing does not change the life conditions causing emotional pain, but engenders hope, acceptance, release of trapped psychic energy, resolution of internal conflicts and new insights (Kakar, 1982). Healing will not be enduring till the painful emotions are acknowledged, worked through and released from one's system.

Siegel (1991) says: 'When you put your feelings outside, you may heal inside. And you will certainly heal your life, if not your disease'; 'for emotional repression prevents the healing system from responding as a unified entity to threats from inside or outside' (p. 188). 'Anger, anxiety, depression, fear and many other feelings are unhealthy only if they remain buried inside, unexpressed and not dealt with' (p. 191). When one goes beyond one's surface emotions and begins to acknowledge one's real fears, one can break through the resentments and disappointments one holds, and herein begins the process of true healing. True healing, in this sense, means one's ability to become 'whole' again, to gather together the many fragmented pieces of one's life and make peace inside. True healing means one's ability to discover oneself and one's sense of purpose and meaning in this life. This is a painful and difficult process and what Campbell (1968) refers to, as '*the hero's journey*'.

Taylor (1997) contends that forgiveness forms the very basis of healing. One cannot 'pretend' to forgive oneself or others. One needs to courageously go within and feel one's hurt and sadness and grieve one's losses; acknowledge one's failures and mistakes, even when one may feel they were justified or deserved; forgive oneself through the hard and difficult path of self-disclosure and honesty. One can find one's true strength and healing only by acknowledging and accepting one's own humanity, one's vulnerabilities and one's limitations (Dalai Lama, 1992). The healing process (of any type) is an emotionally charged experience (Frank and Frank, 1984), and the salience of any social or spiritual practice lies primarily in their ability to elicit healing emotions.

Scientific evidence for the healing power of self-disclosure of emotions and honest self-examination comes from the work of James Pennebaker (1991). Pennebaker found that writing about traumatic experiences for as little as 15 minutes a day for four days can reduce physician visits for illness, improve serum immune function and enhance work performance up to six months' time. That is to say, that sharing one's true feelings and needs helps one to unlock the power of one's healing system. Why does this disclosure improve one's health and trigger one's healing system? The disclosure is a deep and sometimes painful exploration of one's deepest thoughts and feelings involved in the traumatic event. Somehow, when one moves one's disturbing thoughts, feelings, fears, hurts, disappointments and resentments onto paper, one takes that energy 'out of our bodies' in an appropriate manner (i.e., not dumping it onto others or kicking the cat) and begin to 'free up' one's own internal healing energies.

The present study has relied on the narrative approach to illuminate the process of healing emotional pain. Narratives are life stories. Narratives are about the past happenings of one's life, which are reconstructed as a sequence of events in a story form. Because narratives are constructed retrospectively, they also reflect the ways in which the narrator has come to understand his/her own experience (Jacobson, 2001). While talking about one's personal experiences, a narrator endeavours to move from confusion and meaninglessness to greater clarity (Jackson, 1994). Thus, a life narrative is more than a simple description of past events. It is a process through which events are construed as having a meaningful and coherent order, through which events and experiences are interpreted and through which the narrator acquires an identity, like a character in fiction (Good, 1994). Under conditions of adversity, individuals often feel a pressing need to re-examine and re-fashion their personal narratives in an attempt to maintain a sense of coherence and identity. The self is, thus, reconstructed through narrative.

The narrative analysis respects and upholds this self of the narrator in responding to crisis predicaments in a creative manner. When a layperson constructs and communicates through the narrative of one's personal experience, one does so within cultural settings, which provide specific forms of language, values, role expectations and modes of living. As Kelley (1994) has noted, 'people develop a sense of self, and attempt to construct a public identity for themselves on the basis of the way they talk about coping' (p. 6).

The narratives are compelling because not only do the narrators convey their emotional pain, but they attempt to reconfigure their experience and wrest meaning from the same. Healing narratives amount to reliving painful memories and trying to find meaning in the experience of traumatic events. Williams (2000) argues that healing narratives provide insights into how people reconstruct some sense of purpose in their lives. In this exploratory study, a narrative of a woman who went through severe emotional pain was taken, to systematically follow the trail of self-healing.

METHOD

The narrative discussed in this chapter is Madhur's life story. Madhur is a 50-year old woman who has three grown-up children, two married daughters and a son looking after the family business. Madhur hails from a traditional upper middle class background. She got married in a joint family when she was just 17. Her husband was the eldest son and was involved in the family business. A few years after her marriage, Madhur underwent a series of life crises (marital distress, bereavement and illness in family). When she was contacted for an interview, she had considerably recovered. She was willing to talk and share her inner experiences of having lived through the various upheavals of her life.

Madhur was interviewed at her residence. Despite the fact that it was the first time that I was meeting her, she was very cooperative, willing and gave her very best in sharing her most innermost feelings and experiences. She was quite eager and forthcoming in her narration, and there were places where she became emotional. But due credit goes to her for recounting all her experiences from the very beginning and reliving her pain and all the associated feelings of those experiences. It seemed, as though, she was pouring out her heart without any attempts to withhold or conceal anything. The researcher was not without some guilt for having raked up her past memories, but towards the end of the interview, it was reassuring to learn that Madhur had happily graduated from her past crises. It was an exceptionally intense session that continued for almost four hours.

The interview was recorded after taking Madhur's prior consent. The language of the narrative was a mix of both Hindi and English, and was transcribed verbatim. In the narrative discussed here, the names, locales and backgrounds have been altered to preserve anonymity of the narrator. The effort was to stay as close to the narrative as possible and to use the closest possible English translation of the Hindi language. Wherever it was felt that the translation would alter the meaning or sense of the expression as the narrator had used it, the Hindi word/expression was retained as it was.

Analysis and Interpretation

The narrative script was chronicled in the order the events unfolded. As far as possible, the events were documented along with the context in which they occurred. Efforts were made throughout to make sense of the narrative from the narrator's perspective. The main focus was: on the emotional pain which Madhur suffered in her relations and bereavement, on her search for an anchor in her own self, on her release from her emotional cocooning and on subsequent attaining of inner peace and tranquillity. Madhur's narrative provides an insight into the way emotions play a pivotal role in reorganizing the self to efficaciously deal with life crises. The attempt has been to stay with the flow of her narration to delineate the process of emotional healing.

The experience of emotional pain

After marriage, Madhur gave herself fully to her husband's family and tried to live up to everyone's expectations. She earned an enviable place for herself in the family, so much so, that her father-in-law would often seek and act upon her opinion in family matters, much to the chagrin of her husband, who did not enjoy as much say. Some time later, when Madhur discovered her husband's infidelity, she was very distressed. She felt she had lost all grounds with her husband. Her sense of failure multiplied when she confronted the indifference of her (in-laws) family. She had served and catered to them as her own family, but none of them stood by her when she needed their support in the time of her crisis. In response to her husband's illicit relationship, which was an event almost 20 years in the past, she narrated her plight as if it had happened yesterday.

> I used to be very upset, I could not sleep in the night. I suffered from insomnia and became dependent on sleeping pills, for without them I couldn't sleep in the night. I used to keep awake the whole night ... I told the family members also, but no one helped me ... Then I realized that perhaps this is no one else's problem, this is only my problem ... Then I started finding faults in myself that there is something lacking in me and so he's doing this (having a relation outside marriage). I used to ask him also that do you also (find something lacking in me)? He used to say, 'No, there's nothing wrong with you, please don't think in this manner ever' ... I started looking for a reason, that is there something lacking in me, but I found nothing lacking in myself ... Gradually I started understanding that perhaps he was suffering from some complex, and was unable to take my goodness and my abilities in a positive manner and was taking them negatively. This was my own psychological analysis that stands till today.

She further added: 'Suddenly one day something came up in our conversation (between husband and wife), it must have been for just a minute, and I went into severe depression, and I was drowned in that for two and a half years ...' She continued:

> He mentioned his friend's name—he said something, exactly I don't want to remember, and I got such a shock, like (I'd been hit by) an electric current, and I felt that I am drowning in it ... deep inside ... and I won't be able to come out of it ... I had that feeling inside ... and the feeling that I've become a failure in life ... that after doing all this (for everyone) I have become a failure ... I tried a lot that somehow he gets improved, but his heart was not in his business ...

It was an emotional trauma for Madhur and she plunged into an abyss of depression. Her self-esteem was badly bruised. She found her world crumbling, both within (herself) and without. Her emotional investment in her husband and his family was so intense that she felt cheated and dejected. Her depression left her emotionally drained and washed-out. She lost interest in household work and was mostly confined to her room, brooding over her failure in life. She had no one to share her problems with, and slowly became a recluse.

As Taylor (1997) observed, the initial phase of depression entails a feeling of loss and isolation, and one is mired in unresolvable emotional conflicts. One may feel incapable of expressing any kind of emotion and may find it difficult to relate with people in one's social world. One experiences constant pain that has no boundaries. All one knows is that one cannot bear these feelings, yet, must continue to endure them.

In Madhur's own words:

> I started feeling that the family members were not my own. Slowly I started feeling that all are selfish, this whole world is selfish, and that I have to fight my battles myself. Most of the time I would feel my children to be a burden. How do I look after them, what do I do? I was so warped in my own problems that I didn't understand what guidance to give them ... I used to do the household work but I used to get very tired. I used to feel that its better that I die. Many times I had suicidal tendencies, but I always resisted the impulse, that if I attempt suicide then I would be faced with a question mark. If I commit suicide then I would be at peace, and somewhere I felt that I would take revenge from the family members also, but ... then what will happen to my children? It would be a stain on their lives forever, i.e., that their mother has committed suicide. So I could never take that step. But from inside there was great anger brewing, which could never come out, and it became so intense that I went into depression ... It was such severe depression that the whole day I would just keep lying down, would not get up, and it took me two and a half to three years to come out of it ... I did not want to discuss this thing outside. I never discussed it outside. Even my parents never came to know ...
>
> I started getting the sympathy due to a sick person. And I don't know, maybe when that sick person gets mentally sick, so his/her body mechanism also becomes such that it begins to seek sympathy, and it begins to get solace in this. Or, I used to feel that perhaps my bodily and mental mechanism would work in such a manner that I may get my husband's attention. Because I was always an analyzing person, so I used to feel that (perhaps) this was my attitude that I wanted his attention, therefore I was sick. But that had got so deeply entrenched within my body that despite my desire to get well, I was not improving.

Reclaiming the self in depression

Madhur emotionally intended to use her depression and misery as a way to seek attention and sympathy of her husband, who, she thought, still loved her very much. Instead, he started avoiding her. That was probably the turning point. Madhur was not the one to give up. She took the cudgels in her hands to salvage herself from drowning in the quicksand of depression. It was during this period that she indulged in a lot of introspection, auto-counselling and cognitive reappraisal to derive meaning out of the existing situation, because somewhere this realization had dawned on her that she only could help herself; if she relied on outside sources for help, she would be left wanting. This conviction indeed helped her to come out of her chronic depression. Depression has the effect of putting a person into a form of painful hibernation where one becomes aware that there is something wrong with one's life and where one has a chance to discover what is wrong and to put it right (Rowe, 1982). She was rediscovering her inner strength to become self-reliant in dealing with her life situation. This episode of her life, as though, set the stage for self-reflection and greater maturity.

> I became a totally different person ... I took treatment on my own, I nursed myself, reasoned out with myself slowly and gradually, every day—when I used to be lying down, I used to (think), that I have to get out of this. There was a lot of anger also, but I have to get out. I cannot change him; now I only have to get out of this situation. May the Lord give enough strength that I come out of this (situation). When the depression lessened, I began understanding things; that I cannot change him ... I felt that both of us were so good and as a couple we did not deserve this ... But I never wanted to take that step, that I divorce him—it was not palatable to me. I loved him very much ... despite everything, till date, no one has ever been so dear to me as he was to me, because I loved him very much.

But, she continued: 'I have my own integrity, I have my own identity. Why should I trouble myself over this? I became matured by then.'

> ... slowly I began to prepare myself to take on all the responsibility on myself; I look over the complete care-taking of my children ... I withdrew myself from the (larger) family because my energy was limited; I could either give to myself or to the family ... This was again a new chapter for me, that you try to equip yourself in such a manner that you are the only person who can manage all this. To prepare oneself each day is a very difficult thing, and without sharing this with anyone, and without anyone's guidance. These were all my own thoughts, and these seemed right.

Certain things were brewing in the family that forced Madhur to come out of her shell and take stock of the situation. It was about the family and business. Despite her depression and sickness, she was sensitive enough to perceive that these developments were not favourable for both her husband and herself. Seeing them preoccupied elsewhere, other family members were attempting to usurp the family business and her husband was getting marginalized. She also noticed that her husband was developing depressive symptoms and was losing interest in his business. She offered him her unstinted support in his work and personally as well.

Her husband's misery and depression somehow became instrumental in facilitating her re-emergence into the world. In the experience of her own pain and agony, she had gained certain insights and had become sensitive enough to realize the seriousness of her husband's predicament. Putting aside all previous grudges, she jumped into the arena to rescue her husband from the throes of his depression. He was holding his father responsible for his failings in the business and used to be very angry with him. Alarmed by his suicidal tendencies, Madhur took him to a psychiatrist. She approached her father-in-law and other family members, voicing her apprehensions and pleaded for some urgent action. But help was not forthcoming. Once again, Madhur stood disillusioned.

> Again it was very painful for me, that what is the use of family ... what is the use of me and my sacrifices, what did I get in return?

Tormented by his anger, bitterness and depression, Madhur's husband, having given several hints, committed suicide. Madhur had had a strong premonition about the same, and despite her best efforts could do nothing to avert it.

> I don't know how, somewhere inside ... I was getting this sense that some day he would do something and I would be left alone ... I would lose him ... as though my conscience from within, like my sixth sense, or you may call it my intuition—there was such a strong intuition that later people told me that yes, you had said this, which I don't remember.

Although her husband's death was not very unexpected, yet Madhur was deeply pained. She was pained by the inaction and insensitivity of her family. For her, it was the most tragic thing to happen.

> When this happened, I went to the hospital and the doctor declared that he's no more. He died ... I was left speechless ... I was deeply pained and I fell that I have lost the whole thing, and I have lost my battle.

Paradoxically, whereas on one hand her husband's death was painful for Madhur, perhaps in some remote corner she felt confident that she could make a new beginning. Now she had to think only for her immediate family and was no longer bound by the expectation of the larger family. She could take her own decisions and was not constrained or helpless as she was when her husband was alive. She had a sense of freedom from all emotional and social bondages.

Janoff-Bulman (1992) writes extensively about the growth that people may experience after coming to grips with tragedies and the shattered assumptions that result from them. From these losses, one may develop new and more realistic assumptions. Essentially, one may learn to be tougher about the nature of life and how it regularly involves losses for oneself and others. That is just the way it is. To successfully adapt, one has to learn to make the best of it.

> My husband passed away ... I lost everything ... but deep inside in my heart, on one hand I was crying also, was feeling upset also, but deep inside, somewhere there was this feeling that I will live it up ... What has happened has happened, the worst that could happen in anyone's life has happened ... My suffering was very much there, but somewhere it was going on in my mind that whatever had to happen, now this chapter of my life is closed. I have to begin a new chapter of my life now. In that new chapter I don't know where my destination is, and I don't even know the way ... and I didn't even know how much support I'd get. But I had immense confidence in myself, which was my inner strength. I was questioning myself, I searched within myself, there were no regrets anywhere, till date I have no regrets ... I was very confident that despite having lost everything in life, I still have something within me! I had this strong feeling inside which I could not share with anyone ... I had this faith within myself, I will not lose from life, and I will live it up and show it to them what living means!

Closeting emotions to brave the world

Madhur took upon the new and changed situation as a challenge and began to invest all efforts in the direction of dealing with the same. She did not allow her pain of losing her husband to weaken her resolve or act as a shackle in any way. She did not want her vulnerability and her weak moments to become apparent before the world!

> My pain was there, but my mind was working on the lines that what do I have to do now ... Then I thought that I have to break this emotional barrier myself, because one becomes helpless at the hands of one's emotions only ... If anyone else attempted to break this barrier it would hurt me ... suddenly this realization dawned on me ... Let me put all this aside and explore other possible avenues.

Somewhere, Madhur's single-handed struggle during her depression days and a certain amount of preparedness about what was going to ensue (regarding her husband's suicide) had instilled a great deal of confidence in her to take on life and whatever the situation at hand was, as a challenge. She was not prepared to let others control her and her children's lives.

> I said, either everything will get ruined or I'll get everything back—it was a gamble. But it will only happen when I'll do something.

A month after her husband's death, against the wishes of her in-laws, Madhur started going to her husband's factory and learning the trade. She knew nothing about the business but had the confidence that she could manage it. She immersed herself in her work so deeply that she withdrew from everything else.

> I thought that like a labourer who toils every day and earns his meal, and doesn't know what will happen about his meal the next day, I'll also think likewise. I work today, I come back, have my meal and go to sleep, get up in the morning and go to work again ... I used to keep taking my sleeping pills so that I'm able to work in the morning, not that I forget everything.

Madhur suffered from insomnia and could not sleep without the aid of medicines. But now her orientation and approach was problem-focused rather than self-indulgent, i.e., her reason for taking sleeping pills was to enable her mind to function properly.

Simultaneously, she used to keep counselling herself that if she had that spirit to learn, she would be able to pick up the skill probably better than the other workers. She never let her ego become a barrier in enabling her to learn the tricks of the trade from anyone and everyone who knew it better than her. She kept her target in sight that she had to stand up and make it on her own, together with tending to her children.

> I became a stronger person, a very firm person gradually. I used to think that I have to do my work—that was my target—I have to do my work and prove myself and give my children everything by the dint of my efforts, in a right manner ... I never felt deprived. I used to feel that this is my world and I was satisfied with it.

Sublimation of the emotional self

When her husband committed suicide, Madhur was very upset with God.

'I used to feel really angry at God that you have done all this with such a true and honest person as me. I had stopped going to the temple.' But her faith remained intact. 'I used to earnestly pray to Him whenever in trouble, that if you are really there, then you tell me what to do now.' She had challenged God: 'If there is God then let him ward off (this pain). If He's there, let Him save (me), we'll see how He saves. I felt that one who is alone and has no support, He is there with him/her.'

She would keep giving herself these messages to reinforce her faith and confidence. After putting in all her efforts and mind when the results were not forthcoming, Madhur surrendered before Him. Surrendering cannot come as a result of cognitive appraisal and efforts—it is very essentially a manifestation of overwhelming emotions, a feeling and realization of utter helplessness and an implicit faith in the Supreme Order.

> When I actually surrendered before God that you only have to do whatever is to be done—this I surrendered when everything slipped away from my hands, when I had failed completely, then God said, 'see this can happen in this manner'. My vision cleared and I saw that this is also possible (and) acceptance came. Maybe it was then that I felt God's presence.

She continued:

> When I didn't know my way around, the family members were also the same, the circumstances were more difficult, and there were so many problems, then ... there was some power which was pulling me along. My inner strength was there, but ... I feel (*mera man*) that it was God's power only ... the strength that He gave me, means the present situation was absolutely opposite of the earlier circumstances ... I lost everything, I lost my husband, love had gone out of my life and I had lost faith in life and truthfulness ... Still I had so much faith in myself.

Madhur's share of trials were not over as yet. About four years later, Madhur almost lost her son in a tragic car accident, in which her father-in-law died and her son was battling with life itself. That was another juncture of her life when her faith in God got reinstated.

> The night the accident took place, I felt that neither money, power, doctors, facilities, nothing mattered at that juncture. Only one thing works here, and that is God ... That night I literally handed him (her son) over to God, because even if I had gone and placed all my wealth there, and would have used all the powers of the city, and would have done everything possible ... I didn't know whether I could have saved my son ... I was sitting in

the night (in the hospital)—I said, 'O God now I have handed him to you—I don't know what is appropriate for me. My heart would wish that my son stays with me but what is right for me, this you decide. If it was in my hands I would spend all my wealth, even if I finish off everything, still I don't know whether I will be getting him back or not ... I was sitting alone and praying ...' Now you decide what is to be done with him (her son)' and I kept sitting like that that whole night.

For almost a fortnight, till her son was out of danger, Madhur did not sleep a wink. For all those people who helped her during that period, she felt they were all god-sent. When her son started responding to the treatment that was being given to him, and the doctors proclaimed him out of danger and promised to return her son as he originally was, Madhur put in all her best efforts and energy in nursing him and attending to all his needs herself. Once again, her faith in God got a fillip. It was a significant day for Madhur when her son returned home. Such great was her satisfaction and happiness that she admitted forgetting everything related to her past suffering and never missed her husband after that. Somewhere it gave a boost to her confidence also that despite the entire trauma that she suffered, her strength did not weaken and held her in good stead through it all.

Release of emotions that healed

Healing never takes place unless emotions are healed. Madhur's is a good example of such emotional healing. After her husband's suicide, Madhur had seemingly taken hold of her situation. She had immersed herself totally in her work. It was a lopsided existence that she was leading—in the sense that she had neglected herself totally, and a certain emotional isolation and apathy had set in. She had almost stopped crying after her husband's death. In the process of making herself strong, she continued to bury her pain deep inside.

> I never used to cry. But because of that the pain kept accumulating inside, I was upset from within, but it didn't show apparently.

It was when she joined a preliminary course of *The Art of Living* and practised meditation as part of the course, something happened which took her by surprise. In one of the sessions she broke down and cried as she had not cried in years. Madhur shared that she cried so bitterly, profusely and so loudly that she could not stop crying for almost 15 days. It seemed as though all the emotions that she had been suppressing all these years burst forth with a vengeance, as though a dam had broken free. All the pent up pain, fury, bitterness, frustration and anguish of so many years, as though, got washed away in her tears. When a person suddenly confronts her pain, she becomes overwhelmed by the realization that her numbness was protecting her from her deep hurt, and that she had not healed as yet (Taylor, 1997). She continued:

> 'I broke down and it seemed as though a storm was let loose.' I remained disturbed for about 15-20 days. I went into a sort of depression. But all my emotions which had been suppressed, they surfaced ... I had started becoming very dry. I used to feel very irritated (*chid*), a kind of detachment was taking hold.

When she did the advanced course, she again had those crying spells:

> I was feeling that the more I was crying the lighter I was feeling, means, as long as I sat for meditation, my tears were flowing continuously. But after that advanced course, I danced so much, the first day I sang a *bhajan* ... (Earlier) I just could not listen to *bhajans*, *kirtans* and harmonium ... There was a transformation and I felt as though I became very light from within. Then I realized that indeed my emotions had been suppressed and they had surfaced now.

Feeling buoyant and relieved, when Madhur sang *bhajans* and danced as she had never done before, it was the expression of her inner self which had experienced the release after such a long period. According to Madhur, '*everything goes through a process*'. Some years back, she had such hatred for her family members that she would curse them. Today, Madhur claims that there is no bitterness, anger or complaints within her; rather, there is forgiveness in her heart for all those who had wronged her. Instead, she is at peace with herself, and it was visible in her countenance.

As Atwood and Martin (1991) commented, one's pain and suffering can be a vehicle for helping one to connect with one's sensitivity. This acknowledgement and acceptance of one's limitations without attempting to raise any defences loosens up the blocked flow within one's innermost layers of consciousness. It is a humbling and an elevating experience at the same time. Therein begins the healing process. Thus, the crisis situation has not changed, but the individual experiencing it has, in attitude, orientation and emphasis. In such a scenario, there is evidence to show that the faith in the goodness of humankind and hope in the benevolence and justice of the Higher Order, all give credence to the fact that the experience of emotional pain does not often maul their spirits—rather, they resurface from its depths, enriched and peaceful. Kakar (1982, 1991) has written extensively about how shamans and gurus transform the self of the person and radically change one's perception that facilitates a feeling of well-being.

In another study, Anand, Srivastava and Dalal (2001) also found that one of the major outcomes of the healing process is a sense of liberation. The perception about oneself changes from that of a helpless victim to that of a person who is in control of one's life, and develops better insights into one's problems and conflicts. Considering healing as a spiritual experience, Taylor (1997) argues that personal loss can be the springboard for transcendence and a sense of freedom.

Concluding Remarks

This study attempted to examine the experience of emotional pain and subsequent reconstrual of the self in the process of healing. Madhur's narrative provided rich insights about how such healing takes place. Emotional pain for Madhur was quintessentially the outcome of a loss of an intimate relationship and that of a familial world, seriously undermining her sense of self. This resulted in severe depression and anger. Though she silently suffered in her depression, it played its facilitative role by affording the much needed time, solitude and personal space to Madhur for contemplation, self-reflection and reconstrual of her painful experience. This enabled Madhur to enlarge her vista and spectrum of understanding, of coming in touch with her unrealized potential and strength and resultantly reclaiming her natural self. Furthermore, having lived and worked through her emotional pain imparted the keen penetration and insight into the machinations of such suffering and empathic sensitivity to deal with her husband who too plunged in severe depression. Her husband's deteriorating mental state alarmed Madhur and led to her coming out of her self-imposed ostracism. Her anger towards the other family members for having wronged her husband and herself also provided the outlet to come out of her shell. Thus, whereas depression pulls a person inside, Taylor (1997) observed that anger brings the person back in contact with the world outside.

After her husband's demise, Madhur was left alone to face the world and to bring up her children single-handedly. Her self-reflections during her bout of depression had made her aware of her strengths and vulnerabilities. She took it on herself to run her husband's business despite the disapproval of her in-laws. She wanted to prove herself and did not allow her negative emotions to become impediments in her path. She emotionally insulated herself and effectively managed to keep her inner and outer worlds separate from each other.

It was during the next traumatic phase of her life, when her son met with a near fatal accident and was battling with life that she realized the ineffectiveness of all worldly resources and support systems she had, in the recovery of her son. It was at this juncture that Madhur came face-to-face with her acute vulnerability and helplessness. The acceptance of the same apparently facilitated her surrender before the divine. Because she had sought divine intervention for her son's recovery, it did not lessen the pain closeted in her. But perhaps her confrontation with, and realization of her limitations and vulnerability prepared the ground for subsequent healing which was to manifest later. As Siegel (1991) observes, 'In our acceptance of our vulnerability is our healing' (p. 268). When one is able to confront one's losses and fears, one's pain and incapacities, one acknowledges one's vulnerabilities. This acknowledging the reality of this sense of vulnerability would tantamount to a beginning of healing (Fife, 1994).

With time, when Madhur was able to prove her mettle and started to live life on her own terms and conditions, perhaps she no longer needed the defences that had been erected to prevent the eruption of painful and unpleasant emotions. One day while attending a spiritual discourse, without any forewarning, the floodgates of her blocked emotions opened up and she could not stop crying for days. This, as though, washed away all her negative emotions and healed her.

REFERENCES

Anand, J., Srivastava, A. and Dalal, A. K. (2001). Where suffering ends and healing begins. *Psychological Studies*, 46(3), 114–26.

Atwood, J. D. and Martin, L. (1991). Putting eastern philosophies into western psychotherapies. *American Journal of Psychotherapy*, 45(3), 368–82.

Bakan, D. (1968).*Disease, pain, and sacrifice-Toward a psychology of suffering*. Chicago: Beacon Press.

Bolger, E. A. (1999). Grounded theory of emotional pain. *Psychotherapy Research*, 9(3), 343-62.

Bradshaw, J. (1990). *Homecoming-Reclaiming and championing your inner child.* Toronto: Bantam Books.

Campbell, J. (1968). *The hero with a thousand faces.* Princeton: Princeton University Press.

Dalai Lama. (1992).*Worlds in harmony.* Berkeley, Calif.: Parallax Press.

Fife, B. L. (1994). The conceptualization of meaning in illness. *Social Science and Medicine*, 38(2), 309-16.

Frank, J. D. and Frank, J. B. (1984). *Persuasion and healing.* London: The John Hopkins University Press.

Good, B. J. (1994). *Medicine, rationality and experience: An anthropological perspective.* Cambridge: Cambridge University Press.

Jackson, J. E. (1994). The Rashomon approach to dealing with chronic pain. *Social Science and Medicine*, 38(6), 823-33.

Jacobson, N. (2001). Experiencing recovery: A dimensional analysis of recovery narratives. *Psychiatric Rehabilitation Journal*, 24(3), 1-12.

Jain, U. (1994). Socio-cultural construction of emotions. *Psychology and Developing Societies*, 6(2), 151-68.

Janoff-Bulman, R. (1992). *Shattered assumptions: Toward a new psychology of trauma.* Toronto: Maxwell Macmillan Canada.

Kakar, S. (1982). *Shamans, mystics and doctors.* Delhi: Oxford University Press.

———. (1991). *The analyst and the mystic.* New Delhi: Viking.

Kelley, M. (1994). *Coping with chronic illness: A sociological perspective.* Inaugural lecture. Greenwich: University of Greenwich.

Misra, G. (2004). Emotion in modern psychology and Indian thought. In K. Joshi and M. Cornelissen (Eds), *Consciousness, science, society and yoga* (pp. 314-31). New Delhi: Centre for Studies in Civilizations.

Paranjpe, A. C. (1998). *Self and identity in modern psychology and Indian thought.* New York: Plenum Press.

Pennebaker, J. (1991). *Opening up: The healing power of confiding in others.* New York: Avon.

Rowe, D. (1982). *The construction of life and death.* NY: John Wiley & Sons.

Siegel, B. S. (1991). *Peace, love & healing.* London: Arrow Books.

Taylor, E. (1997). *A psychology of spiritual healing.* Pennsylvania: Chrysalis Books.

Williams, G. (2000). Knowledge narratives. *Anthropology and Medicine*, 7(1), 135-44.

11

Yoga and the State of Mind

R.L. KAPUR

Most psychiatrists would agree that while their profession has done much to alleviate mental illness and emotional distress, they have very little understanding of techniques which would promote mental health and bring about in the individual a more or less pervasive sense of well-being, joy, alertness, energy, etc. Some Eastern mystical traditions claim to do just that and Yoga is one of the techniques used to bring about a state of what may be called positive mental health.

Yoga is a system of concrete steps to attain what Patanjali (Taimini, 1971) refers to as an 'inhibition of fluctuations of mind'. The steps involve some psychophysiological exercises, a conscious control of instinctual demands, a surrender to a higher will, and on the basis of these, a reordering of one's relation with the external world. Though most closely related to the *Samkhya* philosophy, Yoga is flexible enough to enable its insertion into other philosophical systems, for example, *Tantra*, Buddhism, Advaita and also that of the *Bhagavadgita*.

A lot of research has been carried out to examine the effect of Yoga on neurophysiological, hormonal and metabolic parameters, but while it is of interest that Yogis can control their heartbeat or change their brain waves, the crucial question from the psychological point of view is whether they can control their mental fluctuations. Indian tradition claims that the only way to understand the impact of Yoga on the subjective states is by experiencing it yourself.

A few years ago, I took a year off from my work to do just that. I apprenticed myself to a guru and devoted myself to Yoga, spending about five hours everyday on yogic practices, every evening. I would spend an hour or two recording my observations regarding what had happened to my own mental state. After the completion of one year, I once again stood outside my experience and examined whether my daily observations revealed any consistent patterns. It is my understanding that if a few fellow professionals go through similar training and report their conclusions in a similar manner, some commonalities can be culled out to form a body of phenomenological knowledge around the Yoga technique. Walsh has done such an exercise for *vipasana* meditation but I am not aware of any with respect to Yoga.

This chapter gives an account of my exploration. In Section I, I mention some basic principles of *Samkhya* philosophy and Patanjali's Yoga *sutras*, pertinent to my study. It may be noted that while for the sake of clear comprehension I put this section first, in actual fact, my guru allowed me textual research only after the experiential research had been completed—so as not to bias my results. The second section picks up from my diary, in chronological fashion, some details which give a flavour of my experiences. Finally, in the third section, I describe the conclusions of my research.

YOGA CONCEPT OF COSMIC AND PSYCHOLOGICAL REALITY

1. Yoga borrows from the *Samkhya* the concept that reality consists of two opposite but equally substantive principles—*purusha* (self) and *prakriti* (nature). *Purusha* is the pure, timeless, unchanging, qualityless awareness. *Purusha* is not an agent to any happening, but is a witness to all that happens. All change is in the domain of *prakriti*. *Chitta* or the mind-complex is a part of *prakriti* and not of *purusha*, for the mind is ever-changing. While all the emotional and cognitive activities occur in the mind, the witness function of the *purusha* is essential to an awareness of the mental activities. *Purusha* is like a light in a room full of things: while it does not alter anything in the room, without it the contents of the room remain invisible.
2. *Prakriti* is composed of three genetic constituents called the *gunas*. These are the *sattva*, *rajas* and *tamas*. *Sattva* is the element of enlightenment, *rajas* of activity and *tamas* of torpor, sloth and destruction. The human psyche also contains these three elements which balance each other. While *sattva* helps us to achieve understanding and ethical behaviour, it is the *rajas* which pushes the *sattva* to activity,

when the need arises. Further, *tamas* is also essential because of its destructive qualities: only by negation and destruction can the new be created.
3. In an ordinary existence, the *purusha* is tainted by *prakriti* in such a way that the mind does not understand the difference between the two. This is the cause of all *kleshas* or miseries. These miseries include egotism, attractions, repulsions and fear of death.
4. Naturally, one would like to end miseries. This desire leads people to different actions or *karma*. All actions leave residues in our existential core besides producing their effect in the world. These residues or *samskaras* rise up as *vasanas* or personality traits and determine the manner in which we relate to the world.

Samkhya and Yoga accept the theory of reincarnation. What gets reborn is this collation of *samskaras* and *vasanas*. What follows from the above is that: (*a*) our personality is determined by our actions; (*b*) each new action interacts with the previous collation, modifying the personality accordingly; and (*c*) our future actions (in this life and the life after) get determined by our personality.

While it is impossible to cancel the effects of *karma* once performed, it is possible through Yoga to make our future actions inert (i.e., not leave any *samskaras* or *vasanas*). One reaches a state of *moksha* (liberation) when all the accumulated *karma* has had its effect.

Yoga practices for liberation: The oft-quoted aphorism in the Yoga *sutras* is '*Yoga Chitta Vritti Nirodha*'. Translated, it means: 'Yoga is the inhibition of the fluctuations of the mind'. Patanjali talks of inhibiting not only the emotional fluctuations but also cognitive fluctuations. The most important conditions for achieving this aim are *abhyasa* or constant uninterrupted effort and *vairagya*, i.e., detachment from desires. The highest point in the practice is to achieve a state of *Samadhi* or one pointed concentration.

The path of Yoga is not easy. There are many obstacles or *vikshepas* in the way of those doing it. These are disease, dullness, carelessness, laziness, greed, a tendency to misjudge and misinterpret, mental instability and distractability. These obstacles may cause despair and nervousness. The first step in Yoga is to carry out practices to remove these *vikshepas*. These can be removed through: (*a*) actively cultivating the attitudes of friendliness, compassion, gladness and equanimity; (*b*) taking long breaths; (*c*) concentrating on happier experiences of our past; (*d*) thinking of those who are themselves steady of mind; (e) by self-realization which comes through an examination of one's sleep and dreams.

Once the *vikshepas* are attended to, one starts modestly on the path of Yoga by performing *kriya yoga*, a preliminary set of practices. These include certain austerities, a contemplation of what goes on in one's mind and development of an attitude of surrender to a higher being. The last would mean that whatever happens to you, good or bad, is ascribed to a higher will. This higher will is that of *ishwara*, which must not be equated with God. The description which follows is, in the *Yoga Sutras*, more that of an ideal state of being than of being itself.

Once a certain degree of comfort is acquired in the path of *kriya yoga*, one launches into what may be called Yoga proper or *ashtanga*—the eight-limbed path. It is not clear from the *Yoga Sutras* whether the eight directions are to be taken one at a time in a certain order or simultaneously. Commentators vary in their interpretation. In my view, one may start with any one, whichever seems easier and then go on to the others.

The *ashtanga* or the eight-limbed path of Yoga is as follows:

Yamas are the vows of self-restraint. These include abstention from violence, falsehood, sexual continence and acquisitiveness.

Niyamas are the vows of observances. These include purity, contentment, austerity, self-study and self-surrender to a higher will. Together the *yamas* and *niyamas* may be considered the essential ethical dos and don'ts.

Asanas or physical postures are an important element in the practice of Yoga. While certain other kinds of Yoga, for example, *hatha yoga* have developed an elaborate system of bodily postures, Patanjali asks one just to 'sit in a steady and comfortable posture with relaxation of effort and concentrating on the concept of endlessness'.

Pranayama consists of sophisticated techniques of breath control developed in *hatha yoga*, but Patanjali says only that 'Pranayama is the practice of temporary cessation of breath in inspiration, expiration or between inspiration and expiration'.

Pratyahara is the withdrawal of senses from objects. According to Patanjali—when separated from objects, the senses follow as it were the 'nature of mind'. I understand this as the deliberate cutting off of the processes, which provide meanings to the objects—meanings derived from our previous experiences and conditionings.

Dharana, *dhyana* and *samadhi* are the three stages of one continuous process, which may be roughly equated with meditation. *Dharana* is the concentration of mind on a limited area, be it an object, mental image, word, syllable or a concept. When *dharana* continues without interruption for a long enough time, it becomes *dhyana*. When in *dhyana*, the 'I' disappears and only the object remains, it is *samadhi*. In the deepest of *samadhis*, called the *nirbeeja samadhi*, even the object disappears and what remains is pure awareness.

With regular practice, the Yogi acquires *sidhis* or special miraculous powers. By concentrating on an object or an event in deep *samadhi*—a process called *samyama*—the Yogi can manipulate it. Amongst other things, one can gain knowledge of the past and future, meaning of sounds produced by all beings, knowledge of what goes on in the minds of others, the ability to be invisible, strength equal to that of elephants, etc.! Patanjali insists that there is nothing unnatural about it and that these activities are inherent in all of us—only that in normal consciousness they are blocked, just as the natural flow of water in a channel is blocked if we put an obstruction. Doing *samyama* is like removing an artificial obstruction—so that the natural abilities start flowing again.

A Yogi is advised not to remain attached to these special powers. If he is able to resist this attachment, he gradually becomes aware of the separateness of *purusha* and *prakriti*. This leads to his supremacy over all states and forms. A non-attachment to this supremacy produces a sense of bliss or *kaivalya*. This bliss is transcendental, and in this state there is the cognition of all objects simultaneous and there is a conquering of space and time. A non-attachment to this bliss leads to the *dharma-megha samadhi* or liberation.

AN EXPERIENTIAL ACCOUNT

One year is too short a period to reach *moksha* or even to understand what it means. However, one can, in this period, attain some deeper understanding of the mind and experience psychological state(s) which is closer to what may be defined as positive mental health and which could, with constant practice, become a permanent part of one's being.

'The first step is to create some order around yourself', said my guru when he took me on.

> Order—not for its own sake—but to get things so well arranged that one could leave them anytime and walk away. Order gives freedom. So-called spontaneity is chaos. Real spontaneity arises after an order has been created. Your room should be kept clean. Your books should be properly arranged. You should order your sleeping, eating and work habits.

He went on to say that order was firm though not rigid. Order and flexibility were complementary.

> When friends come, entertain them by all means. However, if you visit others less, less people would visit you. I do not want you to cut out your social life entirely, but cut away the unnecessary. You know what is necessary.

It took me a month to painfully understand how difficult it was to keep up the discipline, simple though it seemed. After this, my guru started teaching me Yoga practices. Initially, I carried out those practices for about half to one hour a day, but by the end of three months, I was doing these practices for about five hours a day. The practices I learnt were some *asanas*, *pranayama*, meditation, *tratak* and *yoga nidra*.

The first three months were very difficult. The Yoga practices made me more aware of my own personality characteristics—both good and bad. I was tormented by the discovery of my negative characteristics. I became aware of my physical infirmities, my jealous nature, my suspicious mind which doubted even my own research. 'What are you doing in a game like this? How will you show your face to your colleagues if nothing comes out of this research?' I became aware of my pathological concern for justice but an insufficient courage to do something to bring it about.

A dream during this period illustrates my state of mind. I am walking on the road with friends. Four people catch hold of others walking on the road and mercilessly chop them with cutlasses. The bits and pieces of bodies are strewn all over. The others on the road just look and go away. I try to scream but my friends stop me, saying it will not help to scream. When I point out that what was happening was terrible and the killers must be punished, I am told that it would not help me to agitate because no one will respond. There is also a threat in the air that if I say anything, I shall be the next victim. The assassins smile after the act, even laugh loudly, and I cry with impotent rage.

All these experiences caused a lot of depression and had my guru not been there, I would have abandoned my Yoga. I feel that this increased 'self awareness' is the reason why most people leave Yoga practices after a month or two, and I believe this is the reason why a guru is so necessary.

After this period of predominant depression, there were days when I would become overconfident. During these periods, I had sudden desires to eat a lot or indulge in sex. This period, which I would call the period of 'mood swings', lasted for another month or so, after which I entered a period which I can only call 'letting go'. I became more and more able to just watch my emotions without reacting to them. My guru described this as adopting a 'witness attitude'.

During this phase, my thinking slowed down. There was less pressure of thoughts and less background chatter. My need to talk, eat and sleep became less. I became more tolerant, felt less tired and became less sentimental. I was more able to postpone decisions till I could examine all aspects of a situation, but decisions once taken became less prone to doubt. My need to consult others about my decisions diminished and the compulsion to explain myself or apologize for my mistakes became less. Some incidents during this period illustrate my state of mind quite well.

In the first case, I had gone to see a friend at his invitation. When I reached, the guesthouse where my friend stayed, I found him busy with someone else. He asked me to wait in the next room. When 10 minutes passed without his appearance, I took out my diary and started writing. The friend came in after two hours and tried to explain that he was handling a crisis situation. Previously I would have fidgeted, felt hurt and angry and perhaps walked away. But now I had no rancour in my mind and we took off from there.

Another incident occurred when an internationally renowned scientist who is a close friend rang up and said that he had consulted an astrologer and the latter had suggested floating six coconuts in moving water to prevent a future mishap! Previously I would have got annoyed and told my friend off for believing in an astrologer in spite of being a renowned scientist. We left at 4 am, for a stream 50 kilometres away, and floated the coconuts at 7 am. We even giggled like school girls because the coconuts got stuck in the muck and we found ourselves 50 kilometres away from home, watching people at their morning ablutions!

Dreams during this period contrast well with the dream described earlier. In one dream, there is a party going on. A number of children are playing, running about and knocking each other down. I am also playing. Suddenly I find my dog dancing gracefully. I find a few people taking a freshly cut tree in a truck. My heart feels sad and I wonder how the tree would be feeling. Suddenly, a tiger jumps out of the truck right in front of me and becomes nervous of the moving traffic. I am more concerned with the possibility of his being run over rather than his attacking me. I pet him and take him to safety across the road.

This stage was followed by a period when I would get ideas as if they had freshly jumped onto my mental screen without any chain linking them to past thoughts or future anticipations. Often, these would appear very profound to me and had great emotional significance. I call this period the stage of 'insights'. For example, 'It is humiliating for me that my happiness should depend on the actions of others. From now on I shall determine my own mental state', or 'an awareness of failure is not necessarily harmful for it leads to self-surrender. Self-surrender in return neutralises the sense of failure'.

I also had some 'unusual experiences'. Previously I used to say to my friends: 'All of you have had miraculous experiences—why don't miracles happen to me?' During this period, things happened which did not look like chance happenings. For example, I phoned a friend whom I had not met for a very long time. No one answered the telephone. After some time my phone rang and I had a conviction that the call was from the same friend—and it was. I went home excitedly to tell my wife what had happened. Before I could open my mouth, she told me that since morning she was thinking of 'synchronicity' and what Jung had written about it. Such experiences occurred when my mind was still, i.e., when the thinking was slow, there was less background chatter, emotional reactivity was less and receptivity to external stimuli was more.

The Yoga experience was not uninterrupted bliss. There were ups and downs. I do not know whether it was my own rhythm or whether Yoga itself is a discontinuous process with the mind needing a rest before going on to the next stage.

I have given a few glimpses of my personal experiences. Now let us look at the conclusions I have drawn.

Effects of Yoga on Subjective Mental States

1. All Yoga exercises increase self-awareness *asanas*, slowly and properly carried out increase the awareness of the body in relation to space. *Pranayama* increases the awareness of breath and the related autonomic activities. Meditation increases the awareness of our thoughts and feelings while *yamas* and *niyamas* increase the awareness of our temptations and failings.
2. Self-awareness induces self-examination. There is no choice but to look at one's self and this proceeds even when one is not actively

involved in the practices. One looks at one's life and one's shortcomings. These do not go away but the *yamas* and *niyamas* do come to one's help by setting up ideals towards which one could move in a conscious manner.

3. There is a slowing down of the thought processes and feelings, a reduction of internal dialogue and a greater willed control over the direction in which thoughts move. Consequently, there is a reduction in impulsive thinking and behaviour. This slowing down is brought about mainly by meditation and *pranayama*, but even the *yamas* and *niyamas* help by restraining desires.
4. Because of the slowing down of the thought processes, there is a reduction in worries about the past or anxieties about the future: one lives more in the present.
5. There is an increase in perceptual sensitivity and hence a greater attention to the events around oneself. While these events are registered, there is a reduction in the conditional responses to these perceptions in terms of associative memories, rise in emotions and stereotyped behaviour.
6. Because of the reduction of internal dialogue and fluctuations of thoughts, it seems there is more 'space' in the mind to receive and process new information. This leads to more accurate decisions.
7. With the slowing of thoughts, an ability to control the movement of thoughts and emotions, success in the pursuance of *yamas* and *niyamas*, there is a subjective experience of an increase in will power.
8. There is a feeling of relaxation both physical and mental.
9. There is less of a need to talk, eat and sleep.
10. The combined experience of relaxation, perceptual sensitivity, mental alertness, reduced impulsivity and a sense of stronger will produce a sense of joy and an emotional 'high', which is noticed by oneself and by others.

To sum up, I have described the results of one year of intense Yoga practice. I have subsequently conducted Yoga, though less intensively, and have used Yoga in clinical work as well. Yoga has clinical uses: as a relaxation therapy, as an exploratory technique and as a method of personality reconstruction, so that one lives more in harmony with other human beings and the cosmos as a whole.

The ideal, according to the *Bhagavadgita*, is to reach a state of mind when one follows one's own *svadharma*—one's own code of conduct, but the person is so much in tune with the universal will that at the same time one is fully autonomous and fully in consonance with the cosmos. This ideal will perhaps never be reached, but through Yoga, one can start understanding what this means.

REFERENCE

Taimini, I. K. (1971). *The science of yoga*. Madras: The Theosophical Publishing House.

12

Psychotherapy and Indian Thought

ALOK PANDEY

Introduction: The Two Approaches

If psychotherapy is the science and art of changing the psychological patterns that give rise to mental distress and disorder, then it must be rooted in the comprehensive understanding of the nature and potentials of human being. Much of psychotherapy is however based on what a human being was, either in his remote and hoary past as a race (a pack of animals that can speak and think as some would say) or in his more recent yesteryears of infancy and childhood. Tracing the roots of the present problem in this fashion, it tries to put a corrective by setting things right there. The principle sounds good in its own right but there are two fundamental difficulties with it. First, how far back does our past go? Second, is the goal of psychotherapy to return the client to his past when he was healthy or his present maximum possibility? Or is it to utilize his crisis for an evolutionary journey towards a more meaningful future? That is to say using the crisis as a learning experience for growth and progress. It is here that we come across divergent worldviews of man and his goal that offers a different understanding of man's past and future. Broadly, these can be divided into two main categories:

1. Man is a creature of the mud formed by a process of chance evolution. He is essentially a physical or perhaps a chemical being. Psychologically, he is nothing more than an outgrown animal or worm that has managed to form itself through a series of mutations.

There is no essential goal or purpose of his life except to struggle and survive as other creatures do, and this tussle between his individual instinct to save himself and the social or collective instinct to save others the source of his inner conflict. The crude animal is his past, the refined animal his maximum scope.
2. In contrast, the other view holds man as a creature of heaven fallen here upon earth, though high and sublime in his origin and parentage. Psychologically, he is a soul, a miniature divinity shut in the prison house of matter seeking for release and escape. His goal and purpose is to find his true and spiritual self. An animal in his nature but divine in his essence, he is a cross between the two and that is the secret of his difficulty and conflict. The animal nature is the trap; freedom from this trap is his hope of salvation.

As we can see, so different are these two views and so disparate their understanding that to think of a reconciling synthesis becomes near impossible. Therefore, they have existed side by side in each civilization and culture in one form or another, but without any reconciling station. There have been some compromises here and there, such as the one attempted by Descartes himself, giving each idea its scope in its own domain. Sometimes their fortune seesawed. The Sophists of old, the later day positivists and the modern materialist try to explain everything on the basis of our material sense perception and the struggle of animal life denying every other experience as a hallucination or poetic imagination. Equally strong has been the rejection of material life as a vanity of vanities, a delusion and nightmare of the soul by the anchorites and the ascetics.

THE NEGATIVE VEDANTIN SOLUTION TO PSYCHOLOGICAL SUFFERING

This view of the *mayavadin*[1] and the illusionist rejects the problem in toto by labelling it as something non-existent, a fever and malady of the soul which can be cured by abolishing the world along with the problem. The solution, therefore, becomes a greater problem for those who are left behind, the cure so radical as to fell the body along with the disease. All

---
[1] One who believes that the sense of the world and all its attendant experiences are a state of delusion.

life is summarily dismissed as a painful illusion, and escape from it is the sole remedy. In its radical extreme outlook, birth is seen as an illness, the grand sire of all illnesses and human life a supreme opportunity to escape from this cycle of birth and death and all that lies in-between. The soul or whatever else (for some views do not admit the possibility of an individual soul, though they do not deny it either) will continue to experience some form of psychological suffering as long as it chooses to be born upon earth. The reasons attributed to this suffering may be construed different in different doctrines. Some blame it again on the past, not on the individual past of this life alone, but other lives as well. Others blame the root cause of suffering to a larger than individual, a cosmic principle of ignorance, *avidya*.[2] It is this child of *maya* that clouds the soul and keeps it a slave and prisoner of *ignorance* with its natural consequence of suffering. Still others speak of the cosmic principle of desire that is the source of all misery and a cessation from desire, the state of blissful calm and freedom or nirvana. It may be noted that suffering according to these conceptions is not only the one that is consciously experienced, but a deep unconscious and greater suffering experienced by the soul because of being trapped in this world of *ignorance*. Yet, so long as the soul chooses to be part of this *avidya*, it will continue to suffer in some way or the other.

The task of a counsellor of this type, if there is one, is to awaken the soul out of this earthly nightmare reminding it of its essential nature. The only solution is to cease from birth. The experience of conscious suffering is only used as a strong point of support, a lever to develop *vairagya*, a state of detached indifference towards life and world leading thereby to non-affliction. It is a kind of desensitization or de-addiction programme for our world-addiction and craving for material happiness that brings much suffering in its wake.

In actual practice, however, one does not take this extremist approach. The mind of the client is led through a cognitive framework, starting from his present crisis, to reveal the transient rather than illusory nature of this world and all its events. The mind is made to see the utter impermanence of things that are today, and tomorrow will be not, the riches and wealth, the position and the fame, the women and children one has, the fortune no less than the misfortune, all are too little to grieve for. To this, the God-believer adds that the only thing worth in life is that which is eternal and imperishable, the soul in man and the Divine above, or as some roll both

---

[2] The principle of division leading to the sense of multiplicity, separativeness and partial or incomplete knowledge.

these individual and universal aspects of the Divine into a single formula, *Brahman*.[3] *Brahman*, however, should not be confused with this or that god though all gods and everything else originate from It. *Brahman* is rather the stable, unchanging and eternal basis of all existence. *Brahman* alone is the object of our pursuit and not this that men seek hereafter, *tadevabrahman tvamviddhi, nedamyadidamupasate*[4] (know That to be the *Brahman* and not this that men seek hereafter). Another Upanishad, the *Katha*, describes through a beautiful verse the transient nature of worldly goods attachment to which brings only grief and suffering and in the end death. Death in these passages of exquisite beauty lauds Nachiketa, the young aspirant for his choice of *shreyas*, the truly worthy good of the soul, over *preyas*, the momentarily pleasant and the transient worldly good.

Thus, through examples and narrative, drawn both from everyday life of the client, the dress he wears and the crisis he has faced and passed through, as well as from the cultural context, the person is led gradually away from the psychological suffering and helped to focus his attention within, towards the true and ultimate goal. In its partial forms, even the first step is regarded as good enough, since by impressing upon the mind the transience and impermanence, he is able to detach himself from his malady and feel lighter and freer.

But one may proceed a step further, depending upon the readiness of the client. One may, for example, help the person view the problem more objectively, since he is now detached from its emotional and other effects. A certain distancing is always known to help us see better and understand the situation more clearly. This impermanence far from being a cause of grief becomes a positive thing, since it also means that grief and unhappiness, tragedy and fall, sorrow and suffering are not an eternal damnation or a permanent doom. They are only a temporary setback. The journey of the soul does not stop with temporary stations but goes on and will go on till one has found the goal.

This much is common to all Vedantic systems. That is to say that this world is not what it seems to be. And that our values are misplaced and wrong due to the mind's conditioning through centuries and millenniums of evolutionary process (series of births and rebirths). The psychotherapist corrects this cognitive error through a dialectic process involving thought and utilizing the experiences of the person to demonstrate this. But there

---

[3] The Supreme Reality, the stable, unchanging and eternal basis of this ever-changing, phenomenal world.
[4] The Kena Upanishad.

is a later divergence too. It is in the goal put forward before the soul after it has thus disengaged itself and is able to look at the problem and enigma of human life and its events dispassionately.

Useful as this method is for a certain class of problems, it has its own drawbacks. First, it presumes a certain degree of intellectual development, though perhaps less than is required, for understanding the complex dynamics of the classical Western models of psychotherapy. The second and even more serious difficulty is that this system proposes that most souls are trapped in the snare of worldly *maya*. So how can the blind lead the blind or the trapped rescue the trapped? Only that has a convincing value which is deeply lived by oneself. The rest touches only the surface and the outer mind, and cannot bring about the inner and radical change. Third, the solution if taken to its logical extreme may induce a tendency for a total indifference towards the world. While this may be appreciated by certain extremist schools, yet the seers who propounded this thought were careful enough not to create confusion in the minds of the average person. An overemphasis on this other-worldliness may well lead to inertia justified under the holy name of *vairagya*.[5] One often enough finds such escapists who have joined the nirvana[6] bandwagon to avoid responsibilities.

Therefore, there is an insistence by the wise ones not to delude the minds of the average man who is not ready for this by enrolling all and sundry into the list of candidates for such a counselling, *na buddhibhedam janyedajnana karmasanginam*.[7] He who is established in the *knowledge* (true knowledge or *jnana*) should not create confusion in the minds of the ignorant (who are still attached to their egos and not yet ready). In other words, the doctrine requires such a high degree of inner development of the counsellor that even many a theoretical pundits would be considered unfit to impart or facilitate an effective psychotherapeutic process through this.

It is important to understand here that the far ancient Indian thought saw in this experience of impermanence only a passage towards a higher Permanence. The illusion was to be understood and torn only to find the Real and not to rest in the midway house built upon the sands of nowhere. But that other thing needs effort, a strong predisposition, a positive seeking which few can command. Yet, if the psychotherapist of this type can take this final and crucial step of turning a negative experience into a

---

[5] Non-attachment.
[6] Release from the cycle of birth and death and rebirth.
[7] The Gita.

positive seeking for the eternal, then it would mean a great and a true release of the client. An example of this type of counsel appears in the classical treatise of *Yogavasistha* wherein the sage Vasistha counsels Rama, while the latter is experiencing a state of utter non-involvement towards life in the world.

This form of counselling, while useful for a select group of clients who mainly suffer from depressions arising due to life situations, is of little use in other forms of psychological disorders, though it may have utility in counselling for those who suffer because of the psychological suffering of their near and dear ones. To take just one example among many, the depressed and suicidal mother of a mentally handicapped was asked how she would have reacted if this child was her sisters and she had yet to bring him up for some treason or the other. The reply was evident. She would do all that she was doing now, perhaps a few things more but without the touch of depression, perhaps even with a joy born of doing a selfless good for someone. As she replied, she could see the obvious, to live in this world without a sense of attachment or possessiveness. A single short session was enough to change her self-view and worldview. She actually recovered and remained so for years to come.

Be it as it may, Indian thought is not only about *mayavada* and illusion. Despite the current emphasis on other-worldliness, there have been other equally powerful and positive streams of Indian thought. From a psychotherapeutic point of view, it is these that can be even more effective in dealing with human problems of the mind. Some of these major trends can be roughly classified into the following.

The Ideal of Inner Purification

According to this thought, psychological pain and suffering is the twin of pleasure and thrill. They are two sides of the same coin. To strive after thrill and vehement egoistic form of pleasure is to invite suffering in return. What is necessary, therefore, is moderation and balance through an enlightened reason and discrimination, *sattvasudhi*. This is actually in a sense the ideal of a sane moderation, something similar to Aristotle's golden mean. It is a conscious and deliberate cultivation of positive qualities of the mind and heart which help one grow into *sukham* or gladness and *prakasham* or light of wisdom. The source of human misery according to this view comes at a certain middle stage of our psychological evolution that is called the *rajasic*. To put it in a nutshell, the human soul evolves through at least three levels in its several rounds of birth before it is ready for the highest spiritual good. The lowest of these three levels is the *tamasic* or the darkened state of inertia, obscurity and utter resistance to change. Here he is driven by the law of the masses, the rule of the herd like a subconscious beast or a half-conscious man.

Next comes the *rajasic* or the state of kinesis and dynamic movement. This second stage can be further subdivided into two. One, the preliminary or the predominantly *rajo-tamasic* wherein the being is engaged in self-flattering gross indulgences of every kind. The other is the *rajo-sattvic* wherein the individual begins to seek some ideal rule of inner law to govern his unruly nature, which he begins to perceive as the source of internal disturbances. Finally, the third or *sattvic* stage wherein the individual learns to subordinate his ego and take from life only what is rightfully his. He seeks instinctively for harmony and is balanced in his conduct and the distribution of life energies.

Now in the primitive or the *tamasic* stage, there is not much conscious suffering to the individual, though he may be the cause of suffering to many others. The need for violent sensations to feel just a little alive drives some of these people towards alcoholism and violent acts and practices. Others simply sulk as in depression, refusing to budge or outgrow their state. The second stage is one of fiery pleasures and equally swift swing to the blues. An inordinate self-seeking, an excess of ambition with its natural fallout of anger, fear, hope and expectations and frustrations, bring in its wake opposite reactions from their environment and this egoistic narrowness makes them extremely susceptible to misery. This suffering is actually a corrective of nature and helps them to push forth here and there to find a way out of their miserable existence. So, lastly comes *sattva*, the great balancer after the soul has experienced these lesser rungs of existence and grown through them.

A counsellor who works along these lines will first roughly place the scale at which the individual stands in his inner evolution. Elaborate descriptions abound in ancient Indian thought especially the *Gita* and the Ayurveda as to the type of inner personality and constitution according to the three *gunas* as these three evolutionary stages are better known. It may be mentioned that all of us are a mixture of the three, but there is a predominance of one or the other *gunas* which leads to physical and psychological afflictions. The kind of therapy and advice given is according to the scale. Thus while a *sattvic* person who may also suffer due to his attachment to idealism and sympathy with others is advised and helped and encouraged to develop a still deeper and spiritual outlook, the *rajasic* man of a higher type advised to do his work with trust in God and according to the right inner law of his nature, *svabhava* and *svadharma*. The lower type of *rajasic* man is counselled and helped towards moderation in life habits and outlook, to tone down the excess onrush of desires that torment and trouble him feverishly. The unruly and excess uncontrolled energy that bursts in his nature is channelled into healthy activities like sports and vigorous games. One has to learn from the army how well they use the *rajasic* type of man and channelize his energies for war. But to the lowest type of man, very little works by way of counselling unless something shakes him up, some terrible misfortune of sort which affects him personally and arouses the sleeping energies in him. Anything, almost anything that can stimulate in this type a will to do work with concentration and perseverance is a good counsel. Fine crafts, manual work that requires physical concentration helps this state as is seen in some psychotics and extreme forms of depression. Also, anything that can stimulate in them a sense of joy, like eating a dish they relish or simple things that give pleasure. The last thing to be advised to this lot is spirituality of the meditative ascetic type. They immediately hold on to it and as mentioned above, use it as an excuse to stay a recluse or to justify inertia and addictions to drugs that easily transport us to altered realms without any inner effort.

The Harmony of Body and Mind

If illusionism is most commonly (mis)understood as representative of Indian thought, then some kind of mind-body harmony through Yoga exercises is the most commonly sought after for therapeutic purposes. Especially the special forms of *hatha yoga* exercises[8] (better termed as *asanas* or *yogasanas*), *pranayama*[9] and meditation are among some of the most well-researched importation from India that has already found a place in the modern psychotherapeutic systems. Many researches done in the East and the West right from the 1960s (perhaps even earlier) has demonstrated the efficacy of these simple stress buster techniques.

In *hatha yoga* and *pranayama*, the practitioner tries to first regulate and then still the otherwise restless physical and vital energies. But this is a preliminary first step. The next and more important is that he tries to in-gather and concentrate these energies so as to reach their divine source

---

[8] *Hatha yoga* exercises are not merely physical exercises, according to the Indian system, but means to open up subtle channels within the body for smooth flow of energy.

[9] *Pranayama* or the science and art of mastering the breath, and through the breath, the life force which uses breath for its effective exchange and interchange.

and bring out their deeper divine possibilities. Once this divine possibility comes out, and even much before that, the energies of the body and life force become forceful, effective, balanced, harmonious and thereby curative. This is excellent for those who are not so psychological-minded and for those less inclined towards an esoteric spirituality. It is besides quite effective and has been used with considerable success in treating psychosomatic disorders. The disadvantage is a technique dependency. These methods to be fully effective have to be practised regularly. They consume a lot of time and need often the supervision of a qualified expert. They are best used as an adjunct in a wide range of disorders including psychotics.

Meditation is however slightly different, even though it comes under the broad categories of 'techniques' evolved by the Eastern paradigm though nowhere with the wide range and variation as in India. It is a vast subject in its own right and one need not go into all the details of the different techniques and their relative efficacy. But suffice it to say that one of its well-known effects recognized now world over is in toning down the response of our SNS. This way it creates a sense of calm at the most physical level. There may be deeper reasons, though since the nervous system, more specifically the autonomic nervous system, is a sort of interface between the gross physical energies and the energies of life and mind pouring upon matter and influencing it.

Two meditative techniques are specifically helpful. One, the Buddhist method of a witnessing self—reflection and introspective meditation. This technique is quite useful for undoing certain habitual nervous responses, anxiety states, obsessive patterns of thoughts and behaviour, anger management, even in studying oneself and thereby controlling oneself. The essential steps here are thought observation, witnessing, control and mastery. But this is a little more difficult, usually demands some isolation on the part of the practitioner and needs a somewhat developed mind to be able to separate one part of it from another. The other and more popular, easier-to-do yet very effective, technique is that of dynamic meditation and its scientific child guided imagery. This method relies on the faculty of imagination and can be considered a first cousin of autosuggestion. In fact, the two are often combined together. The role is again largely in psychosomatic disorders, anxiety disorders, etc.

The Integral Thought of the *Gita*

The *Gita*, unlike many other similar scriptures, is an attempt at synthesis of various truths known till then. In addition, it adds something unique and profound and new, enriching the old with a fresh insight. Its key *sutras* are as follows:

1. The truth that *man is essentially an imperishable soul* who uses the body as a charioteer uses the chariot. It reverses the heavy dependence of man's psychological states on his physical events and happenings by constantly reminding us that we are first and foremost eternal and imperishable souls that assume a transient body as a person wears a dress. This doctrine has had so much impact on the ages to come that till date there is hardly any more effective counselling for grief and pain of death. Millions of people have used the *Gita* in times of their crisis, especially loss events and found solace and strength. This is the first thing to remember that we are essentially souls that cannot be destroyed by the catastrophes of life and of nature.
2. The soul is not merely an article of faith (though faith is a great power, the blind man's indispensable staff till he has begun to see the higher truths). He can discover this soul and out of the many ways that the *Gita* would outline for different categories of people, one such is the *enlightened use of his intelligent will*. Instead of turning it constantly outward and downward to satisfy our desire, this intelligent will in man can be turned upward and inward to discover our own sublime realities which free us from bondage to grief and error and suffering and pain.
3. We are not abandoned helplessly upon earth without support and God Himself is concerned with *the march of civilization* towards some ultimate *good*. What that ultimate *good* would be is left unsaid or only hinted but it incites us to take it as a word of God that He is concerned intimately with earth and men. Each element of the universe has hidden within it a divine superconscient (not the superego or the conscience which are human things, aspects of our mind and ego's constructs) and not just a subconscient animal principle (instincts as the base of everything) as much of Freudian psychology at one time asserted. The *Gita* clearly hints that divinity dwells within the human being and it is the task of each one to bring it out and be guided by it, rather than stifle it.
4. War and conflict are unavoidable evolutionary necessities so long as earth and mankind is imperfect. Our inner conflicts are essentially *evolutionary conflicts*, our inner and outer crisis are essentially a cry for an evolutionary change. Man can choose to remain in his darkened state in which suffering pursues him till sense is knocked into

his head and he once again takes the path to the eternal good, which is also the collective good. The *Gita* elaborately describes towards the closing chapters and in great detail the nature of the powers of light and of darkness. Thus man if he wants to be free of error and grief has to consciously cultivate the qualities of light and truth.

5. According to the doctrine of *nishkama karma*, our everyday actions, even the most trivial, can lead us to a glad and happy state of being if we do them in a selfless spirit of dedication to the Divine Master and remain equal to the fruits that they may bring. This stress upon a tranquil mind equal under every circumstance, in the seemingly pleasant and the seemingly unpleasant, in success and victory no less as in failure and defeat is a great liberating principle of the *Gita* that takes the wind out of much of our everyday psychological and even physical suffering. This equality is not indifference but a state of equal joy by dwelling constantly in The Lord's remembrance and abiding solely by His Will. *Equanimity* is therefore anther very practical method prescribed by the Gita to free us from the stress of everyday life.

But the greatest and crowning word of the *Gita* comes towards the end with the great assurance that God will deliver us from all fear and evil if we can learn to *surrender* ourself in His hand. Now modern psychology born of a sceptic temper suited to material pursuits has little sympathy with the idea of God. Nay, it may even regard it as blasphemous to talk of God in matters of science. But we must remember that psychology is not a physical science. It does not deal with physical but psychological phenomenon and whether we like it or not, due to our own individual biases, the fact remains that God and seeking for divinity and good, faith and surrender are very much psychological phenomenon as ancient or even more ancient than the roots of our hills, at the same time modern and as modern as the quantum theories of the space and the universe. It will be a great loss to psychology if this great body of our psychological self-experience is left unutilized because, well, one does not know why.

The Path of *Tantra* or an Inner Technology

And yet reconciliation is possible. The first attempt to reconcile the two, the material and the spiritual, is that great and now lost tradition of the *tantra*. The *Gita* seeks to reconcile life in the world (the problem of the practical man) and spiritual realization. The *tantra* seeks to reconcile the energies moving this cosmos (the field of the scientist) and the Supreme Energy from which these lesser forms and forces and energies derive themselves. If that be so, then it is possible to master or conquer the lesser energies by the stronger and greater ones. This is the fundamental principle of *tantra* to understand, possess, control and master forces and powers of nature as well as of supernature. Seen thus, it is closer to our conception of science though with a much wider application.

Thus, while science studies and tries to master physical forces and energies of matter, *tantra* goes deeper to study and master other occult energies beyond and behind the play of our material universe. It sees physical phenomenon as a by-product or final end result of still deeper and occult events happening at other levels of our consciousness. In the field of illness, for example, it sees entities and beings and forces of disruption and disintegration on whom one can act directly if one has the occult knowledge, thus curing one of an illness without physical means of intervention. Unfortunately, modern insistence on physical causes alone has done much damage to this highly developed science which has its own rationale of working. *Tantra* itself fell into disrepute since few occultists and *tantrics* had the required inner purity to handle such intense forces. Many fell into the by-lanes of inner life falling into the corridors of power.

When we turn to psychiatry, there is a lot that *tantra* can offer, not by way of our modern misreading of its hieroglyphs through the lens of psychoanalysis, but in understanding the subtler causes of illness. Thus, according to the *tantric* knowledge, frank insanity is due to possession by certain entities from the dark and hostile worlds. These turbulent energies first enter into the atmosphere of a person who is susceptible to them (through affinity of some parts of nature). This is the prodrome stage when the first line of occult prevention can be done. Next, they cast an influence which usually takes one or the other forms, viz:

1. Early influence leading to some personality changes (towards loss of faith and will, doubts, depression, confusion, perverted religiosity, excessive self-vanity, sexuality and other appetites, uncontrolled impulsiveness, etc.).
2. Epilepsy, which is more characteristically due to resistance by the effected person's being against the force.
3. Hysteria, especially possession states, dissociation, multiple personality, etc.
4. Active communication with these dark entities through voices and other means.

5. Finally, frank possession/incarnation of one of these stronger dark entities leading to a total perversion of thought and feeling and will and action and speech creating the cruel tyrant, the psychopath and the outright pervert.

Now the *tantric*, the occultist, the *shaman*, the thaumaturgist, call him whatever, knew about these forces and ways to neutralize them just as a modern scientist would know about the forces of wind and rain and fire and know how to handle them. These can be further subdivided into two main types. The lower type who have within their control some powerful entity of the same plane, which would execute their will for good or for evil purposes. Others have mastered the higher energies through sufficient purity and self-control. These then can neutralize the lower beings with the power of *light*. Naturally, this latter type is not only preferable but more permanent so to say, but then this type is rare since it requires too much inner austerity on the part of the practitioner.

The lost knowledge of *tantra* is now recovering itself, though in another form more suited to the scientific temper of our times. *Reiki*, *pranic* healing, working with body energy and mind energy, a study of the effects of thoughts and other vibrations upon the body and mind, a systematic study, etc. It is strange that for all the assault of our infant science, this grandmother of sciences is not dead. It is rather seeking a rebirth through the parapsychology and other such newer sciences. Physical science itself has entered the threshold of the occult and it would not be surprising that in times to come, the old ghosts return in the garb of new names and the buried are raised in a different attire.

The Grand Synthesis and More

It is here that Sri Aurobindo steps in with his new Yoga that stretches the line of experience of the way of knowledge as well as of the way of power to its utmost height where they reconcile and find their supreme unity. His Yoga then flows from these remote and inaccessible Himalayan heights as the Ganges running down from its icy caves to the fertile planes of India to bring out that which is already concealed within the bosom of our earth. But the Ganges is not simply the melted ice and snow but something else and much more. So also, Sri Aurobindo's Yoga is not an eclectic combination of different ways and paths though the highest knowledge possible to the Vedantin and the greatest power possible to the *tantric* are included in it. And yet there is more, something much more not found elsewhere. What is that and how we can help us in our knowledge and practice of medicine and psychiatry to that we can turn now. As we know, Sri Aurobindo has shed light on practically every sphere of life. But for our present purposes, we shall confine only to the problem of psychological well-being and see it in the background of ancient Indian thought by way of summing up the main issues involved.

First, man himself. Sri Aurobindo confirms the ancient knowledge that man is not just an aggregate of physical cells or chemical reactions. He is that only in his outer material basis. His true self-identity is that he is a soul. Sri Aurobindo does not use the word soul in a vague general sense. There is a universal self of all but there is too an individual soul that has been projected from the one Self into the drama of our earthly life. This individual soul, called the psychic being, is an important key to our psychological well-being. The psychic being is our true being, the secret divinity in us. Its very essence is peace and harmony and joy. It has a natural attraction for the true, the good, the beautiful. However, it is veiled in human beings for a long time by the surface nature and its movements. But even in the crudest of human natures, it exists behind as a ray of light and hope, a little spark of undying truth covered by a heap of darkness.

The one source of our psychological maladies springs from our inability to dwell in the *psychic consciousness*. We live mostly upon the surface of our nature where there is, as of now, nothing but confusion and disorder. Our surface nature, unable to have a sure light of guidance, depends heavily upon our outer mind and sense data. The fancy of our desires and the pull of our emotions and passions further corrupt this imperfect partial and broken knowledge (called ignorance). The result is a falsification of knowledge, a crass ignorance about ourselves and others. This wrong identification with the *ignorant* movements of nature as if that is 'me' is the origin of our subjective sense of the ego, which appears so very real. With this sense of the surface 'me' comes also the sense of what is 'not me', since no real unity or harmony is possible with the ego; only at best some accommodation, tolerance and adjustment. This is one source of our conflict with all that is not perceived as myself, whether it be as seen in others or hid in our own subconscient depths, which in essence is the same thing. For we almost instinctively see in others a reflection of ourselves. We also wish to see in others the perfection that we secretly desire but have not yet arrived at.

To put it more truly, *the outer conflicts of man are the reflection of his inner conflicts*. The real inner conflict is a tussle between what we are and what we secretly aspire to be, between our animal past and our godlike future. There is no part of human nature that can truly resolve this conflict. Reason, even at its best, very often leaves us in a quandary as happens in the case of Arjuna. What is the thing to be done and what should not be done leaves often the sages too perplexed, says the Master of the *Gita*.

Not content with theorizing alone, Sri Aurobindo and The Mother have given abundant practical methods for the *discovery of our psychic being*. To discover and uncover the psychic consciousness is to break through *ignorance*, towards our own true nature and unleash the knowledge and power of the soul. But this is only a first great step. Sri Aurobindo affirms once again the ancient truth of rebirth but he gives it a totally new and unique significance. From birth to birth and through experience to experience, the soul in us grows till it is ready to manifest its inherent divinity upon earth. *Mukti*, which essentially amounts to an essential freedom from our lower nature and its reactions, is only a preliminary step towards something higher to take place in matter. It is the manifestation of a higher supernature upon earth. Though our soul is inherently divine and its discovery helps us immensely in recovering our true inner poise and outlook upon things, yet the nature that the soul wears as a robe around it is not a perfect one. As long as our nature that we wear around us as a cloak remains fallen and obscure, life on earth shall remain a field of error and suffering and a hazardous experiment. Our individual soul realization will no doubt save us from personal affliction of misery, but the common universal problem will continue with its effects of disease and disorder on the body and mind. It will be like being a king in a kingdom of rogues or the owner of a decrepit estate!

So the next thing is to *ascend to higher and higher levels of spiritual consciousness* beyond the mind and with each ascent to take up the lower levels and elevate it to a higher quality by the touch of the higher descending into the lower. This is the evolutionary aspect of life. Behind the outer evolution, there is going on a parallel evolution of consciousness. In animals it is an unconscious process, but in human beings it begins to assume a more and more conscious process. In other words, we are not just helpless and mute witnesses or unconscious automatons in nature's hands being shaped by struggle or whatever else towards a higher and higher development. We are and can be active participants; our choices can help or hinder the evolutionary pace, though it cannot stop the inevitable outcome. Our evolutionary journey stretches through many lives and it is here that we discover the real significance of rebirth, that much talked about mystery in Indian thought. Our illnesses are not the result of some punishment for bad deeds; they, as indeed everything else, are simply a kind of learning process, an inner growth through learning the effects of different types of responses to different energies put forth by our nature.

Here we discover another source of our *conflict*. The first conflict is a general one, between our true spiritual self and the false ego self. The other conflict is between the different parts of our nature which dwell on different levels of consciousness. This creates an *inner disharmony*. Thus the mind in us may be ready to evolve towards a greater light while the heart may refuse to move and remain shut in its narrow boundaries and fixed formulas. Or the heart too may be ready to widen, but the life impulse may be stuck with lower motives and the body utterly refuses to move due to inertia. This creates an inner disharmony leading to psychological and physical imbalances. If the imbalance is too strong, and especially the psychic development weak, the cosmic forces of disruption and disorder may step in and create more serious imbalances like the ravaging psychotic and the perverted sociopath criminal.

A Terrestrial Divine Perfection: The Complete Solution

To grow in knowledge (the aim of the Vedantic Yoga) and to grow in power (the aim of *tantric yoga*) and through this growth to discover the *ananda* of becoming is the great human journey. The meeting point of these two seemingly different aspects of existence is consciousness, which in the ancient Indian conception is at once knowledge and power, *chit-shakti*. A *growth in consciousness is the aim of human life and also the solution of our human misery and suffering*. The more we grow in consciousness (i.e., towards higher and higher levels of knowledge and power), the more we become progressively free of ignorance and limitation, the more we discover the peace and *ananda* hidden as the base and support of everything.

Illness, in this sense, is a barometer, if we like, to discover our hidden weaknesses or points that need to be developed and perfected, or to use the Darwinian language, challenges thrown across the soul by nature to uncover its own inherent divine potential. Each illness represents as it were the obverse side of some potential yet to be discovered. Each shadow of the body or mind taking the form of illness is a concealment of some possibility of light yet to be born. Our illnesses are therefore evolutionary challenges, our crisis and conflict a means for greater self-discovery. Nature utilizes our pain and struggle so that a greater being of delight and strength may be born within us. And it is the task of the therapist to assist this evolutionary process.

How shall he do it? What will be his means and tools and instruments? The first and most important tool and instrument in this catalytic process is the therapist himself. It is the consciousness of the therapist interacting with the consciousness of the client that effects this change. The main task of the therapist is to induce this faith in a higher grace or power and awaken in him the will and the possibility of a change. Till that happens, the therapist becomes a kind of spiritual midwife to assist the delivery of the client in his dark and painful passage through the womb of nature. The task is indeed a delicate one, hanging between dependence to something outside him to his discovery of the only true and authentic freedom, independence or autonomy (call it whatever) possible, that of handing oneself in the hands of the divinity within. This was the original conception of the guru provided for in the Indian thought and on which so much stress is laid. The guru according to the ancient Indian conception is a representative of the Divine who is now veiled to the eye of humanity. He reveals humanity its own higher part, the spiritual self which is covered by our surface consciousness.

The guru's light also unmasks the hidden weaknesses in the disciple without undergoing the more painful and difficult way of disease and crisis, that is the method of nature. It is this growth in sincerity through the guru's intervention, this stripping off of our subconscious defences (rather than strengthening them), so that we may see ourselves as we are and then, with the guru's help, grow into our own divine nature that is forever free from afflictions and imperfections, full of harmony and peace and *ananda* that is the crucial movement of inner growth. In the ancient Indian conception, it is not the ego defences (mature or immature) that are strengthened, but the strength of the soul that is cultivated. The ego, however necessary it was at a stage of our evolution, becomes a pain and a prison at another stage and must be replaced by the soul principle. This does not mean a defeatist attitude of inaction as those who know of no other identity but the surface ego identity suppose. That is only a warped alter ego. It means an exchange of our surface orientation, superficial understanding and, therefore, limited responses with a deeper, truer and more powerful understanding and response to life and people and the world.

The counsellor in other words leads the client through a progressive deepening, heightening and widening of his consciousness using every experience as materials for the evolutionary process. Towards this end, he may use any and every means again depending upon the client's readiness of acceptance, his natural bent and temperament, most of all, his constitution and faith. All the methods mentioned above under different approaches can be used provided of course that the counsellor knows something about them himself. In certain situations he may even refer the patient for a particular technique as a temporary aid to one who is an expert in that field, say for *yogasanas* or *pranayama* if that be felt necessary. But he must know that these techniques are merely temporary devices. One needs to outgrow them as one needs to outgrow all devices. The goal of the psychotherapeutic journey is not just a warding off of the present symptoms but the discovery of the inner healer who can heal not only this but all other anomalies of life in all times to come. It is this inner discovery of the true soul, this ascent to our own higher summits of consciousness that will progressively reduce the outer dependence on the outer form of the guru since one would have discovered the same guru within.

THE COUNSELOR–CLIENT RELATIONSHIP IN INDIAN THOUGHT

It must be, however, noted that the guru–*shisya* form of counselling that often took place in the ancient Indian setting was not just a ritualistic formula or a method but simply a statement of fact. Not everyone could be a guru but only the realized man, one who had at least moved far on the path of self-realization or God-realization, as the case may be. The guru is not an erudite scholar trained in spiritual dialectics or a master in spiritual philosophy. He may or may not be these things. He may not be a trained psychologist or perhaps even a man of letters, though if he were also these things, it would be an immense advantage. He must at the least be a man who had found his true soul and was living consciously in it. If he can transmit this soul experience to another, then so much the better. This is important to note because the modern mind often misreads in the guru–*chela* relationship, either the dependence of a Freudian type or else a convenient device to facilitate the psychotherapeutic process through faith alone. Faith is no doubt important in the Indian setting, but the emphasis on faith is not by way of sanction to blind and irrational obscurantism but as a necessary precondition to arrive at knowledge. It is an enlightened faith that is necessary, a faith that is consistent with reason that if there is a divine sense and purpose in this world then surely there must be a means to discover it; that if there is a soul that can help heal and succour, then surely there must be a means to find it; that if one man has found it, then, given the right means and method, others too can find it. Above all, a faith that if there is at all a diviner guidance in this world behind the so-called anomalies of life, then there must be a purpose in each trial and tribulation of life, behind each crisis and failure, behind every stumble and fall. The guru aids and assists in this process of discovering the real meaning and significance of the crisis, and through it the meaning of our own life in this seemingly meaningless universe. Faith and surrender to the guru's guidance is the starting point of this discovery, will and effort and aspiration the middle term, knowledge and union with the truth that is found are the third and last term of this process. According to the Indian tradition, the counselling ideally does not stop with the immediate recovery of the perceived distress but is carried beyond till the person has gone beyond all possibility of distress. The distress is only an outer excuse that the soul in us uses to start the great journey. Its end is not a temporary relief from the transient stresses and satisfactions of life but the establishment of a permanent peace and an unfading joy in the being, a radical cure from all our present, past and future ills.

And since we are at it, this needs to be mentioned that the spirit of counselling is not commercial at all. If we go back to the ancient Indian thought, there was only one criterion that the guru used in taking his disciple. It was the readiness to evolve along the lines in which this master had gained his expertise, the *adhikara bheda*. But once accepted, all commercial and other considerations were put apart. If the disciple offered something out of his own sweet will, it was another matter. Indeed, the disciple was expected to offer something by way of *guru dakshina* at the end of the course and it may be something as small as a penny or as big as an empire or an object held dear to him. The disciple gave it in faith and gratitude trusting that the master knows best. This gift of love at the end of the course of instructions was good for the student since of all the lapses of life the worse was considered to be ingratitude towards the master since his debt one can never repay. Instances are on record how some masters took upon themselves the entire outer and inner burden of the disciples not only for one life but for all lives to come.

We may ask as to the relevance of all this in modern scenario, and even if it be a wonderful thing, whether it is practicable at all. Here, we must understand that the whole drift of ancient Indian thought was to make the ideal pragmatic and practically possible and it can be so since throughout the ages, the spirit of ancient India is not dead. No doubt it is reeling temporarily under the wave and storm of materialistic thought that has blinded our hearts and clouded our vision, but this, I believe and hope, is a temporary phenomenon. Even now, such teachers, instructors, counsellors and masters exist who continue to go about their task silently without any outer considerations of money or fame. The gift of knowledge and the help provided by it is the highest that one can envisage. By the very fact of it being a gift, it becomes one with love and the two are the most potent powers to effectuate a deeper change, which is the goal of all authentic psychotherapy.

The Goal of Psychotherapy

The goal of psychotherapy can be no different than the general goal of mankind in its great evolutionary journey. The crisis is only an incidence pushing us further towards the goal through a dark and hasty tunnel dug in emergency. The psychotherapist is only a catalyst helping towards this journey from darkness to light, providing support through authentic love and compassion one with wisdom and strength. The end point is not just a temporary restoration of the original status quo but a growth through the process, a growth in consciousness towards a greater wisdom, a greater love, a greater freedom, a greater harmony that come by our ascent out of animality into divinity, by the discovery of our secret soul.

In Conclusion: A Question of Faith

The role of the psychotherapist is not to convert or convince the sick and suffering to any particular form of belief, though that may well happen incidentally in the process. That is only natural, for man instinctively develops faith in something that has helped him in his darkest moments of crisis. Faith, we may also say, is not only the common denominator in the Eastern but also in the Western, the ancient as well as modern systems. A philosophical doctrine remains ineffective for life unless it can seize and hold not only the mind's interest but also the heart and faith and will in man. Therefore, the first thing necessary in the practical application of ancient Indian thought is that the psychotherapist will live in a wide catholicity utilizing the intrinsic faith of the patient as an essential means of support to start his work. And if he finds the faith insufficient to support the change, then he will work towards instilling and widening it along the lines of the client's natural bent and past evolution rather than trying to convert or win over an argument.

Faith works best when it arises from within, as a flower springs from a bud. It works poorly when it is superimposed from without, as the scentless artefact of a flower. This blossoming of faith is a very important and crucial element in all psychotherapy without which everything else remains incomplete. So common is loss of faith in psychological problems, especially depression, that one may well say that most crises of life are actually deep within a crisis of faith.

Faith is a very important element in life, even more than reason and one must say with good reasons. For in spiritual things that exceed and transcend the mind, it is necessary to suspend mental judgements and begin with faith. It is said and rightly so that in the end, this faith is fulfilled and justified with knowledge that comes by direct and authentic spiritual experience. In a sense it is true of everything else, including science. One begins with faith in a proposition or a method and works patiently till one discovers that towards which one's inner intuition was calling. That is why we choose one out of so many possibilities to labour and strive for.

Belief is something outward. It is a system of thought held by our surface mind or a heart, and will condition to respond to certain movements by man and society. It belongs largely to the outer man, at best only to a fringe of his inner being. Faith is more intrinsic; nay, it is the very grain and mark of man, as the *Gita* says. It is the spontaneous cry of the soul often buried within a heap and mass of dead rituals, mechanical beliefs and professed creeds. It is the task of the psychotherapist to patiently extract this intrinsic faith as a careful anatomist extracts the minutest nerve rather than the way of the surgeon ready to excise and mutilate in order to relieve. Faith is in essence the inner scripture hid in every heart. It is this inner scripture that the psychotherapist has to open for the patient and help him to read it. This is the Indian version of cognitive therapy approaching his mind, not through the mind but through the soul of the client. To change from within outward, by using the client's own faith, is therefore the method used by the therapist.

Towards this end, he naturally moves from the surface to the deeps from outer and professed beliefs and non-beliefs towards that which is yet hidden and concealed in the secret spaces of the soul. The therapist in this process uses the helpful materials offered by the client's mind and heart and will. He works patiently, through timely suggestions and an intuitive guidance, upon the materials that resist this recovery of faith. And it is in this process that we find the role of cognitive and other aspects of the patient's inner constitution.

Despite the enormous complexity and many-sidedness of Indian thought, the common cognitive and emotional structures supporting the belief as the case may be fairly simple. It can be chiefly summarized as a belief in an individual soul, in a personal Divine (whether outwardly professed or not in the corresponding philosophical school), a belief in rebirth with its attendant reward and punishment theory, a belief in the existence of cosmic forces that help or harm us, and finally a belief in *mukti* or liberation as the final goal to which all shall one day arrive. At the same time, the Indian mind has had one great advantage of this complexity; it has become very catholic in its approach since it accepts more readily than other faiths that there can be diverse approaches to truth and freedom and God. The Indian mind is more ready to accept the word of an enlightened man without much argument. It is not because of credulousness as is commonly supposed but because of the nature of its inner being. The inner being of most Indians is awake to subtler and deeper realities and knows that the mind must subordinate itself before the spirit. It knows instinctively that the way of arriving at truth is not through reason and analysis but through faith and practice. Most of all, he believes that God's grace or the intervention of a highly developed person can help us bail out of difficulties, inner or outer. The therapist can use these cognitive structures and emotional bonds already deep rooted in the human psyche of the Indian type.

Truth is not only an external objective reality but even more an intimate subjective reality, false perhaps to the one who does not experience it but deeply real to the one who is identified with it. And of all realities known to mankind since he began exploring the truths of his own life and of his earth, there is none more insistent attractive and universal than the experience of the Divine within and around us as the one single simultaneously objective and subjective experience. To deny it in the name of an artificial science is to deny the very roots of life itself; nay, it is to deny man and his total existence. To drown it amidst the noise of our superficial material research may do temporary good to some vested interests but it will be at a great and permanent harm to the further progression of the human race and its hope in conquering pain and evil for good. The limits of our sight are not the limits of light!

> Our science is an abstract cold and brief
> That cuts in formulas the living whole.
> It has a brain and head but not a soul:
> It sees all things in outward carved relief.
>
> But how without its depths can the world be known?
> The visible has its roots in the unseen
> And each invisible hides what it can mean
> In a yet deeper invisible, unshown.
>
> The objects that you probe are not their form.
> Each is a mass of forces thrown in shape.
> The forces caught, their inner lines escape
> In a fathomless consciousness beyond mind's norm.
>
> Probe it and you shall meet a Being still
> Infinite, nameless, mute, unknowable.
>
> —Sri Aurobindo: 'The Discoveries of Science'

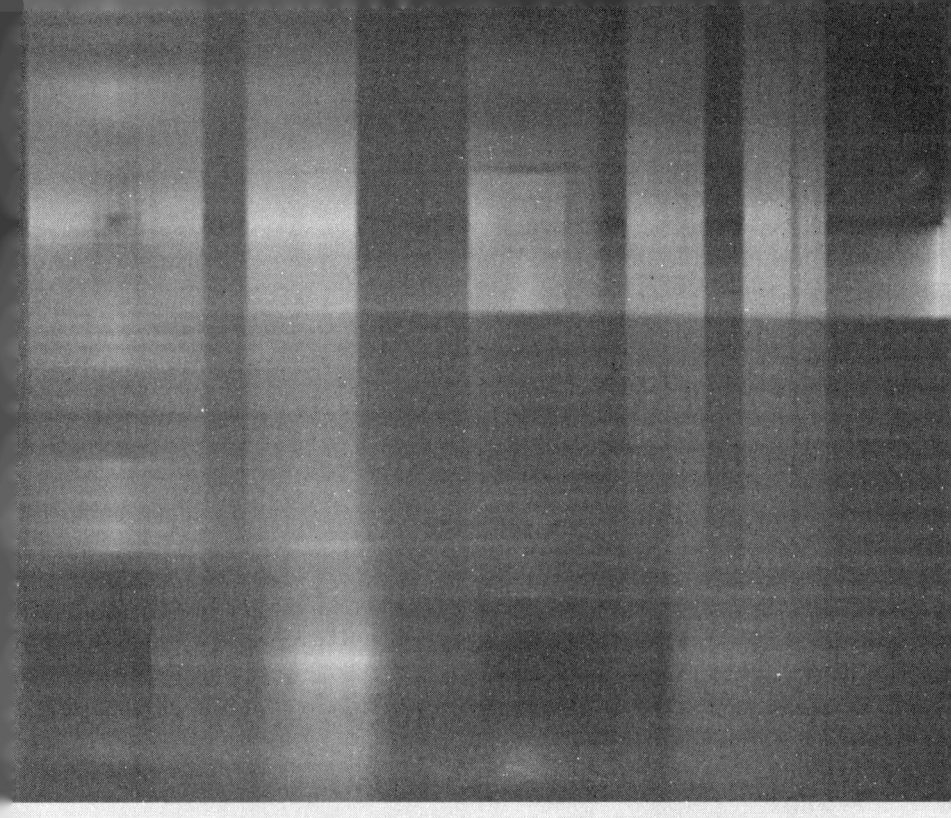

Part IV

OVERCOMING DISTRESS

Introduction

Stress has become an important and inevitable ingredient of contemporary life. In course of everyday interactions, people frequently encounter situations in home, at workplace and at social gatherings that create a threat for well-being. As a concept, 'stress' has proved to be one of the extensively researched themes. Today, it has become a very handy label to voice any unwelcome state of being. In psychological literature, stress has been considered as a major threat to health and well-being of people. As a result, coping with stress and managing it has become an important aspect of interventions in professional and community circles.

The study of stress and related phenomena has been carried out in different traditions and has provided considerable data on its antecedents and correlates (Pestonjee, 1992). In general, psychologists converge on the position that the perception of an event and its appraisal determine the way we respond to it. The same situation, however, may be appraised as threatening/harmful/challenging depending on one's resources, availability of support, perception of control and psychological makeup (for example, temperament, presence of optimism, hope, resilience, etc.). Thus, there is no one-to-one correspondence between the properties of a stimulus situation and the mode of our response to that. There are people who have high degree of stress tolerance and resilience. They grow out of stressful situations and display high degree of adaptability and performance. This kind of picture has emerged from a variety of studies across different cross-sections of people.

The studies also indicate that the happenings at individual and societal levels are correlated. For instance, the conditions of unemployment, social displacement, gender disparity and inequity in relationships often lead to problems of adjustment causing threats to health and well-being. The past research brings out the centrality of the way people cognize their life situations. It is critical for health outcomes. People's beliefs and attributes often mediate and moderate the relationship between stressful situations and its impact on health. This section presents Indian contributions that sample different types of stressful situations, varied age-groups, diverse methodological strategies and a variety of psychological attributes that shape our responses to stressful situations and make us less or more vulnerable leading to differential experiences of well-being.

In the first contribution, Namita Pande and R. K. Naidu describe a study of an indigenous concept of *anasakti* (non-attachment) and its implications for health. The perspective is rooted in the *Bhagavadgita*. They note that the purpose of life is liberation from suffering and realizing the identity of self with the ultimate reality. Disengagement of consciousness from immediate outcomes and desires is called *anasakti*. Desire leads to sense organs attachment that leads to ego's *asakti* or *mamatva*. Anasakta or detached action is one when the actor undertakes action without a concern for the outcome. This makes the emotional response to success and failure different. It is held that no desire can lead to mental serenity. The key features of *anasakti* identified and operationalized by Pande and Naidu include *effort orientation, emotional equipoise* and *weak concern for external reward*. Anasakti relieves one from the anxieties of success and failure. Resistance occurs. The study empirically explored the relationship of *anaskti* with stress and strain in a sample of young adults. The results showed that *anaskti* had a negative relationship with distress. It is recommended that progressive detachment may reduce stress and lead to better performance.

How do people respond to a long-term illness was the subject matter of the meta-analytic study conducted by Ajit K. Dalal. This contribution examined the relationship between cultural beliefs about illness and psychological adjustment to a chronic disease. The findings of five studies were meta-analysed. In all these studies, hospital patients suffering from various types of health problems were interviewed at different points in time, and measures were used to assess their psychological adjustment. The findings revealed that patients' in Indian hospitals consistently attributed their illness to *karma* and God's will. These cosmic beliefs were found to influence patients' treatment-related decisions. However, no consistent linkages were unravelled between patients' illness beliefs and their psychological adjustment. It was conjectured that these cosmic beliefs acquire different symbolic meaning when illness and social context change. The chapter argues for an integrated health care system combining the strengths of traditional healing and biomedical practices.

Near-death experiences (NDE) are the focus of the third contribution. In this work, Satwant Pasricha examines two major issues—the prevalence of NDEs and their characteristics in a part of the Karnataka state in South India. In all, 16 NDE cases were reported among an estimated population of 17,192, showing a prevalence rate of about one case per thousand. The 16 subjects were interviewed for details of their experiences. Interviews revealed that 71 per cent of the subjects seemed to have been to the 'other realms', where they were taken by some messengers or deceased relatives or some religious figures. The subject appeared before Yama (God of Death), his book (containing a report of one's deeds during one's terrestrial life, which forms the basis of judgment for ones next destination) was opened, a mistake was discovered and hence he was sent (or asked to go) back to his terrestrial life. A comparison was done between these NDE experiences and those reported by Sabom on an American population which revealed that six (out of 12) features were reported exclusively by the Indian subjects. The differences seen within and across cultures may be due to actual variations in experiences of persons living in different geographical regions, or due to differences in the methods of investigation. However, it is possible that some of the variations may be due to the differences in the understanding or interpretation of an experience in a particular cultural context. The commonality in the content of features in different cultures is perhaps indicative of a phenomenon which is shaped by, but transcends, cultural beliefs.

In the final contribution to this section, Sweta Srivastava and Arvind Sinha have dealt with an aspect of positive psychology which looks at the human strengths in a systematic manner. The experience of well-being is central to their concerns. They tried to examine the linkages between well-being, self-esteem and happiness in an adult sample. They introduced experiential training and found that resilience is positively related to well-being, self-esteem and happiness. Experiential intervention using 'T' group type training was found to be effective.

REFERENCE

Pestonjee, D. M. (1992). *Stress and coping: The Indian experience*. New Delhi: SAGE.

13

Anasakti and Health: An Empirical Study of *Anasakti* (Non-attachment)

NAMITA PANDE AND RADHA KRISHNA NAIDU

The study investigated the role of *anasakti* in the stress process because control of emotion and emotional equilibrium are integral components of *anasakti*.

According to almost every system of Indian philosophy, whether orthodox or heterodox, realistic or idealistic, the purpose of human life is to achieve liberation from suffering and realize the identity of self with the Ultimate reality. To be able to achieve the goal of self-realization, disengagement of consciousness from desire is necessary. Desires, which are directives of the senses, spring from the identification of self with the ego and its concerns of ambition, pride, attachment (*asakti*) and insistence on mineness (*mamatva*). For this study, description of *anasakti* given in the *Bhagavadgita* was examined. The reason for selecting the *Bhagavadgita* over other sources was simple. The *Bhagavadgita* describes *anasakti* in great thoroughness and works out the various conceivable ramification of the concept in all their details.

In the *Bhagavadgita*, the ideal of *anasakti* embodies the principles of spiritualism as well as exhortations to pragmatism and action orientation. *Anasakti* (the end state) has been explained in terms of *anasakt* action or *niskamakarma* (which implies to achieve that end state). *Anasakti* action does not refer to physical abstention from activity. It is an intense, though disinterested action, performed with a spirit of dispassion, without nurturing concerns about success or failure, loss or gain, likes or dislikes.

This results in a complete unification of the actor with the act and a consequent task excellence. According to the *Bhagavadgita*, task excellence comes about only when the actor has understood that his concerns lie only in actions and not in their results, that actions should not serve any personal motives and that these cognitions should not imply inaction. Being wedded to the piece of work at hand only implies that while an individual is at work, he is allowing his abilities to run to waste in mental preoccupations and fears pertaining to the results and consequences. Such an attitude towards work significantly affects the emotional response to success and failure. Following the relinquishment of desires, mental serenity is acquired and the individual maintains greater emotional equipoise in the face of consequence, be it good or bad, desirable or undesirable. In other words, by way of recommending commitment and total absorption in the task, the doctrine of *anasakt* action offers an excellent way by which our worldly endeavours can become more effective. A theoretical analysis of these and other psychological concepts embedded in the *Gita* is presented by Thapa (1983). Thapa analysed the dimensions of the concept, traced their linkages with current motivational concepts and came up with the first draft instrument for assessing effort and outcome orientations as an individual difference variable.

THE BEHAVIOURAL REFERENTS OF *ANASAKTI*

The qualities defining the *sthitaprajna* helped in the identification of the behavioural referents of *anasakti*, which formed the core of items of the *anasakti* measure. These behavioural referents will be presented in terms of characteristics which an *anasakta* individual is likely to manifest in the conduct of his degree of *anasakti* will:

1. Perceive his work as duty. He is likely to discharge his duties scrupulously without mental attachment to the consequences.
2. Show a lack of concern for the consequences of action. An *anasakta* person is likely to act without much insistence for rewards.
3. Appraise his success and failure in objective rather than in egoistical terms.
4. Be less governed by external standards such as social approval or censor. His behaviour will be guided by his own internal standards about correctness of conduct and excellence in performance.

5. Not experience strong negative emotions such as passion, fear or anger ('*vitaragabhayakrodhah*', 2: 56).
6. Not insist on seeking pleasure and avoiding pain. At the physical level, an *anasakta* person is expected to show greater endurance for pain than others. At the social level, he is expected to overcome temptations and resist hedonistic compulsions. As a result of these, it is anticipated that an *anasakta* person would be able to exercise ethical choices more readily against various appetites and aversions (Naidu, Thapa and Das, 1986).
7. Show an absence of egotism or sense of mineness. He would perhaps be able to replace his smaller personal motives by larger impersonal goals.
8. Maintain an emotional equipoise in the face of positive as well as negative experiences. He would maintain equanimity of emotions while facing the desirable and the undesirable and would remain unperturbed by success or failure, auspicious or inauspicious, pleasant or unpleasant events.
9. Show total absorption in the task at hand. He would manifest complete involvement in all kinds of tasks that he may undertake, dissolving the past fears and future expectations (Swami Chinmayananda, 1975).
10. Show heightened concentration. An *anasakt* person would be able to focus on the task at hand and would not be easily distractible. He would concentrate on any task with a relative ease, regardless of what be its affective value for him.
11. Make an effort towards achieving task excellence. Under no circumstance an *anasakt* person would compromise with lower standards of task excellence.

MEASURING ANASAKTI

The *Bhagawadgita* is not only a metaphysical treatise (*darsana sastra*) but also a treatise on ethics (*nitisastra*). The *Samkhyan* metaphysical dualism, which the *Gita* embodies, explains material phenomena of the manifest world (*jagat*) as modifications (*vrittis*) of the primordial matter (*prakriti*). *Prakriti* reinforces a sense of mistaken identity (*imithya bodh*) with matter (*anna*), mind (*manas*), intelligence (*vijnana*) and egotism (*ahamkara*); perpetuates ignorance (*avidya*) and renders the recognition of the real self (*purusa*) improbable. However, it is the ethical conduct of life which the teachings of *Bhagawadgita* systematically deliberates that has made its philosophy more comprehensible to the common man. Elabording Karma Yoga, the *Gita* prescribes *anasakta* (non-attached action) to spiritual seeker which can help him avoid bodily excesses of indulgence and resist external distractions to become harmonized (*yukta*) with his actions and get detached from all desires for fruits (*karma phalasa*).

The *Gita* contends that action performed with a sense of duty enables man to achieve control over the modifications of his mind. Besides explaining the ideological imports of this prescription, the *Gita* portrays the characteristic attitudes, feelings and actions of the *sthitaprajna* (the man of stable wisdom) who is the ideal practitioner of *anasakti* or *niskama karma*. The *sthitaprajna* is human being who has transcended the usual human levels of experience and behaviour. To operationalize *anasakti*, descriptions of the attitudes and behaviours of the *sthitaprajna*, as set forth by the *Bhagavadgita*, were examined. This description also formed the source for the items of the *Anasakti* Scale.

ANASAKTI AND MENTAL HEALTH

The causal linkage between *anasakti* and health can now be explicated. It can argue that the doctrine of *anasakti* action conveys a message, which is central to coping with life stressors. This argument is based on the psychological literature which demonstrates the significance of cognitive and attitudinal systems in determining the manner in which stress-inducing situations are confronted (Pearlin, Liberman, Menaghan and Mullan, 1981).

The distinctive characteristics of *anasakti* are effort orientation, emotional equipoise in the face of success and failure, a relatively weak concern for obtaining extrinsic rewards and an intense effort to achieve excellence. Therefore, those high on *anasakti* are expected to experience lesser and exhibit fewer symptoms of strain. These arguments will be extended on the basis of conjectures and empirical evidence.

Frankl (1963) stated that people engage in an active search for meaning even in their sufferings. While studying the nature of stressors and coping strategies of the physically handicapped children, Srivastava (1981) noted that in spite of the various disadvantages that the physically handicapped children face, they still view own condition and that of their fellow beings more positively. It is also seen that commitment to some higher goal in life enables people to meaningfully reconstruct even those experiences which can be described as damaging. In the light of these facts, *anasakti* action seems to offer an important coping resource. It may be reaffirmed here that *anasakti* action is not without a goal; rather, it has a very definite goal—the goal of self-realization. In performing actions in an *anasakt* manner, the more familiar and common goals are subordinated to the less familiar and less common ones. This results in recognizing the spiritual value of action in addition to its material significance. If the goal is fixed inwards, the emotional impacts of external success and failure are minimized. Once this happens, the consequences—good or bad—will be cognized as milestones in the path to self-realization rather than as reflections of personal capabilities.

Since these intrusive cognitions and emotional excitations are crucial in the reaction to stressors, it can be argued that greater concentration and absorption in the task at hand will eliminate task-irrelevant thoughts such as anticipations about the nature of outcomes. This will perhaps result in task excellence. On the other hand, emotional stability acquired through mentally dissociating oneself from the outcome will protect the individual from emotionally succumbing to the experience of failure. Therefore, it seems that *anasakti* will help the individual in such a way that he does not perceive life events as stressors. It may also serve as a significant 'resistance resource' (Antonovsky, 1980) and increase his physical and psychological resistance to distress.

Tripathi, Naidu, Thapa and Biswas (1993) studied the impact of various professional and personal life stresses on the health and performance of police personnel in Uttar Pradesh. This study was supported by the Bureau of Police Research and Development. Attachment to the immediate surroundings was measured by a brief five-item scale. It was found that those high on attachment were characterized by higher Type A Personality scores, greater depression, fear and guilt and reported more daily hassles.

A cross-cultural study of the moderator role of *anasakti* was conducted by Naidu and Roseman (1992). In this study, 140 American and 287 Indian university students served as subjects. The *Anasakti* Scale had 22 items. For both the American and Indian samples, it was found that *anasakti* was associated with lower level depression and anxiety. Though *anasakti* did not account for a major part of stress–strain relationship, it did buffer it to a small but significant extent. The report of this study is still under preparation. Currently, work is in progress, which examines the relationship between *anasakti* and mood fluctuations, and further work on the impact of this attitude on performance of certain physical and mental tasks is at the stage of planning.

It was, therefore, hypothesized that attachment would enhance the desired outcome and moderate the adverse effects of stress.

Method

Sample

The data were collected on 465 adults in the age range of 30–50 years, with minimum education up to matriculation level. Of these subjects, 230 were males and 235 females. The males represented various professional groups such as doctors, engineers, lawyers, businessmen as well as those employed in public sector undertakings. The mean age of males and females were 38.14 and 32.44 years, respectively.

Instruments

The Measure of Anasakti. A scale measuring *anasakti* was developed to assess the degree to which people show *anasakti* in the conduct of their daily lives. The scale (in Hindi) consisted of 28 items, which were based on the description of *sthitaprajna* (a man of steady wisdom) given in the *Bhagavadgita*. These items were related to five factors of *anasakti*. These factors were: Outcome Vulnerability, Attachment, Effort Orientation, Endurance and Equipoise, and Physical–Sensual Non-identification. Subjects were asked to report the extent to which behaviour described under each item was applicable to them on a five-point rating scale ranging from one (not at all applicable) to five (entirely applicable). The minimum and maximum *anasakti* scores were 28 and 140, respectively. Details relating to the construction of this scale are reported elsewhere (Pande, 1990).

The Measure of Stress. The stress scale used in this study included 76 items which covered major events as well as minor ongoing hassles. These items were grouped in the following categories of stressors: Stressful Events, Ongoing Stressors, Financial, Health of Others, Bereavement, Work/Occupational, Interpersonal, Ego, Family, Separation, Personal Setbacks and Major Changes. Subjects were required to report events during the past one year. A five-point rating scale was provided for each item. Subjects used this scale to indicate the extent to which they had experienced distress when a given event occurred in their lives. The scale points were one (no distress at all), two (a little distress), three (average distress), four (much distress) and five (too much of distress).

The Measure of Strain. A symptom checklist-cum-rating scale to assess ill health was used. The scale comprised 45 items; some of these items were taken from a health scale constructed by Caplan, Naidu and Tripathi (1984), while others were framed to assess the mental and psychological health of subjects. These items were related to nine factors of strain, which were: Depression, Physical Vitality, Positive State, Self-image, Anger, Digestion, Flu, Sleep-lethargy and Inadequacy. Subjects were asked to indicate on a four-point rating scale how often they had experienced each of the symptoms in the past two weeks. The scale points were: one (did not happen at all), two (happened on a few occasions), three (happened many times) and four (continued for almost all the time). The minimum and maximum strain scores were 45 and 180, respectively.

Computation of *Anasakti*, Stress and Strain Scores

Anasakti scores were obtained by summating the ratings given by the subjects to all 28 items of the scale of *anasakti*. Reverse scoring was done for items which were negatively rated.

For each subject, three stress scores were computed. The Simple Stress Score (SSS) was obtained by counting the number of stressful life events experienced by the subject. Of the three stress scores, this was the most objective score of stress. The Weighted Stress Score (WSS) was obtained by summating the distress ratings given by the subject to the events which he/she had experienced. This score was a function of both the objective count of events and subjectively perceived intensity of distress. It was a composite score of both the environmental event and subjective perception. The Average Distress Rating (ADR) was obtained by dividing the WSS by the number of events experienced or SSS. It yielded a measure of the average amount of subjectively perceived distress across the endorsed items. Of the three stress scores, this was the most subjective score, the purest measure of subjectively perceived distress.

The strain score of each subject was derived by summating the ratings which he/she gave to 45 strain symptoms included in the strain measure. Reverse scoring was done for items indicative of the subject's well-being.

Results

This chapter reports a part of the data of a larger study which investigated the moderator role of *anasakti* in the stress process. In the section, data pertaining to the correlation between the measures of stress, strain and *anasakti*, comparison of the means of these variables of two extreme *anasakti* groups and the identification of predictors of strain will be presented.

CORRELATION BETWEEN STRESS, ANASAKTI AND STRAIN

Correlations were computed between stress, *anasakti* and strain scores. The coefficients of correlation between SSS, WSS, ADR, *anasakti* and strain have been presented in Table 13.1.

Table 13.1: Coefficients of Correlation between SSS, WSS, ADR, *Anasakti* and Strain

n = 465

	SSS	WSS	ADR	AS	Strain
SSS	–				
WSS	0.94**	–			
ADR	0.22**	0.46**	–		
AS	–0.08	–0.12**	–0.14**	–	
Strain	0.29**	0.33**	0.26**	–0.39**	–

Source: Author.
Notes: AS is *Anasakti*.
$**p < 0.01$.

The three stress scores, i.e., SSS, WSS and ADR were correlated positively with each other. Subjects, who encountered greater number of stressful life events, gave higher distress ratings and on an average felt more distressed. A very high correlation between SSS and WSS ($r = 0.94$) was obtained because the computation of WSS was dependent upon SSS, WSS or the sum of distress ratings of events endorsed constituted SSS. In comparison to the correlation between SSS and ADR ($r = 0.22$), a higher correlation was obtained between WSS and ADR ($r = 0.46$) because both WSS and ADR were related to the perception of distress.

Anasakti was significantly correlated with WSS and ADR but not with SSS. This implied that a higher degree of *anasakti* was related to the perception of lower distress. Compared to the three stress scores, *anasakti* had the highest correlation with strain.

In order to make comparisons between SSS, WSS, ADR and strain scores of subjects who were high and low on *anasakti*, criterion groups of *anasakti* were identified. Subjects whose *anasakti* scores were below 104 (30 percentile of the frequency distribution of *anasakti* scores) were included in the low *anasakti* group and those who had scored above 118 (70 percentile) were included in the high *anasakti* group.

Difference between Means of Stress and Strain Scores

Means of SSS, ADR and strain scores were derived for high and low *anasakti* groups and significance of difference between means was rested.

Table 13.2: Means of SSS, WSS, ADR and Strain Scores of the Criterion Groups

	High Anasakti Group (n = 117)		Low Anasakti Group (n = 115)			
	Mean	SD	Mean	SD	t	p
SSS	12.12	8.42	12.09	8.12	0.03	n.s.
WSS	36.77	29.41	40.29	29.22	0.91	n.s.
ADR	2.89	0.951	3.23	0.890	2.83	<.01
Strain	71.75	15.12	91.01	23.96	7.29	<.01

Source: Author.
Notes: SD = standard deviation.
  n.s. = non significant.

The analysis revealed that the two groups were almost identical on mean SSS and there was a non-significant difference between the means of WSS of the two groups in the expected direction. Thus, WSS failed to reveal a significant difference probably because it was very highly correlated with SSS. The non-significant difference was perhaps a weak pointer towards differences in the manner in which these two groups perceived life events. This feature was brought out more clearly in ADR, which was a purer measure of the perception of distress. ADR was significantly lower in the case of subjects who were high on *anasakti* compared to those who were low on it.

The capacity of the high *anasakti* group to cope with stressors and experience less distress was reflected in the process of somatization also. Subjects high on *anasakti* exhibited fewer symptoms of strain compared to those who were low on *anasakti*.

Identifying Predictors of Strain

A simultaneous multiple regression analysis was done to determine the relative significance of *anasakti* and stress scores in predicting strain. Since SSS and WSS were strongly correlated (r = 0.94), only WSS was entered in the regression equation along with ADR and *anasakti*.

In can be seen from Table 13.3 that *anasakti* had a significant but negative regression coefficient. Anasakti and stress scores accounted for almost 25 per cent of variance in the strain score. The contribution of these three predictors was found to be statistically significant [$F(3,461) = 49.89, p < 0.01$]. All the three-predictor variables significantly contributed to prediction of strain. Comparing the beta coefficients, it can be tentatively suggested that of the three predictors, the contribution of *anasakti* was higher in predicting strain than the contribution of WSS and ADR.

Table 13.3: Multiple Regression Analysis for Total Sample: *Anasakti*, WSS and ADR as Independent Variables, Strain as Dependent Variable

Variables	r	B	Beta	STD Error B	F
Non-attachment	-0.39	-0.547	-0.348	0.064	72.20**
WSS	0.33	0.186	0.253	0.034	30.50**
ADR	0.26	2.08	0.089	1.078	3.74
Multiple R		0.497			
R Square		0.245			
F (3,461)		49.89**			

Source: Author.
Notes: *$p < 0.05$.
**$p < 0.01$.

Discussion

The concept of *anasakti* in the spiritual lore means progressive detachment of consciousness from the psychophysical apparatus. Patanjali's and Shankaracharya's systems envisage five stages of development of consciousness of one who is pursuing the spiritual goal. These five stages are termed *panchakosha* or five sheaths (Swami Ram, Ballentine and Swami Ajay, 1976). The concept of *panchakosha* has a logical consequence for psychology. To understand the experience and behaviour of people in the five different *kosha*, different psychologies are needed.

Most people belong to the *manomayakosha*, which is the middle level of the five hierarchical stages of development. The *manomayakosha* refers to the mental level including the lower and higher minds. The lower mind, or *manas*, serves to coordinate sensory input and motor output after the higher mind, the *buddhi* has adjudged the meaning of the incoming sensory information and has decided on the course of action to be taken.

The *manomayakosha* is a wide band. Those who are primarily at the level of *manas* would exhibit impulsivity and a strong tendency to seek pleasure. Those who are primarily at the level of *buddhi* would be more discriminating. Therefore, this *kosha* represents a stage of intellectually controlled emotionality; a stage where cognitive structures exert controlling influence on emotions. Modern psychological theories, which have relevance within the framework of *manomayakosha*, are cognitive theories of stress (Lazarus, 1975; Rosenbaum, 1988).

One of the aims of this study was to demonstrate the possibility of conceptual bridges between disparate paradigms. Therefore, the findings of this study will be interpreted in terms of the cognitive theories of stress.

Anasakti, Perception of Distress and Strain

The most significant findings which emerged from this study concerned the perception of distress in stressful life events. It was found that subjects high on *anasakti* did not significantly differ from those low on *anasakti* in terms of the number of life events which had occurred in their lives (SSS). When the number of events, which they had experienced, was controlled, the average subjective perception of distress (ADR) was significantly lower for subjects who were high on *anasakti*. The tendency to experience less distress, in general, helped the more *anasakti* subjects to maintain superior physical and psychological health compared to those who were low on *anasakti*.

Stress is a multi-dimensional concept, which necessitates an understanding of its personal and environmental antecedents. Lazarus (1975) has emphasized the significance of threat appraisals in the perception of distress in negative life events. Another important fact of appraisal refers to the meaning which is assigned to those events. Negative life events can be more deleterious if they are perceived to be central to one's existence, are considered to be stable and are attributed to global causes (Metalsky, Halberstadt and Abramson, 1987).

These psychological interpretive mechanisms are crucial in determining the emotional reactions to stressful life events. Depending upon whether the situation is interpreted as harmful, beneficial, threatening or challenging, an individual experiences positive or negative emotion. The interpretation of a situation as involving harm or threat generates such affective states as anxiety, nervousness, tension and anger. The affective states, which may be the most ubiquitous emotional reactions to situations to which are appraised as stressful, interfere with cognitive functioning and with coping (Schwarzer, 1984). Two mechanisms of interference have been emphasized. First, a motivational one in which attention is diverted from the task at hand to more pressing emotional crisis, which is perceived to be associated with a situation (Schonpflug, 1983), and second, a cognitive one in which anxiety-related thoughts, which may be unrelated to performance, are nurtured. If, however, a situation is interpreted as presenting challenges rather than threats, more positive emotions are experienced leading to effective coping. Folkman and Lazarus (1988) have suggested that on certain occasions, focusing on the problem, which is causing distress, may lead to an improved emotional state. They refer to focusing on the problem as planful problem solving. According to them, planful problem solving results in an improved person–environment relation, leading to a favourable cognitive appraisal and, therefore, to a more positive emotional response.

Within this framework, the findings relating to the perception of distress can be interpreted. As started earlier, subjects high and low on *anasakti* differed from each other with respect to their subjective perception of distress (ADR) and symptoms of strain. Since *anasakti* is characterized by a strong tendency towards effort orientation, those high on *anasakti* were able to evoke action-oriented self-regulatory processes more effectively than those who were low on *anasakti*.

Self-regulatory processes consist of three phases (Rosenbaum, 1988). When stressful situations are encountered, these phases involve representation, evaluation and action. In the representation phase, the individual reacts emotionally and/or cognitively to stressors which disruption in his daily routine. In the evaluation phase, he evaluates the significance of disruption caused by stressors terms of his well-being. In the action phase, he responds to stressors in such a way that the disruption may be minimized.

Significant mean differences in ADR suggested that individuals high and low on *anasakti* differed from each other in the manner in which stressors were represented. When they confronted stressful life events, they felt differentially distressed. *Anasakti* helped the higher *anasakti* group to evaluate stressful events as presenting challenges rather than threats.

They could evolve suitable coping strategies because of their disposition to remain emotionally poised. In the case of subjects low on *anasakti*, threat appraisals, emotional instabilities and coping ineptitudes may have led to greater perceived distress. These individuals also manifested more symptoms of psychological and physical ill health.

Anasakti: The Predictor of Strain

The relative significance of *anasakti* and stress scores in predicting strain was tested. More than the stress scores, *anasakti* significantly predicated strain symptoms. This finding suggested that dispositional factors increased an individual's susceptibility to stressors more than the situation itself. *Anasakti* represents one facet of human personality which helps individuals remain well-adjusted and healthy, despite exposure to stressors. It was also found that the contribution of *anasakti* in predicting strain was greater than the contribution of stress scores. The psychological processes underlying this finding will be discussed.

As stated earlier, *anasakti* refers to an end state and also a means to achieve that state. The end state is that of self-realization, which can be gradually approached through the performance of actions without attachment to their consequences. One who has achieved this end state, the *siddha*, becomes spontaneously *anasakti* by terminating his identity with the 'empirical self' (Tart, 1975). He enjoys a state of profound peace, which cannot be altered by any crisis. One who aspires to achieve that state, the *sadhaka*, remains in peace because he voluntarily relinquishes all egoistical desires and practises *anasakti* as a means to achieve his goal.

Even the Western literature on stress admits that perception regarding thwarting of desires constitutes major category of stressors and presents potential dangers to an individual's well-being. Housten (1987) has defined desires as longing for something which one does not have and keeping something which one already has. Desires emanate from attachment. Individuals experience distress when their attachment to people or things is threatened. Stronger the attachment, greater is the desire to protect and preserve, and higher will be the feeling of agitation if that desire is thwarted.

Coping with negative life events is influenced by an individual's 'assumptive world' (Parkes, 1975). This world consists of his strongly held assumptions about the world and about his own self. Epstein (1984) has asserted that an individual's personal theory about reality acts as a conceptual tool for solving life's fundamental problems. According to him, this theory incorporates a world theory and a theory regarding self. It may not exist in his conscious awareness but as a preconscious conceptual system; it may structure his experiences and direct his behaviour. Implicit in the ideal of *anasakti* is a worldview in which self-realization is considered to be the goal of human life and identification of self with the material world to be a major impediment in the path of self-realization. This worldview perhaps helped people in changing the perception of life events from stressful to being, reducing egotism from strivings and hence softening the impact of many stressors.

REFERENCES

Antonovsky, A. (1980). *A call for the study of autogenesis*. Paper prepared for the national Academy of Sciences, Ben-Gurion University of the Negev, Beersheba, Israel.

Caplan, R. D., Naidu, R. K. and Tripathi, R. C. (1984). Coping and defending: Constellations versus components. *Journal of Health and Social Behavious*, 25, 303–20.

Epstein, S. (1984). Controversial issue in emotion theory. In P. Shaver (Ed.), *Review of personality and social psychology: Emotions, relationships and health*. Beverly Hills, CA: Sage Publications.

Folkman, S. and Lazarus, R. S. (1988). Coping as a mediator of emotion. *Journal of Personality and Social Psychology*, 54, 466–75.

Frankl, V. E. (1963). *Man's search for meaning. An introduction to logotherapy*. New York: Washington Square Press.

Housten, B. K. (1987). Stress and coping. In C. R. Snyder and C. E. Ford (Eds), *Coping with negative life events: Clinical and social psychological perspectives*. New York: Plenum Press.

Lazarus, R. S. (1975). A cognitively oriented psychologist looks at biofeedback. *American Psychologist*, 30, 553–61.

Metalsky, G. I., Halberstadt, L. J. and Abramson, L. Y. (1987). Vulnerability to depressive mood reactions: Towards a more powerful test of the diathesis-stress and causal mediation components of the reformulated theory of depression. *Journal of Personality and Social Psychology*, 52, 386–93.

Naidu, R. K., Thapa, K. and Das, M. M. (1986). *On measuring detachment: An example of a scientific analog of an indigenous concept*. Unpublished manuscript, University of Allahabad, Allahabad.

Naidu, R. K. and Roseman, I. (1992). *Data on anasakti*. Unpublished report, University of Allahabad, Allahabad.

Pande, N. (1990). *Studies on differential vulnerability to stress: The impact of detachment on health.* Unpublished doctoral dissertation, University of Allahabad, Allahabad.
Pande, N. and Naidu, R. K. (1992). Anasakti and health: A study of non-attachment. *Psychology and Developing Societies,* 4, 89–104.
Parkes, C. M. (1975). What becomes of redundant world models. A contribution to the study of adaptation to change. *British Journal of Medical Psychology,* 48, 131–37.
Pearlin, L. T., Liberman, M. A., Menaghan, E. G. and Mullan, J. T. (1981). The stress process. *Journal of Health and Social Behaviour,* 22, 337–56.
Rosenbaum, M. (1988). Learned resourcefulness, stress and self-regulation. In S. Fisher and J. Reason (Eds), *Handbook of life stress cognition and health.* New York: Wiley.
Schonpflug, W. (1983). Coping efficiency and situational demands. In G. R. J. Hockey (Ed.), *Stress and fatigue in human performance.* New York: Wiley.
Schwarzer, R. (Ed.). (1984). *The self in anxiety, stress and depression.* Amsterdam: Elsevier.
Srivastava, O. P. (1981). *Stress and coping mechanisms of physically handicapped children.* Unpublished doctoral dissertation, University of Allahabad, Allahabad.
Swami Chinmayananda. (1975). *The Holy Gita.* Bombay: Central Chinmayanand Trust.
Swami Ram, Ballentine, R. and Swami Ajay. (1976). *Yoga and psycholotherapy: The evolution of consciousness.* Honesdale, Pennsylvania: The Himalayan International Institute of Yoga Science and Philosophy.
Tart, C. T. (1975). *Transpersonal psychologies.* New York: Harper & Row.
Thapa, K. (1983). *Effort-consequence orientation as a moderator variable stress-strain relationship.* Post-doctoral dissertation, University of Allahabad, Allahabad.
Tripathi, R. C. (1984). Unpublished MS. 'The measure of strain: A symptom checklist-cum-rating scale', Department of Psychology, University of Allahabad, Allahabad, India.
Tripathi, R. C., Naidu, R. K., Thapa, K. and Biswas, S. N. (1993). *Stress, health and performance: A study of police organization in U.P.* Unpublished report, Department of Psychology, University of Allahabad, Allahabad, India.

14

Living with a Chronic Disease: Healing and Psychological Adjustment in Indian Society

AJIT K. DALAL

The psychological adjustment of people suffering from chronic diseases is an area of research in which a series of hospital studies were conducted by Dalal and his colleagues at Allahabad University. These studies were conducted on hospitalized patients who were seeking treatment for various types of chronic diseases. The major objective of this research is to examine the causal attributions which patients make for their illness, and the way in which such attributions are related to their health behaviour. The relationship between cultural beliefs about illness and psychological adjustment is explored. General conclusions based on the findings of five studies are presented.

The prevalence of chronic diseases has increased rapidly in last two or three decades. Increase in life expectancy, lifestyle, dietary habits, occupational and environmental stresses along with a host of other factors have led to a fourfold increase in the occurrence of chronic diseases in the twentieth century. The WHO Report (1996) observed that whereas deaths due to acute and infectious diseases had declined from 36 per cent in 1900 to 6 per cent in 1980, deaths due to chronic diseases had increased from 20 per cent to 70 per cent during the same period. For instance, if an individual is above 50 years of age, chances are more than 80 per cent that he or she would be suffering from some chronic disease. Chronic diseases, particularly those like cancer and heart attack, are now central to the modern consciousness of what illness means.

By definition, chronic diseases are long lasting, often lifelong. The symptoms may not be present all the time, but the chances of recurrence of the symptoms suggest that the prospects of recovery are limited. In most cases, therapeutic intervention is limited to symptomatic treatment with little possibility of complete cure of the disease. Because of the long-drawn nature of the disease, a person is required to integrate the disease into his or her daily life. The disease becomes a part of a person's existence. The meaning it acquires in a person's life largely depends on factors intrinsic to the disease, such as the nature of the disease, its severity and spread, as well as on factors intrinsic to the social status of the person—age, gender, nature of occupation, achievements and obligations, etc. The afflicted person is required to comprehend the significance of the disease in terms of the nature of adjustments that he or she is expected to make to live with a disease in the world of healthy. Obviously, the person suffering from a chronic disease is expected to assume the major responsibility of managing his or her own disease. The person would be required to identify the symptoms, monitor progress of the disease and control its debilitating side effects. It becomes the responsibility of the afflicted person and his or her family to manage the medical, occupational, social and psychological after-effects, and to restore the person's sense of self-worth and meaning in life. The person is not only expected to live with the illness but also to continue to participate in everyday life, not as a patient but as a social being.

It is obvious that the medical model of health care has failed to provide effective services in these cases. Medical treatment, as we know, is best suited for the treatment of acute, infectious diseases, and has very little to offer to people with chronic diseases, apart from some palliative treatment. Whereas medical procedures treat patients as passive recipients of the treatment, long-term care in the case of chronic disease calls for the active involvement of the afflicted person. Any such therapeutic programme has to take into consideration the person's own understanding of the disease and has to deal with his or her social–psychological problems as well.

Much of the personal initiative to manage one's own disease depends on the way one understands the experience of illness and its causes. People need to be made aware of the causes of their illness to keep their world predictable, where things do not happen accidentally. Quite often the initial reaction to the diagnosis of a chronic disease is one of shock and disorientation, threatening their earlier mode of believing and living. A causal understanding of the problem is reassuring that they still live in a stable, predictable world. Bulman and Wortman (1977) and other researchers have shown that people who have an answer to the question 'why me?' are much better off than those who have no answer to this question. Such knowledge is often essential to formulate a course of action and to make treatment-related decisions. Beliefs about causality as well as recovery are often part of the implicit theories about the disease and its treatment. Leventhal (1984) noted that patients with malignant lymphoma seemed to gauge the effectiveness of chemotherapy by monitoring the size of their tumours. Paradoxically, patients whose tumours reduced dramatically expressed a much higher level of distress during therapy than those whose tumour showed a more gradual remission. In the latter case, patients could attribute their remission to the treatment they were receiving, while in the former case, no such reasons were available. They, thus, had no way to predict the future course of their recovery from the understanding of the disease (Bishop, 1991). A knowledge of the factors which caused their disease and of the factors which would contribute to recovery from it, facilitates in long-term adjustment to the chronic problem. Again, an understanding of the causes gives people a sense of personal control in the prevention of its occurrence in future or in containing the debilitating consequences of the disease.

Two factors contribute to the stability of such beliefs about causality and recovery from the disease. First, these health beliefs represent a shared understanding of the disease in particular and of human suffering in general. These beliefs are ingrained in the social consciousness of people in every culture and shape their health practices. Such health beliefs are mutually reinforced and sustained by the social support system on which people in crises depend upon. Second, a chronic disease gives people enough opportunity to test these beliefs in the long duration of the illness. The beliefs which are substantiated during this period are likely to be enduring.

The causes to which people attribute their disease are often at variance with the medical causes. This is specially true in traditional societies with alternative health care systems. The work of Arthur Kleinman (1988) in Asian countries has shown that more than 90 per cent of the illness instances are managed at the family and community level. In these countries, cultural beliefs about the disease play a crucial role in making health-related decisions. As the works of Kleinman and Kakar (1982) have evidenced, the metaphysical causal beliefs constitute the core of the Asian cultural belief system. These beliefs find manifestation in the traditional healing practices of a society. Studies have reported differences in the health beliefs of Euro-American and Indian societies. The works of Blaxter (1983), M. S. Joshi (1995) and Taylor (1983) have shown that in the West, people more frequently attribute chronic illnesses to heredity, germs and environment, whereas Indians make attributions to metaphysical causation, such as God and *karma*.

Not only are there wide cultural differences in the metaphysical beliefs which people have about the world and their own disease, but also these beliefs in a complex way affect the health status of people. Levin and Vanderpool (1991) reviewed a long list of nearly 300 articles published in this area in epidemiological, gerontological and behavioural sciences supporting a linkage of religious beliefs and practices with physical health outcomes. These studies have highlighted both the deleterious and salubrious effects of religion on health status. Most of these studies were descriptive in nature and no clear patterns of results were obtained. A process-oriented approach may perhaps be more appropriate in this field to make sense of the resulting relationships between religion and health (Dull and Skokan, 1995). The spiritual experience being multi-dimensional and context-specific, the issue of relationship between religion and health has to be addressed within the larger domain of spiritualism and its relevance for an individual.

In traditional Indian society, metaphysical beliefs, i.e., beliefs in *karma*, God and fate are presumed to be important determinants of many happenings in one's life, including illness and suffering. The theory of *karma* is invoked as an explanation for an array of undesirable life events. This theory holds that good and bad deeds accumulate over all previous lives and if people have done some wrong in this or previous births, then they have to bear the consequences. The present suffering is frequently attributed to one's own misdeeds of this and previous lives. Another metaphysical belief—God's will—is also frequently used as an explanation for many events in life. Differing from the principle of *karma*, God is seen as an external agent who controls reward and punishment, not always according to what one deserves (Paranjpe, 1984). A person's bad deeds may be condoned by a benevolent God. The belief in fate implies that all life events are predestined and one can do little to change their course. Though conceptually different, these metaphysical beliefs are quite often used interchangeably in everyday parlance.

In this paper, an effort is made to draw general conclusions from a series of five studies conducted on hospital patients. In these studies, factors to which people suffering from various health problems attributed both causality and the subsequent recovery were examined. These studies further explored how such illness beliefs were linked with patients' health-related decisions and responses, which in turn affected their psychological adjustment to their chronic disease.

INTERVIEWING HOSPITAL PATIENTS

In all the five studies, the samples were drawn from different government hospitals in Allahabad city. These patients were undergoing treatment for orthopaedic problems, tuberculosis (TB), cervical cancer and myocardial infarction (MI). Most of the patients studied were Hindus, from lower socio-economic strata and rural background, and a majority of them had no formal schooling.

The patients were interviewed in the hospital setting using an open-ended schedule. With doctors' permission the patients were asked questions related to their perception of the illness and were given measures of psychological adjustment/recovery. All the patients were interviewed on at least two occasions. The time taken to complete the interviews varied from 30 to 85 minutes.

ABOUT THE STUDIES REPORTED

The five studies were conducted at different points in time by Dalal and his colleagues. One of the major objectives of these studies was to examine the beliefs patients had about their own illness, particularly beliefs related to causes of the disease, factors contributing to recovery and beliefs about personal control. The linkages of these beliefs with affective reactions, psychological and medical recovery were also examined. The focus was on understanding the process through which these health beliefs influenced recovery outcomes for the patients who were passing through an acute phase of the disease, necessitating hospitalization. In all these studies, disease and recovery were studied from the patients' perspective.

The first of these studies (Dalal and Pande, 1988) was conducted on orthopaedic patients who were victims of some major accident. These patients were categorized by the attending doctor as permanently disabled (such as amputees) or temporarily disabled due to an accident. They were interviewed two weeks and one month after the accident to record their health beliefs and recovery from the illness. The second study (Dalal and Singh, 1992) examined TB patients convalescing in a local hospital. These patients were asked questions about the perceived causes of the disease and beliefs about recovery. Their psychological and medical recovery was also examined. The third study (Agrawal and Dalal, 1993) investigated the recovery process of MI patients. Their recovery was monitored at three time points, twice during hospitalization and later at home. The aim was to investigate the relation between their disease-related beliefs and the recovery process. The fourth study (Kohli and Dalal, 1998) was conducted on cervical cancer patients to examine their explanatory models and psychological recovery. Women at different stages of treatment for cervical cancer were interviewed to understand their metaphysical beliefs about the disease. In the last study (Dalal, Kohli and Agrawal, 1999), perception of the hospital environment and its relation with the affective state of the patients undergoing treatment for various types of chronic diseases were examined.

MAJOR FINDINGS

In this paper, the major findings of these five studies are collated to delineate the overall pattern of the relationship between health beliefs and recovery from the disease. Since different questionnaires and measures were used in these studies, for purposes of comparison the findings were in some instances subjected to some transformation. Again, not all measures were included in these five studies and the comparisons were made wherever it was possible.

Causal and Recovery Beliefs

The mean ratings of causal and recovery attributions were rank-ordered to compare findings across the first four studies conducted on different groups of patients. The highest mean rating was given the rank of 1 (see Table 14.1).

The trends of ranks in Table 14.1 show that patients' health problems were most frequently attributed to God's will and *karma*, except in the case of MI patients. Others' carelessness was the least cited category of causes, except by accident victims. MI patients attributed the blame more to themselves than to any other factor.

The pattern was not very clear in the case of recovery attributions. Recovery was most frequently attributed to the attending doctor, perhaps because all the patients were hospitalized. After the attending doctor, recovery was most frequently attributed to God. The other recovery attributions were contingent on the nature of illness.

Table 14.1: Rank Order of Causal and Recovery Beliefs as Reported by the Patients

	TB n = 70	MI 70	Cancer 114	Orthopaedic 41
Causal Beliefs				
Own Carelessness	3	1	5	4
Other's Carelessness	6	5	6	3
Family Conditions	5	3	4	5
Fate/Chance	4	–	3	–
God's will	1	4	2	1
Karma	2	2	1	2
Recovery Beliefs				
Self	5	4	4	–
Family	7	2	5	–
Money	4	–	–	–
Fate/Chance	3	–	6	–
God	2	3	2	–
Karma	6	5	3	–
Doctor	1	1	1	–

Source: Author.

Treatment Decisions and Affective Reactions

The actual ratings of causal attributions as reported in Table 14.1 in the case of cancer patients were categorized along three causal dimensions and were correlated with delay in seeking treatment and perception of the hospital environment. The three causal dimensions were internal (own carelessness), external (other's carelessness, family conditions) and cosmic (fate, God's will and *karma*). The correlations of these causal dimensions with other variables are reported in Table 14.2.

The results show that in the case of cancer patients there was greater delay in seeking treatment when these patients attributed their illness to internal and cosmic factors. It was also observed that the hospital environment was perceived as less threatening when the disease was attributed to internal factors, and more threatening when causal attributions were made to cosmic factors.

Table 14.2: Correlations[+] of Causal Dimensions with Delay in Seeking Treatment and Perception of Hospital Environment

Causal Dimensions	Treatment Delay[++]	Hospital Envir. Perceiv. Threat
Internal	0.29*	–.21*
External	–.12	0.27*
Cosmic	0.37**	0.25*

Source: Author.
Notes: *$p < 0.05$
**$p < 0.01$
[+] Perceived severity was partialled out.
[++] Only cancer patients.

The findings of the last study (Dalal et al., 1999) are presented in Table 14.3. The table depicts patients' perception of the hospital environment and its correlations with their affective reactions. The findings revealed that female patients expressed more anger and anxiety during hospitalization, whereas male patients more often resorted to mental disengagement (thinking of something else) and transcendence (thinking beyond the mundane). It was also observed that patients who perceived the hospital environment as threatening, more frequently experienced anxiety, depression and helplessness.

Table 14.3: Affective Reactions of Hospital Patients

Affect	Male (n = 88)	Female (n = 34)	Overall (n = 122)	Corr. with Hosp Threat[+]
Anger^	1.56	1.87	1.64	0.23
Anxiety^	1.75	2.17	1.87	0.51**
Depression	2.44	2.66	2.50	0.38**
Helplessness	2.58	2.72	2.62	0.47**
Disengagement^	2.30	1.96	2.20	–.13
Rationale^	2.83	2.56	2.75	0.09

Source: Author.
Notes: n = 122
*$p < 0.05$
**$p < 0.01$
[+] Perceived severity of the health problem was partialled out.
^ Males and females differed on these affective reactions.

Illness Beliefs and Psychological Adjustment

The two types of beliefs (causal and recovery), as used in some of these studies, were correlated with measures of psychological adjustment[1] of the patients. The indices of psychological recovery varied in these studies, but common among all the four studies were items related to disease appraisal, hope, mood state and positive attitude. The simple correlations between beliefs and psychological adjustment are given in Table 14.4.

Table 14.4: Correlation of Health Beliefs with Psychological Recovery/Adjustment Measures

	TB	MI	Cancer	Orthopaedic Temp	Orthopaedic Perm
	n = 70	70	114	20	21
Causal Beliefs					
Own Carelessness	0.22	0.30**	−0.10	0.30	0.01
Other's Carelessness	−0.24**	0.01	−0.14	0.11	0.25
Family Conditions	0.26**	0.02	−0.31***	−0.06	−0.14
Fate/Chance	−0.15	−	−0.03	−	−
God's will	−0.09	−0.37***	0.15	−0.05	0.29
Karma	−0.06	−0.19	−0.10	0.39*	0.29
Recovery Beliefs					
Self	0.05	0.24*	0.28***	−	−
Family	−0.03	−0.06	0.16	−	−
Money	0.08	−	−	−	−
Fate/chance	−0.28"	−	0.11	−	−
God	−0.29**		0.29**	0.09	−
Karma	0.18	0.29**	0.02	−	−
Doctor	−0.12	−0.18	0.00	−	−
Control Beliefs					
Self	0.40***	0.21	0.04		
Disease	0.18	0.33**	0.29**		

Source: Author.
Notes: *p < 0.10
 **p < 0.05
 ***p < 0.01
 Temp = Temporary; Perm = Permanent

---

[1] In some of the studies reported here the terms 'psychological adjustment' and 'psychological recovery' are used interchangeably.

The results show that, in general, the correlation between causal attributions and psychological adjustment was low and there was no consistent trend across different samples. Only in the case of MI patients, self-blame was positively correlated with adjustment. Attribution to family conditions was positively correlated with adjustment in the case of TB patients and negatively in the case of cancer patients. Cosmic beliefs also did not show any consistent pattern. On the other hand, for MI patients, attribution to self, God and *karma* was positively correlated with adjustment. The pattern of correlation was reverse in the case of TB patients. The two measures of control, i.e., control over self and over the disease, had significant positive correlations with the psychological adjustment of the patients.

Linkages between Psychological and Physical Recovery

The measures of psychological recovery/adjustment and medical recovery varied for different categories of patients. Medical recovery was assessed from the doctor's report, which also made note of the use of pain killers and sedatives. The measures of psychological recovery were correlated with doctors' reports of medical recovery. As shown in Table 14.5, only in the case of MI patients, significant correlations were found between these two types of recovery. In the case of TB patients, there was no relation between psychological and medical recovery. Reports of medical recovery were not available in the other studies.

Table 14.5: Correlation of Psychological Recovery/Adjustment with Medical Recovery

	MI	TB
Time 1	0.30*	0.07
Time 2	0.36**	0.16

Source: Author.
Notes: *$p < 0.05$
 **$p < 0.01$

Discussion

The findings of the five studies reported here clearly revealed that patients in Indian hospitals attributed their illness to cosmic factors. This finding was consistent across all the four groups of patients. That Indian patients attributed their chronic health problems to *karma* and God seems to be a fairly robust finding. The other factor to which causal attribution was more often made was 'own carelessness'. Patients appeared to blame themselves for their own misfortune. On the other hand, they rarely blamed others for their problems.

In this context, it is interesting to note that attributions to *karma* and God did not emanate in an open-ended inquiry. Rarely did patients talk about it on their own. Only when they were directly asked did they mention God and *karma* as the most important causes of their present suffering. M. S. Joshi (1995) also noted in her study in a hospital in Bombay that patients rarely mentioned about their cosmic beliefs, unless they were categorically asked about them. In the hospital setting, the patients were probably shy of sharing such beliefs, lest they were laughed at for being ignorant and superstitious. In fact, as was observed in an informal chat with the patients, a large number of them were seeking some kind of alternative healing, along with the medical treatment.

How do patients reconcile with this contradiction? In fact, most of the patients did not see any contradiction in it. They wanted to try anything which would work. In his work on health practices in the Garhwal region, P. C. Joshi (1988; 2000) reported that the local people made a distinction between *bis* and *bimari*. For *bis*, which is primary and a metaphysical cause, they visited a local traditional healer. For *bimari*, which is secondary (bodily symptoms), they sought the services of a medical doctor. The patients had intuitively learnt to keep these two aspects of the disease separate. Kleinman (1988), in his studies in China and other Asian countries, found that in all these countries traditional healing and biomedical treatment co-exist and are not perceived as contradictory. What lies at the core of the Indian (Hindu) belief system is the principle of *karma* as an explanation for suffering in one's life. Though this principle of *karma* acquires different meanings in varying contexts, in general, belief in *karma* and cosmic causation inculcates in the individual an attitude of acceptance of his or her own and other's suffering. Belief in *karma* and fate, and the consequent attitude of acceptance has its basis not only in the religio-philosophical background, but also in the climate that characterizes the Indian subcontinent (such as unpredictable rains on which the economy depends) (Sinha, 1988). This belief keeps the faith in a just world alive even under very adverse conditions, and sustains the hope that good deeds will ultimately result in good outcomes (Paranjpe, 1998).

Attributing illness to metaphysical factors such as God's will, *karmaphala* and fate also provides patients a convincing and socially acceptable explanation for their illness. Whenever people face a crisis, care-givers (such as family members) also invoke these cultural beliefs to explain suffering. In other studies conducted on diverse samples from the Indian population, it was reported that the poor (Sinha, Jain and Pandey, 1980), the disadvantaged (Misra and Misra, 1986) and the depressed (Jain, 1988) frequently made attributions to metaphysical factors.

The findings of these five studies, however, did not unravel consistent linkages of causal beliefs with affective reactions and psychological recovery. Attributions to God's will had a negative and *karma* had a positive relationship with psychological recovery. Fate was not correlated with psychological recovery across the different groups of patients. In the case of recovery beliefs, however, significant correlations were obtained between cosmic beliefs and psychological recovery/adjustment in the case of MI and TB patients. When MI and cancer patients attributed recovery to their own efforts, their actual recovery was better. What these findings suggest is that though Indian patients have shown a propensity to attribute their physical suffering to cosmic factors, there is no direct and linear relationship between these beliefs and the recovery process. Two postulates can be advanced to comprehend the findings. First, *karma* and God's will are part of the complex cultural belief system, their folk meaning varying in different social-psychological contexts. For example, the subjective meaning of belief in *karma* may range from a fatalistic attitude to hope and expectations; from a sense of helplessness to faith in action (Gokhale, 1961). The same can be said about attribution to God. Second, the relationship between cosmic beliefs and health status is mediated by many other social-psychological-environmental factors. Research studies which take into consideration a host of these variables can probably unravel the missing links between beliefs and recovery. To our knowledge no such work has been done in the past. We are only beginning to understand the role of cultural and personal belief systems and it is a long way before we can make any definitive statements.

What conclusions can be drawn from these studies? Some of the findings clearly stand out, providing useful insights into the way Indian rural, poor, uneducated patients deal with their own health problems. First, all these patients are actively engaged in constructing the meaning and causality of their problems. Many of their explanatory models are rooted in the cultural belief system, which clearly determines how they will deal with the crisis. Second, the patients' own representation of the disease is not only contingent on its medical aspects, but also on the cultural meaning of the illness experience. They rarely attribute their health problems to factors like virus, heredity or environmental pollution, as was observed in Western studies, but viewed it as a transcending experience. Third, it is against this backdrop that the traditional healers play an important role in the psychological well-being of patients. India has more than 5 million faith healers and their services in providing relief to people suffering from chronic diseases cannot be overlooked. Faith healing in combination with biomedical treatment can be a potent treatment regimen for chronic diseases. However, it remains to be seen how medical services and traditional medicinal/healing services can be integrated into a unified health care system.

REFERENCES

Agrawal, M. and Dalal, A. K. (1993). Beliefs about the world and recovery from myocardial infarction. *Journal of Social Psychology*, 133, 385-94.
Bishop, G. D. (1991). Understanding the understanding of illness: Lay disease representations. In R. T. Croyle (Ed.), *The mental representation of health and illness* (pp. 32-59). New York: Springer-Verlag.
Blaxter, M. (1983). The cause of disease: Women talking. *Social Science and Medicine*, 17, 59-69.
Bulman, J. R. and Wortman, C. B. (1977). Attribution of blame and coping in the 'real world'. Severe accident victims react to their lot. *Journal of Personality and Social Psychology*, 35, 351-63.
Dalal, A. K., Kohli, N. and Agrawal, M. (1999). *Reactions to hospitalization*. Unpublished manuscript, University of Allahabad, Allahabad.
Dalal, A. K. and Pande, N. (1988). Psychological recovery of the accident victims with temporary and permanent disability. *International Journal of Psychology*, 23, 25-40.
Dalal, A. K. and Singh, A. K. (1992). Role of causal and recovery beliefs in psychological adjustment to a chronic disease. *Psychology and Health: An International Journal*, 6, 193-203.
Dull, V. T. and Skokan, L. A. (1995). A cognitive model of religion's influence on health. *Journal of Social Issues*, 51, 49-64.
Gokhale, B. G. (1961). *Indian thought throughout the ages: A study of some dominant concepts*. Bombay: Asia Publishing House.
Jain, U. C. (1988). Attribution-behaviour relationship in the context of learned helplessness. In A. K. Dalal (Ed.), *Attribution theory and research* (pp. 98-111). New Delhi: Wiley Eastern.

Joshi, M. S. (1995). Lay explanations of the causes of diabetes in India and the U.K. In I. Markova and R. M. Farr (Eds), *Representations of health, illness and handicap* (pp. 163-88). Chur, Switzerland: Harwood.
Joshi, P. C. (1988). Traditional medical systems in Central Himalayas. *Eastern Anthropologist*, 41, 77-86.
——. (2000). Relevance and utility of traditional medical systems (TMS) in the context of a Himalayan tribe. *Psychology and Developing Societies*, 12 (1).
Kakar, S. (1982). *Shamans, mystic and doctors: A psuchological inquiry into India and its healing traditions*. Delhi: Oxford university Press.
Kleinman, A. (1988). *The illness narratives: Suffering, healing and human condition*. New York: Basic Books.
Kohli, N. and Dalal, A. K. (1998). Culture as a factor in causal understanding of illness: A study of cancer patients. *Psychology and Developing Societies*, 10(2), 115-29.
Leventhal, H. (1984). Behavioural medicine: Psychology in health care. In D. Mechanic (Ed.), *Handbook of health, health care and health professions* (Vol. 2, pp. 709-43). New Jersey: Erlbaum.
Levin, P. and Vanderpool, D. (1991). Physical illness, the individual and the coping process. *Psychiatry in Medicine*, 22, 156-68.
Misra, G. and Misra, S. (1986). Effect of socio-economic background on pupils' attributions. *Indian Journal of Current Psychological Research*, 1, 77-88.
Paranjpe, A. C. (1984). *Theoretical psychology: The meeting of east and west*. New York: Plenum Press.
——. (1998). *Self and identity in modern psychology and Indian thought*. New York: Plenum Press.
Sinha, D. (1988). The family scenario in a developing country and its implications for mental health: The case of India. In P. Dasen, J. W. Berry and A. Sartorious (Eds), *Health and cross-cultural psychology: Towards applications*. Newbury Park: Sage.
Sinha, Y., Jain, U. C. and Pandey, J. (1980). Attribution of causality to poverty. *Journal of Social and Economic Studies*, 33, 435-41.
Taylor, S. E. (1983). Adjustment to threatening events. *American Psychologist*, 38, 1161-73.
WHO. (1996). *World health report*. Geneva: WHO Publications.

15

Near-death Experience in South India: A Systematic Survey in Channapatna

SATWANT PASRICHA

Some persons after recovering from a close encounter with death from illness or other life-threatening situations, report unusual affective, cognitive and seemingly transcendental experiences. These have been frequently referred to as 'near-death experiences' (NDEs).

In the past two decades a number of reports on NDEs have been published from the West—(Greyson and Stevenson, 1980; Moody, 1975; Ring, 1980; Sabom, 1982; Owens, Cook and Stevenson, 1990; Morse, Conner and Tyler, 1985) as well as from India—(Osis and Haraldsson, 1986; Singh, Bagadia, Pradhan and Acharya, 1988; Pasricha and Stevenson, 1986; Pasricha, Forthcoming). Most (Greyson and Stevenson, 1980; Moody, 1975; Ring, 1980; Sabom, 1982; Owens, Cook and Stevenson, 1990; Morse, Conner and Tyler, 1985; Osis and Haraldsson, 1986; Singh, Bagadia, Pradhan and Acharya, 1988) of these researches are based on hospital populations consisting of specific groups of patients or volunteers. However, there is a general paucity of studies concerning the prevalence of NDEs. Except for one survey each from India (Pasricha, Forthcoming) and the US (Gallup, 1982), there are almost no reports of epidemiological studies, as far as the literature shows, published from any part of the world. The present paper is another contribution in this direction and reports the prevalence and characteristics of NDEs in an area of the Karnataka state of South India.

MATERIAL AND METHODS

The Population

In order to determine the prevalence rate of NDEs and to study the features of subjects of the identified cases, a systematic survey was conducted in taluk Channapatna, district Bangalore, of the Karnataka state. Channapatna is one of the eleven taluks (roughly corresponding to tehsils in North India and counties in the US and UK) or subdivisions of the Bangalore district; it is situated 60 kilometres south-west of Bangalore on the Bangalore–Mysore road. This taluk was chosen for (a) the nature of its population (it consists of both rural and urban populations) and (b) operational feasibility (it was easily accessible from NIMHANS). Channapatna consists of 145 villages, of which 12 have been listed as uninhabited (Census of India, 1981). By using appropriate sampling techniques, 17 survey villages were drawn from the 1981 census lists. The outcome of the survey in 13 villages[1] will be reported in the present paper.

Two thousand four hundred and thirty-nine households were chosen by using voters' registration lists; one member from each household was designated as the target respondent and interviewed. The person interviewed was usually the head of the household, but a younger member was interviewed when the target respondent was not available. Of the 2,439 target respondents, 232 had either moved out of the village or were not available at the time of our visits (the respondents who were not available on two call-backs after the first scheduled visit, were not contacted further). Hence, a total of 2,207 respondents were available for the interviews. Before conducting the individual interviews, the school teachers and village leaders were contacted to explain the purpose of our visits, to enlist their cooperation and seek their consent for conducting the survey.

Demographic Characteristics of the Respondents

The ages of the respondents ranged between 16 and 90 years; 1,321 (60 per cent) of them were males. One thousand seven hundred and six

---

[1] Due to some operational difficulties, the survey was discontinued after completion of work in four villages. It was resumed after a gap of about 18 months. Hence, the findings of four villages surveyed earlier have been separately reported elsewhere (Pasricha, Forthcoming).

(77 per cent) were illiterate or functionally illiterate, 111 (5 per cent) had attended a primary school, 170 (8 per cent) had gone to a middle school and 253 (10 per cent) had education up to high-school or beyond (28 were college graduates).

Four hundred and nine (64 per cent) of the respondents were cultivators, 190 (9 per cent) were housewives, 392 (28 per cent) were labourers and 46 (2 per cent) were caste labourers,[2] 63 (3 per cent) had a shop or had their own business, 41 (2 per cent) were in some service (government or private sector), 22 (1 per cent) were not engaged in any occupation due to old age and 13 (0.6 per cent) were students.

A majority of the respondents (60 per cent) belonged to the lower middle socio-economic class, 211 (10 per cent) to the middle or upper middle class, while 664 (30 per cent) came from the lower socio-economic class. The socio-economic status was appraised by using a standard tool developed for the rural population of India (Pareek and Trivedi, 1964).

The Interviews

The interviews were conducted in two stages. First, with the target respondents for the identification of the NDE cases, and subsequently with the identified subjects and/or their relatives to learn at first hand the details about the experiences.

An interview schedule was administered to each target respondent. In addition to eliciting the usual demographic data, it solicited questions about the respondents' belief, familiarity and knowledge regarding cases in which a person had apparently died and revived. Respondents, who knew of such cases, were asked to give specific information about the location of the subjects. Later, these subjects were interviewed in detail about their experiences; in addition, informants who were present when the subject revived or narrated his experiences were interviewed in as many cases as available. Most of the interviews lasted between 15 and 50 minutes. If the respondents did not have any knowledge of or familiarity with a case, only their demographic details were noted down, which did not take more than 15 minutes; on the other hand, if they knew of some cases and details about them or when the informant happened to be a subject or a subject's relative, the interviews lasted for 50 minutes or longer.

---

[2] For example, a person belonging to the dhobi (washerman) caste did washerman's work and a kumhar (a potter) made pots for his living.

When the subjects were interviewed, they were first allowed to narrate their experiences spontaneously and then specific questions were asked regarding their NDEs. Initially, the subjects were not asked about the possible features; subsequently a checklist was prepared (on the basis of earlier experiences and the previous studies) to elicit specific information about all possible features not mentioned spontaneously.

Criteria for Inclusion of NDE Cases

For determining the prevalence rate of NDEs, the following criteria were applied: (a) the subject must have reported some unusual experiences he had while unconscious or ostensibly dead, (b) the subject must have been a resident of the survey village at the time when the survey was conducted, and (c) the subject must have been alive at the time of the survey.

RESULTS

Belief Familiarity and Knowledge of Revival[3] and NDE Cases

Four hundred and forty-eight (20 per cent) respondents believed that it was possible for a person to die (or almost die), recover from death (or unconscious state) and remember unusual experiences he had had during that time. Four hundred and thirty-six (20 per cent) respondents had heard of one or more such cases, but all of them had not known of specific cases; only 161 (37 per cent) of these had heard of cases in their own village and 70 (16 per cent) of them in other villages. In all, they made references to 42 cases in the survey villages; 15 of the subjects had died long before the survey and one subject had moved out of the village. The remaining 26 subjects were approached for further study, two of whom did not cooperate for interviews. Of the remaining 24 cases, eight (33 per cent) subjects, although seriously ill or thought to be dead,[4] had no NDEs. Table 15.1 shows the distribution of cases of persons who had seemingly died (or nearly died) and revived, and the number of subjects who reported NDEs.

---

[3] The term *revival* was used to describe the condition wherein the subject of a case had ostensibly died and revived; but it was not known to the informants whether or not he had had an NDE.

[4] The villagers generally decide that a person has died by the following signs: failure to respond when name called, cessation of breathing and other movement, no pulse or heartbeat and pallor of skin.

Table 15.1: Prevalence of Revival and NDE Cases in the Survey Villages

Population/Village	1985 (Estimate)*	No. of Revival Cases	No. of NDE Cases
Kudambhalli	3,156**	6 (1.8)	2 (0.6)
Arulasandra	1,398	3 (2.1)	3 (2.1)
Jagadapura	858	1 (1.2)	1 (1.2)
Kondapura	1,062	0 (–)	0 (–)
Garkahalli	1,424	1 (0.7)	1 (0.7)
Neralur	2,131	2 (0.9)	2 (0.9)
Anigere	930	2 (2.2)	2 (2.2)
Sankalagere	1,528	5 (3.3)	1 (0.6)
Aralapura	496**	0 (–)	0 (–)
Siddanahalli	845	1 (1.2)	0 (–)
Mallangere	588	0 (–)	0 (–)
Chakkere	2,544	5 (2.0)	4 (1.6)
Nayidolle	232	0 (–)	0 (–)

Notes: Figures within parentheses show prevalence per 1,000.
  *Estimated annual growth (by Arithmetic Progression [Sunder Rao, 1983]) from 1971 and 1981 census figures.
  **A decrease in population was recorded from 1971 to 1981 census.

The Prevalence of NDE Cases

In all, 16 NDE cases were reported among an estimated population of 17,192 (based on annual arithmetical growth projections of the 1971 and 1981 census), showing a prevalence rate of about one case (0.93) per 1,000 population.

The 16 subjects were interviewed for details of their experiences. The relatives or friends of the subjects were available for interviews in six cases. In addition to the questions about the subject's physical condition, they were asked about their version of what the subject had told them (the informants) about his experiences. The versions of the informants who were not subjects agreed, in general, with the accounts given by the subjects.

Physical Condition and Location of Subjects at the Time of NDE

Seven subjects were reported to have been healthy prior to the NDE, while 9 (56 per cent) subjects were suffering from a mild-to-severe physical illness. Their illness included a wide variety of complaints such as high or low grade fever (4), dysentry (2), typhoid (1), cough and asthma (1) and fits of unconsciousness (1). I was able to confirm the physical condition of five subjects from the informants; informants were not available for the remaining cases. One of the subjects was treated in a nearby hospital and had an NDE on the way back from the hospital, all the other subjects had their experiences while at home. The hospital records of this subject were not available as the episode had occurred several years earlier. The subjects who revived at home, almost certainly had no formal measures of resuscitation available to them.

Demographic Characteristics of the Subjects Who Had NDEs

The median age of the subjects at the time of the NDE was 43.5 years (range 9–97 years) and it was 75 years (range 38–108 years) at the time of our first interview with them; the median time lapse between the NDE and the first interview was 20 years (range 2–70 years). Eleven (69 per cent) of the subjects who reported an NDE were females. Most (62.5 per cent) of the subjects belonged to a lower middle class, four (25 per cent) to the lower and two (12.5 per cent) to the middle socio-economic class. Five (31 per cent) of the subjects were housewives, two (12.5 per cent) were caste labourers (dhobis), three (18.7 per cent) were cultivators, two (12.5 per cent) were in government service and four (25 per cent) were not working. Thirteen (81.3 per cent) of the subjects were illiterate, and one each had been educated up to primary, high-school and inter-mediate college.

Main Features of NDE Cases

As the checklist was introduced at a later stage, the subjects were not asked about all the possible features. Therefore, the data are missing for some analyses. Table 15.2 presents the main features of the subjects of the NDE cases identified during the survey.

Experience of 'other realms': Seventy-one per cent of the subjects seemed to have been to the 'other realms' where they were taken by some messengers or deceased relatives or had gone unaccompanied. Some of them reported having met deceased relatives or some religious figures. The subject appeared before the Yama (the god of the dead), his book (containing a report of one's deeds during terrestrial life which forms the basis of

Table 15.2: Main Features of NDE Cases

Features	N	n	%
Seemed to be in 'other realms'	14		
Taken by some messengers or by deceased relative		10	71
Found himself there; seemed to go alone		4	29
Saw his own physical body	11	0	–
Went to 'a man with a book'	10	7	70
Another person said to be due to die instead of subject	9	1	11
Sent back because of a mistake; subject not scheduled to die yet	11	5	46
Met deceased relatives/acquaintances	12	3	25
Brought back from other realms by messengers or by deceased relatives	9	5	56
Apparently revived through thought of loved living persons or own volition	11	2	18
Sent back by a loved one or an unknown figure, but not because of a mistake	9	1	11
Residual marks on physical body after NDE	9	3	33
Change of attitude towards death	10		
Lost fear of death		2	20
Developed fear of death		1	10
No change		7	70

Note: N represents the number of cases concerning whom a particular feature was inquired about; n refers to the presence of that feature.

judgement for his next destination) was opened, a mistake was discovered (about his being in the other realm) and hence he was sent (or asked to go) back to the terrestrial life.

Reasons and means of reviving: Forty-six per cent of the subjects reported that they were sent back because they were seemingly taken to the other realm by a mistake as they had not yet finished their allotted life-span, or some one else was due to die. However, unlike the North Indian cases, the subject in the present series did not mention the name of the person who was supposed to have died. Three of the subjects reported that they were either sent back by their loved ones or revived of their own volition for the love and responsibility towards the living persons, but not due to a mistake.

Other features: Three of the nine subjects reported that they had been branded on their body in the other realm. (I was able to see a mark in one case and the informants corroborated the subjects' claim of a post-NDE mark in all the three cases.) The basis for getting these marks is viewed differently by the subjects of the south and the North Indian cases. In the North Indian cases, the residual marks, as we refer them, are reported to have resulted when the subjects were forcefully pushed down with some instrument (such as a trident) or by hand. This generally happened to the subjects who resisted coming back from the other realm. On the other hand, in the south Indian cases, it is widely believed that a mark is put on every person when he returns back from the other realm to the terrestrial life. This belief, however, is not supported by the available data.

Of the 11 subjects who were asked whether they had seen their physical body while unconscious or ostensibly dead (out-of-the-body-experience or OBE), none of the subjects reported the presence of this feature. In an earlier series (Pasricha, Forthcoming) of investigation of the south Indian cases, however, the OBE was reported by one subject.

Attitude towards death following NDE: In most (70 per cent) of the cases, the subjects reported no change in their attitude towards death as a result of an NDE. Two subjects lost fear of death, while one subject developed a fear of it following the experience.

DISCUSSION

The prevalence rate of NDEs in the present series was about 1 case per 1,000 persons, whereas it was about two cases per thousand in an earlier series (Pasricha, Forthcoming) when a survey was conducted in four different villages in the same general area. No definite explanation can be offered at this stage for the drop in the prevalence rate, although it is not uncommon for results to change when a larger sample is taken.

Of the 26 revival cases in the present series, 62 per cent of the subjects had reported an NDE. In the earlier study in India (Pasricha, Forthcoming), the revival/NDE ratio was 72 per cent, and in the one reported from America by Sabom (Sabom, 1982), it was 43 per cent. The revival/NDE ratio among Indian cases is therefore higher than that of the American cases. Almost all the Indian cases had their experiences while at home, whereas Sabom's patients were treated in a cardiac unit. It is possible that the location of the patient at the time of crisis and the mode of intervention influence the occurrence of an NDE. The question whether a relationship exists between the type of treatment received and the occurrence (and recall of) NDEs may perhaps be addressed if more data are available. These data could derive from a comparison between the experiences of persons who revived as a result of using specific techniques of resuscitation in a hospital setting and those of persons who revived at home without such formal measures. Furthermore, a comparison of features in a larger series of patients who were judged to have died with patients who were judged only to be 'nearly dead' would improve our understanding of the phenomenon of NDEs.

Among the 12 features compared between the American cases (taken from the, for example, Greyson and Stevenson, 1980; Pasricha and Stevenson, 1986) and Indian cases (North Indian and both series of South Indian cases combined), six features were reported exclusively by the Indian subjects. These were: [the subject was] 'taken to other realms by messengers or someone', 'passed on to the man with a book', 'another person was due to die', [therefore he was] 'brought back by messengers from other realms' [or] 'was sent back because he was mistakenly taken there' and the 'presence of residual marks' on the physical body of the experient on return from the other world. Only one feature, namely, 'panoramic memory or review of [one's] own life' at the time of near-death was reported by the American subjects, but never by Indian ones. The remaining five features—('met deceased relatives/acquaintances', 'saw beings of light or religious figures', 'revived through the thought of the loved living persons', 'were sent back [from the other realm] by a loved one', and 'saw their own physical body' while ostensibly dead) were reported by the subjects of both the Indian as well as the American cases. The last two features were, however, missing when features of the North Indian cases were compared with the American cases (Pasricha and Stevenson, 1986).

The content of the NDEs among the North and the South Indian subjects was generally the same, although some features such as seeing the 'being of light' or religious figures were reported only by the North Indian subjects. This feature, although missing in the subjects of the south Indian cases, was reported by some of the American subjects. On the other hand, a feature (seeing one's own physical body) was not reported by the subjects of the North Indian cases but was reported by one subject among an earlier series of the South Indian cases. In other words, features missing in one series of cases may be found in another (perhaps larger) series of cases in the same culture.

The differences seen within and across cultures may be due to actual variations in experiences of persons living in different geographical regions, or due to differences in the methods of investigation. It is also possible, however, that some of the variations that appear to be 'culture-specific' may, in fact, be due to differences in the understanding or interpretation of an experience in a particular cultural context. For example, the features, review of one's own life' (a characteristic feature of the American cases) and 'meeting a man with a book' (a specific feature of the Indian cases), are both concerned with the review of actions of the experient's terrestrial life. The decision for the Indian subjects to return back from the other realm, however, is taken by the god of the dead (Yama), whereas subjects of the American cases themselves decide to return back. The expression of features in general seems to reflect the behaviour of people in the two cultures. The people in India, by and large, evince an attitude of complete submission to, and accept the decision of, their superiors; whereas the Americans assert themselves and exercise their will in taking decisions.

The commonality in the content of features in different cultures is perhaps indicative of a phenomenon which is shaped by, but transcends cultural beliefs.

Conclusions

The prevalence rate of NDEs in a region (of Bangalore district) of South India was about 1 case per 1,000 persons. Almost all the subjects had had their experiences at home. The ratio of revival and NDEs was appreciably higher than in American subjects, many of whom had their experience while under intensive medical care. The type of condition of the patient (clinically dead versus nearly dead) and the mode of intervention may have a significant role in the emergence of NDEs.

The differences in some features were reported among cases from within India and also between the Indian and the American cases. However, on a closer look, all the differences do not seem to be 'hard' differences. For example, the feature, 'seeing one's physical body' while seemingly dead, was reported *only* by the American subjects when compared with an earlier series of Indian cases (Pasricha and Stevenson, 1986). However, the same feature was reported by one of the subjects of a later investigated series of Indian cases (Pasricha, Forthcoming).

The reporting of different features in different cultures might have resulted from a true difference in the experience, from the understanding of the experience in the experient's cultural context, or from the variations in the techniques of investigation. A larger sample and, if possible, the use of more uniform methods of investigation in different countries will help to clarify the origins of the differences (and similarities) between the features of cases across various cultures.

Acknowledgements

The author would like to thank the following: NIMHANS for support of the project; M. Sudhama Rao (research associate) for assistance in data collection and some of the analyses; the Biostatistics Department, NIMHANS, for the computer analysis of the data; Professor Ian Stevenson, University of Virginia, for valuable suggestions for improvement of the article.

References

Director of Census Operations: *Census of India 1981* Series-9, Karnataka—Bangalore District (Paper 3 of 1984).
Gallup, G. Jr. *Adventures in immortality.* (1982). New York: McGraw-Hill Book Company.
Greyson, B. and Stevenson, I. (1980). The Phenomenology of near-death experiences. *American Journal of Psychiatry,* 137(10), 1193-96.
Moody, R. A. Jr. (1975). *Life after life.* Atlanta: Mockingbird Books.
Morse, M., Conner, D. and Tyler, D. (1985). Near-death experiences in a pediatric population: A preliminary report. *American Journal of Diseases of Children.* 139(6), 595-600.
Osis, K. and Haraldsson, E. (1986). *At the hour of death* (Rev. ed.). New York: Hastings House.
Owens, J. E., Cook, E. W. and Stevenson, I. (1990). Features of 'near-death experience' in relation to whether or not patients were near death. *The Lancet,* 336(8724), 1175.
Pareek, U. and Trivedi, G. (1964). *Manual of the socio-economic status scale (rural).* Delhi: Manasayan.
Pasricha, S. and Stevenson, I. (1986). Near-death experiences in India: A preliminary report. *Journal of Nervous and Mental Disease,* 174(3), 165-70.
Pasricha, S. (Forthcoming). A systematic survey of NDEs in South India. *Journal of Scientific Exploration.*
Ring, K. (1980). *Life at death: A scientific investigation of the near-death experience.* New York: Coward, McCann and Geoghegan.
Sabom, M. (1982). *Recollections of death: A medical investigation.* New York: Harper and Row.
Singh, A. R., Bagadia, V. N., Pradhan, P. V. and Acharya, V. N. (1988). Death, dying and near death experience: Preliminary report on surveying the need and developing the method. *Indian Journal Psychiatry,* 30: 299-306.
Sunder Rao, B. S. S. (1983). *An introduction to biostatistics: A manual of health statistics for medical students.* Vellore: C.M.C.

16

Resilience for Well-being: The Role of Experiential Learning

SWETA SRIVASTAVA AND ARVIND SINHA

The present study attempts to make explorations in the relationships of resilience, happiness and self-esteem with well-being. The study also aims to see the effect of T-group type intervention on the change in the average magnitude of the variables in the study. The study may be treated within the purview of positive psychology. What is positive psychology? From one point of view, it is nothing more than the scientific study of ordinary human strengths and virtues. Positive psychology revisits 'the average person' with an interest in finding out *what works, what is right* and *what is improving*. Positive psychology is thus an attempt to urge the psychologists to adopt a more open and appreciative perspective regarding human potentials, motives and capacities. Sigmund Freud gave importance to the animalistic *id*, whereas contemporary terror management theorists accord prominence to the fear of death or decay. It has been argued by the positive psychologists that the psychologists should focus more attention on the positive aspects of human nature. If psychologists allow themselves to see the best as well as the worst in people, they may derive important new understanding of human nature and its ramification.

The mission of positive psychology is to understand and foster the factors that allow individuals, communities and societies to flourish (Seligman and Csikszentmihalyi, 2000). Positive mental health, according to numerous theorists, facilitates approach behaviour (Cacioppo, Gardner and Berntson, 1999; Davidson, 1993; Watson, Wiese, Vaidya and Tellegen, 1999) or continued action. From this perspective, experiences of positive affect prompt individuals to engage with their environments and partake in activities, many of which are adaptive and 'effective' for the individuals, its species, or both.

THE SETTING

The study was conducted at an institute which maintains a very high level of academic pressure through high standards of teaching and learning, as well as high performance and expectations. The students, who were also the participants in the study, come from all over the country and also from abroad. They are usually the very high rank performers at their previous institutions; however, as and when they join their current institute, they start competing with the cohort wherein each person was almost the best in the previous place of study. So, it becomes a competition between the bests. There being a relative grading system, someone will have to stand at the lowest rank in a given lot of performers. This creates a lot of cognitive dissonance as to how an erstwhile best can be a lesser mortal now. Things are made worse due to their not so ripe chronological age and expectations running high both at the institute as well as back home. Such a state of affairs creates a psychological situation of existence that is marked by apprehension, uncertainties, anxiety and a lowered self-esteem. Compensatory behaviours align them to manage a brave face on the surface and defensive reactions are not very uncommon. The whole setting puts a tremendous amount of pressure on the person who has to keep siphoning large amounts of physical and psychological energy in order to roll back to the previous performance level or to maintain a consistency in the self-concept, and this might continue up to four years or even more in isolated cases. There is a very high probability that such a state of existence tells upon the psychological well-being of the person, and consequently there is a need to understand, predict and control the antecedents and consequences of psychological well-being specific to such a setting which is engaged in the commendable task of preparing some of the brightest future scientists, technocrats and other agents of social change. It was with this view that the present investigators got motivated to conduct the study.

Apparently, psychological well-being depends on a number of factors that can be a part of the personality, the personal history of various positive and negative reinforcements or even the genetic configuration. Not all of them could be dealt with in a study like the present one. However, if one tries to find out some of the learnable or trainable aspects of life and the realities around which the course of life is charted, resilience as a variable may be a choice. Resilience is a capability which can be learnt on the person's initiative or training is also possible to be imparted on the institutional initiative. It is plausible to expect that resilience would positively contribute to psychological well-being, self-esteem and happiness. Apart from other possibilities, the T-group learning method is known for its efficacy in enhancing the sensitivity and skills of a person in dealing with affective components of human existence and thereby enabling and empowering the individual to have a more effective dealing with his/her own negativities and the personally relevant aspects of the environment.

THE VARIABLES IN THE STUDY

Well-being

Well-being is a complex construct that concerns optimal psychological functioning and experience. In part, this reflects the increasing awareness that just as positive affect is not the opposite of negative affect (Cacioppo and Berntson, 1999), well-being too is not the absence of mental illness.

For more than 20 years, the study of psychological well-being has been guided by two primary conceptions of positive functioning. One formulation, traceable to Bradburn's (1969) seminal work, has distinguished between positive and negative affect and defined happiness as the balance between the two. The second conception, which has gained prominence among sociologists, emphasizes life satisfaction as the key indicator of well-being.

Keyes, Ryff and Shmotkin (2002) have extended these distinctions, which are referred to as subjective well-being (SWB) and Psychological Well-being (PWB). Their basic suggestion is that the studies of SWB have repeatedly included not only affective indicators of happiness (hedonic well-being), but also cognitive assessments of life satisfaction. SWB consists of three main components: positive affect, negative affect and life satisfaction (Andrews and Withey, 1976; Campbell, Converse and Rodgers, 1976; Diener, 1984). Positive affect consists of pleasant emotions or feelings such as joy and happiness, whereas negative affect consists of unpleasant feelings or emotions such as sadness and fear. Life satisfaction refers to a cognitive, judgemental process—a global assessment of one's life as a whole

(Diener, 1984). Positive effects result from commitment to and striving for positive incentives, whereas negative affect results from the preoccupation with trying to avoid negative incentives. Although both approaches assess well-being, they address different features of what it means to be well: SWB involves more global evaluations of affect and life quality, whereas PWB examines perceived thriving vis-à-vis the existential challenges of life (for example, pursuing meaningful goals, growing and developing as a person, establishing quality ties to others).

Ryff (1989b) suggested a multi-dimensional model of PWB that distilled six psychological dimensions of challenged thriving. In combination, these dimensions encompass a breadth of wellness that includes positive evaluations of oneself and one's past life (self-acceptance), a sense of continued growth and development as a person (personal growth), the belief that one's life is purposeful and meaningful (purpose in life), the possession of quality relations with others (positive relations with others), the capacity to manage effectively one's life and surrounding world (environmental mastery) and a sense of self-determination (autonomy).

Resilience

Resilience is defined as a pattern of psychological activity which consists of a motive to be strong in the face of inordinate demands, the goal-directed behaviour of coping and rebounding (or resiling) and of accompanying emotions and cognitions. It is a dynamic phenomenon influenced by both the internal characteristics of the individual and various external life contexts, circumstances and opportunities. Resilience is not a trait that people either have or do not have. It involves behaviours, thoughts and actions that can be learned and developed in anyone.

According to Kobasa (1979), the secret to successfully meeting life's crises seems to lie in the three personality characteristics, namely: (a) commitment, i.e., a tendency to involve oneself in whatever one is doing; (b) control, i.e., a tendency to feel and act as if one is influential; and (c) challenge, i.e., a belief that life is changeable and to view this as an opportunity rather than a threat. Factors contributing to resilience include: (a) having caring and supportive relationships within and outside the family; (b) the capacity to make realistic plans and take steps to carry them out; (c) a positive view of yourself and confidence in your strengths and abilities; (d) skills in communication and problem solving; and (d) the capacity to manage strong feelings and impulses. All of these are factors that people can develop in them. The interest in research on resilience in relation to well-being continues. Beasley, Thompson and Davidson (2003) suggest a buffering model in which cognitive hardiness is postulated to moderate the effects of emotional coping or adverse life events on psychological distress. Tugade and Fredrickson (2004) used a multi-method approach in three studies to predict that resilient people use positive emotions to rebound from, and find positive meaning in, stressful encounters. They found that the experience of positive emotions contributed, in part, to participants' abilities to achieve efficient emotion regulation, demonstrated by accelerated cardiovascular recovery from negative emotional arousal, and by finding positive meaning in negative circumstances.

Happiness

Happiness is a pleasant emotional experience, the affective component of SWB (Andrews and Withey, 1976; Bradburn, 1969; Campbell, Converse and Rodgers, 1976; Diener, 1984). Bradburn and Caplovitz (1965) conducted a pioneering study on American people's quality of life and their PWB. They found that positive and negative feeling states were not correlated with each other, though both were correlated individually with general measures of happiness.

Empirical studies have led to identification of various factors related to happiness such as self-esteem, internal locus of control, social relationships, being in love and being loved, friendship and spending more time with friends, finding meaning in life, having a job, accomplishment at work, positive evaluation of one's health and even the political system under which people live may influence a person's happiness. There is a fairly impressive and long-established literature on trait correlates of happiness. DeNeve and Cooper (1998) reported meta-analysis of 137 personality traits and SWB. Those most closely associated were: repressive–defensiveness, trait emotional stability, locus of control, hardiness, positive affectivity, self-esteem and leisure.

Self-esteem

Self-esteem is a socio-psychological construct that assesses an individual's attitudes and perceptions of self-worth. Self-esteem refers to the extent to which a person believes him/herself to be capable, significant, worthy, successful and the extent to which a positive or negative attitude is held towards the self (Coopersmith, 1967; Kling, Hyde, Showers and Buswell, 1999). Individual assessments of self-esteem are formed through two interrelated processes. First, individuals compare their social identities, opinions and abilities with others. To the extent that individuals feel that they are inferior to those with whom they interact, their self-esteem will be negatively affected. Second, individuals assess themselves through their interaction with others. People learn to see themselves as others believe them to be. If significant others do not think highly of an individual, that individual will come to think poorly of himself or herself. This is referred to as the 'reflected appraisal' of one's self-worth (Rosenberg and Pearlin, 1978).

A person with high self-esteem is more likely to view an insecure work situation as challenging than as threatening and therefore avoid experiencing job insecurity. Brockner (1988) has advanced a hypothesis that persons with low self-esteem are generally more susceptible to environmental and, in particular, organizational events than are persons with high self-esteem. Ryff (1989a) proposes that some factors of well-being, in particular self-acceptance, environmental mastery and purpose in life, are highly correlated with self-esteem. In occupational stress studies, self-esteem has also been regarded as an outcome variable. As Judge and Bono (2001) have stated, self-esteem may be more susceptible to situational influences than other traits. According to Major, Cooper, Cozzarelli, Richards and Zubek (1998), self-esteem may be thought of as a core resource that contributes to a resilient personality. A person with a resilient personality has a positive view of him or her, a sense of control and an optimistic outlook on the future. Although there could be many correlates of self-esteem, the present research endeavour focuses on well-being, resilience and happiness as its major correlates.

T-GROUP TRAINING (THE EXPERIENTIAL LEARNING)

A T-group (the 'T' stands for training) is a group activity in which one gives and receives feedback about affective or emotional (and other) reactions from others. Participants learn about how they are read by others in affective terms and a lot about interpersonal dynamics in general. This enables participants to better understand their own way of functioning in a group and the impact they have on others, which would enable them to become more competent in dealing with difficult interpersonal situations. An important aspect of group activity sessions is to provide a safe environment in which to foster a level of trust between participants so that they may talk personally and honestly about themselves and each other in a free and open manner without fearing any risk. The group's work is primarily process-oriented rather than content-oriented, with a focus on 'here and now' behaviour. The focus tends to be on the feelings and the communication of feelings, rather than on the communication of information, opinions or concepts. Attention is paid to particular behaviours of participants, not on the 'whole person'; feedback is usually non-evaluative and reports on the impact of the behaviour on others. The T-group experience may also be seen as an application of the Johari Window (Luft, 1969) in the sense of opening up the public area, so making the other three areas (hidden, blind and dark/unknown) as small as possible. This is done by regular and honest exchange of feedback, and a willingness to disclose personal feelings, with occasional help, especially with respect to the unknown area, from the facilitator or consultant.

Sources of Change in Groups

The participants in a group setting are likely to experience some changes, which may be based on the following: (*a*) self-observation; (*b*) feedback; (*c*) insight; (*d*) self-disclosure; (*e*) universality; (*f*) group cohesion; (*g*) hope; (*h*) vicarious learning; and (*i*) catharsis.

To recapitulate, the study aimed at making explorations in the relationships of resilience, happiness and self-esteem with well-being, and the impact of T-group type intervention on these variables. The conceptual scheme used in the study is presented in Figure 16.1.

The conceptual scheme was founded on the following assumptions. First, a state of SWB and happiness is by itself desirable. Besides, such states may have a snowball effect on those who come in contact with people having a high magnitude of SWB and happiness. Hence, it may be worthwhile to explore some of the antecedent variables that might lead to such a state. The antecedents that could be identified and included in the study were resilience and self-esteem.

Second, resilience is not a trait that people either have or do not have. It involves behaviours, thoughts and actions that can be learned and

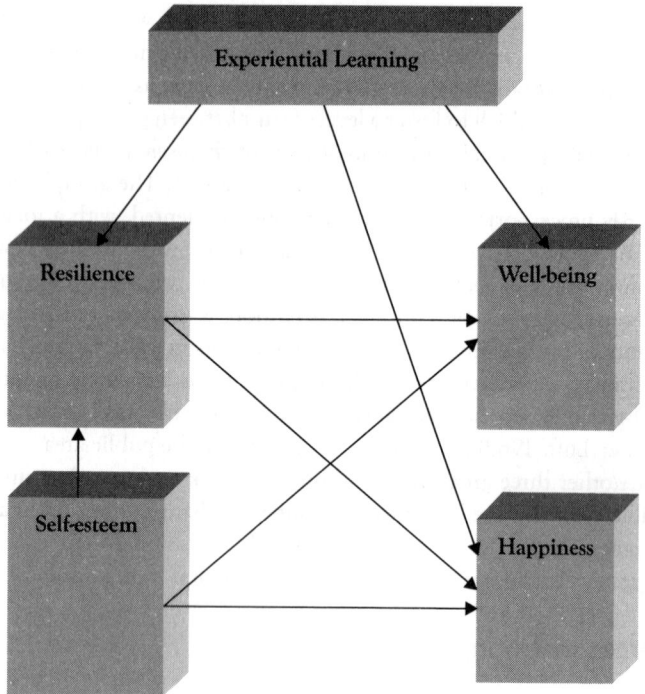

Figure 16.1: Initial Conceptual Schemes

Source: Authors.

developed in anyone. Therefore, it could be regarded as an important variable if it contributes to well-being and happiness because it is amenable to change through learning, training and development, even through self development.

Third, self-esteem refers to an individual's sense of self-worth or the magnitude of a favourable attitude towards the self. It is widely assumed that self-esteem functions much like a trait and is likely to be stable across time within individuals. It was hypothesized that self-esteem may contribute to well-being and happiness and possibly also to resilience. A reason could be that a person having high self-esteem may not easily yield to pressures and thus might develop strategies and skills facilitating resilience, which in turn would contribute to increased well-being and happiness.

Hypotheses and Research Questions

Specifically, the following hypotheses and research questions were postulated:

Hypotheses

1. Resilience would be positively related to well-being.
2. Resilience would be positively related to happiness.
3. Well-being would be positively related to happiness.
4. Self-esteem would be positively related to resilience, well-being and happiness.
5. Experiential learning would significantly increase the magnitude of resilience, well-being and happiness.
6. Experiential learning may not have a significant effect in terms of increase or decrease in self-esteem as self-esteem is conceptualized to be functioning as a trait and thus may remain invariant across time.

Research Questions

In addition to the above mentioned hypothesis, some research questions were also identified to facilitate the course of research and data analysis. They were as follows:

1. Experiential learning would cause a perceived shift (increase or decrease) in variables of self-disclosure, resilience, well-being, self-esteem and happiness.
2. Experiential learning would cause a perceived shift (increase or decrease) in the intensity of group work.
3. Experiential learning would cause a perceived shift (increase or decrease) in the effectiveness of group work.
4. Experiential learning would cause a perceived shift (increase or decrease) in the contribution to the group work.
5. Experiential learning would cause a perceived shift (increase or decrease) in the contribution to the effectiveness of group work.
6. There would be a significant difference between subjective self-rating and group ratings of the individual's self-disclosure, resilience, well-being, self-esteem and happiness.

Method

Sample

The sample consisted of 30 male undergraduate students belonging to a premier technological institution located in North India. [(Mean age = 20.13, SD age = 0.81 (Minimum age = 19, Maximum age = 23)]. All the students in the sample were participating in a course on organizational behaviour in which experiential learning in a T-group setting over a period of nearly 90 days, out of about 115 days of total course duration, was required.

Measures

The data were obtained on two time points with an interval of nearly three months. Data were obtained on the following measures:

Self-esteem. Self-esteem was measured through a 10-item questionnaire with a four-point scale, which was based on Rosenberg (1985). An illustrative item is: 'I am able to do things as well as most other people'. (Strongly agree = 1, Agree = 2, Disagree = 3, Strongly disagree = 4).

Well-being. Well-being was measured through an 85 items scale with six-point response category that was based on the work of Ryff (1989b; personal correspondence, 2003). An illustrative item is: 'I have not experienced many warm and trusting relationships with others' (reverse coded). The response categories were: Strongly Disagree = 1, Disagree Somewhat = 2, Disagree Slightly = 3, Agree Slightly = 4, Agree Somewhat = 5, Strongly Agree = 6.

Happiness. Happiness was measured through a 'face pattern' pictorial measure based on the work of Andrews and Withey (1976). It consisted of seven face outlines representing the feeling states from the most happy to least happy. The participants were asked the question: 'Here are some faces expressing your various feelings. Below each is a letter. Which face comes closest to expressing how you feel about [your life as a whole]?'

Resilience. Resilience was measured through a 29 items, five-point scale, which was based on the work of Klohnen (1996; personal correspondence, 2003). An illustrative item is: 'Several times a week I feel as if something dreadful is about to happen'. (Reversed scored); Disagree Strongly = 1, Disagree = 2, Neutral/Mixed = 3, Agree = 4, Agree Strongly = 5.

Additional measures. In addition to the above mentioned four measures, data were collected on some aspects that are usually considered to be a part of the experiential learning in a T-group type setting. They included the following: realization of 'who am I'; location and identification of the processes (as against content); ability to work with feelings (as against cognitions); ability to focus on here and now (versus there and then).

Further, data were also obtained through the self-ratings on the perception of the extent of the following at the time of first data collection and the second data collection: self-disclosure non-risk variety; self-disclosure risk variety; resilience; well-being; self-esteem; happiness; intensity of group work; effectiveness of group work; my contribution to the group work; my contribution to the effectiveness of the group work. Additionally, perceived group and personal ratings were obtained on the following: self-disclosure; resilience; well-being; self-esteem; happiness.

Procedure

The data were collected through structured questionnaire on two time points, with a gap of nearly three months in between. The participants were participating in a course on organizational behaviour in which experiential learning in a T-group type setting is required. The data collected at first time point provided for the baseline or the initial state of the participants on the variables included in the study. After the first phase data were collected, the participants started participating in experiential learning in a T-group type setting which was facilitated by the instructor who had an experience of nearly two decades in working through experiential learning. Having undergone the experiential learning phase for about three months, the second phase data were obtained from the same set of participants on the initially included variables plus some additional variables pertaining specifically to increased awareness through experiential learning. It may be noted that in phase one, 36 participants participated, out of which three were females. In the second phase, three male participants did not show up on the day of data collection. Besides, since the females constituted a highly disproportionate low ratio of the total sample dominated by males, their responses were omitted at the final stage of data collection.

Debriefing. The participants were informed before the commencement of the course of the possibility of such data collection and they were assured that this will not affect their grades in any way. After the course concluded and the examination results were announced, the participants were thoroughly debriefed about the process of analysis and the overall results. The individual standing vis-à-vis the group was made available to all the participants who desired to know about their status.

RESULTS AND DISCUSSION

It would be recalled that the study included four variables in the main. They are resilience, happiness, self-esteem and well-being. Out of these, happiness was mapped through a single item pictorial measure, whereas the other three variables were measured through multi-item questionnaires.

Exploring the Underlying Dimensions of the Construct: The Factors Analysis Results

The three questionnaires measuring resilience, self-esteem and well-being were subjected to factor analysis (principal factoring with iterations and oblique rotations using the principal axis [PA] two option of the SPSS-X statistical analysis package programme). Factor analysis results may be obtained from authors on request. Brief description of the factors pertaining to respective measures follows.

Form 1: Self- esteem. This questionnaire consisted of 10 items. Factor analysis resulted in two significant factors, which were named as follows: (*a*) Positive Self-esteem (consisting of four items) and (*b*) Feeling of Worth (consisting of four items).

Form 2: Well-being. This questionnaire consisted of 85 items. Factor analysis resulted in six significant factors, which were named as follows: (*a*) Close Relation with Others (consisting of two items); (*b*) Autonomy (consisting of three items); (*c*) Planned_Accomplishment (consisting of two items); (*d*) Purpose in Life (consisting of two items); (*e*) Positive Relation with Others (consisting of three items) and (*f*) Environmental Mastery (consisting of two items).

Form 3: Happiness. As mentioned earlier, this was single item pictorial measure and therefore was not subjected to factor analysis.

Form 4: Resilience. This questionnaire consisted of 29 items. Factor analysis resulted in three significant factors, which were named as follows: (*a*) Tenacity and Self-assurance (consisting of five items); (*b*) Public Self-confidence (consisting of three items) and (*c*) Happy Outlook (consisting of three items).

The study included observations at two time points. Since the changes in the primary relationship among the variables at time point two were not of interest for the present purposes, the basic statistics pertaining to the data obtained at time point one only are presented (Appendix A).

Addressing the Hypotheses and Research Questions

In order to address the hypotheses 1-4, Multiple Regression Analysis (MRA) was used. For addressing hypotheses five and six, and the remaining research questions (1-6), the T-test for correlated means was used. The individual results are sequentially described below. In the interest of brevity of presentation and conservation of print space, the tables are not presented in the chapter. They may be obtained from the authors on request.

Results pertaining to hypothesis 1 showed that: (*a*) Public Confidence is a positive predictor of Close Relations with Others. This indicates that those who are good and confident in public setting are likely to be good in entering into close relationship with others as well. Apparently, maintenance of close relationship provides an additional buffer that may be needed for well-being and here, resilience seems to contribute; (*b*) Happy Outlook and Tenacity and Self-assurance are positive predictors of Planned Accomplishment; (*c*) Happy Outlook is a positive predictor of Positive Relations with Others. Taken together, there seems to be ample evidence to suggest that resilience is a significant variable that might contribute at least to some aspects of well-being. Since resilience is conceptualized as a variable amenable to change through learning and training, it may be a good idea for the individuals to seek opportunities, ways and means to develop resilience and organizations and employers may do well by focusing on resilience enhancement programmes; lastly, (*d*) Tenacity and Self-assurance emerged as a positive predictor of Purpose in Life. Apparently, there seems to be some merit in the old adage 'never ever give up' and 'believe in yourself'. It appears that a tenacious and self-assured stance contributes to Planned Accomplishments, and a sense of Purpose in Life. None of the three factors of resilience turned out to be a significant predictor of perceived happiness. None of the factors of well-being were a significant predictor of happiness either.

Further it was found that: (a) Feeling of Worth and Positive Self-esteem were negative predictors of Tenacity and Self-assurance; (b) none of the two factors of self-esteem turned out to be a significant predictor of Public Self-confidence; and (c) Positive Self-esteem and Feeling of Worth turned out to be negative predictors of Happy Outlook. Additionally: (a) none of the factors of Self-esteem turned out to be significant predictor of Close Relation with Others, Autonomy and Planned Accomplishment; however, (b) Feeling of Worth was a negative predictor of Purpose in Life; (c) Positive Self-esteem was a negative predictor of Positive Relations with Others; and (d) Feeling of Worth was a negative predictor of Environmental Mastery. None of the factors of self-esteem turned out to be significant predictor of happiness. Self-esteem was a variable in the study that seemed to be behaving in an unexpected manner. The findings are baffling and suggest the need to explore further into the nature and dynamics of self-esteem in relation to the other variables in the study, may be with a bigger and varied sample. It may not be said with confidence yet, but perhaps there is a need to evaluate the effect of culture on the relationship between self-esteem and some of its anticipated consequences. There are some indications available in this direction; for instance, Diener and Diener (1995) found that the size of the correlation between self-esteem and life satisfaction was greater in individualistic nations than in collectivistic nations, perhaps because the former place greater emphasis on autonomy and internal feelings.

The results pertaining to the effects of experiential learning on resilience, well-being and happiness showed that all the three factors of resilience, namely, Tenacity and Self-esteem, Public Self-confidence and Happy Outlook registered an increase in the mean score as a result of experiential learning in the T-group type setting. Two out of the six factors of well-being, namely, Purpose in Life and Positive Relations with Others registered a significant increase in their mean scores as a function of experiential learning. There was an increase in the mean happiness score of the participants as a function of experiential learning. By and large, the experiential learning in a T-group type setting seemed to have a positive effect on the mean scores of well-being, as well as resilience and happiness.

The sixth hypothesis was advanced under the assumption that experiential learning will not cause a significant difference in the mean score of self-esteem as self-esteem is normally conceptualized to be functioning as a trait and thus is likely to remain invariant across time. However, the results pertaining to this hypothesis showed that there was a change in the mean scores of the two factors of self-esteem, namely, Positive Self-esteem and Feeling of Worth. Surprisingly, the change seemed to occur in a negative direction, i.e., self-esteem registered a lower mean score after the experiential learning.

After examining the changes in the actual mean score (based on the questionnaire responses obtained at two different time points), it was decided to examine the changes in the mean score of the core variables in the study as well as in a few other variables relevant to a T-group type setting, namely, self-disclosure, intensity of group work, effectiveness of group work, contribution to the group work and contribution to the effectiveness of group work. The results showed that an increase was perceived by the participants on these variables. It may be noted that increase after the experiential learning intervention was recorded on the questionnaire measures as well as the subjective perception measures of well-being, resilience, happiness and self-esteem. This may be taken as a cross check and reconfirmation in the efficacy of experiential learning.

Further Analyses

Additionally, it was also planned to see the differences between the self-ratings and the small groups' ratings on the core variables. The following descriptions are related to these concerns, which pertain to the research questions 1–5.

The last research question, i.e., question six was related to difference between subjective self-ratings and group ratings on self-disclosure, resilience, well-being, self-esteem and happiness. The results showed that no subjective differences were reported on the variables.

After going through the planned analysis according to the hypotheses and research questions, it occurred to the investigators that there could be an alternative way of looking at hypothesis 3, which states that well-being would be positively related to happiness. The results obtained showed that none of the factors of well-being was a significant predictor of happiness. This was difficult to understand for the investigators and therefore it was decided to explore further into the relationship between well-being and happiness. Consequently, regression analysis was done using the factors of well-being as the criteria for happiness as the predictor. This, essentially, was testing the hypothesis 3 the other way round. The results thus obtained showed that happiness emerged as significant positive predictor for three out of six factors of well-being, namely, Close Relations with Others, Autonomy and Purpose in Life. The results seem to obtain support from the work of Wessmen and Ricks (1996) who found that happy men were involved with a large number of goals and purposes, whereas unhappy men were uncommitted to goals and had few long-term prospects. It was interesting to note that rather than well-being predicting happiness, it was the happiness that turned out to be a significant predictor of the three dimensions of well-being. Thus, the results were indicative of the fact that happiness contributes to some aspects of well-being that are rather close to individual, as compared to the aspects of well-being that go beyond the individuals' existence per se and seem to be more related with adjustment with the environment. Although the idea needs to be investigated further, there is an indication that well-being and happiness may require to be treated as two distinct constructs with a directional and positive effect coming from happiness to well-being. Happiness did not emerge as a significant predictor for Planned Accomplishments, Positive Relations with Others and Environmental Mastery. Similar to the above, indications were also observed when the results pertaining to (a part of) hypothesis 4 suggested insignificant contribution of self-esteem to happiness. On the lines of above mentioned approach, it was decided to see the strength of association of happiness as a predictor of self-esteem. The result indeed showed that happiness was a significant predictor of self-esteem. However, it turned out to be a negative predictor.

Again, the results pertaining to hypothesis 2 had shown that resilience was not a significant predictor of happiness. However, further explorations showed that happiness was a significant predictor of all the three factors of resilience, namely, Tenacity and Self-assurance, Public Self-confidence and Happy Outlook. That happiness was a predictor of Happy Outlook may not be a great finding by itself, however, since happiness was measured through a different instrument (a pictorial one), this finding may be at least taken as a validation of the pictorial measure. Nonetheless, happiness did predict the Public Self-confidence, a dimension of resilience, which indicates that happiness may contribute to at least some aspect of resilience. Similar findings have been reported by Klohnen (1996) where she has suggested that some fundamental characteristics of resilience include the ability to be happy and contended with a sense of purpose, a sense of environmental mastery and capacity for warm and trusting relationships.

Regarded as a 'basic building block, a value in terms of which other values are justified' (Braithwaite and Law, 1985, p. 261), happiness may be considered universal but, as stated by Schwarz and Clore (1983), its meaning remains complex and ambiguous. Arguably, happiness deserves further attention of researchers in the area of positive psychology.

Looking at the composite picture presented by the results presented, it appears that happiness is a variable of intriguing nature. Several variables did not seem to contribute to happiness as per the initial hypotheses, however, happiness emerged as a significant predictor of the variables in the study, namely, self-esteem, well-being and resilience. As mentioned earlier, happiness was initially conceptualized to be a 'dependent' variable, which could possibly be enhanced through the direct effects of well-being, resilience and self-esteem, or by way of indirect effects of resilience and self-esteem through well-being. However, the finally obtained results were suggestive of need for a revised conceptual scheme (Figure 16.2).

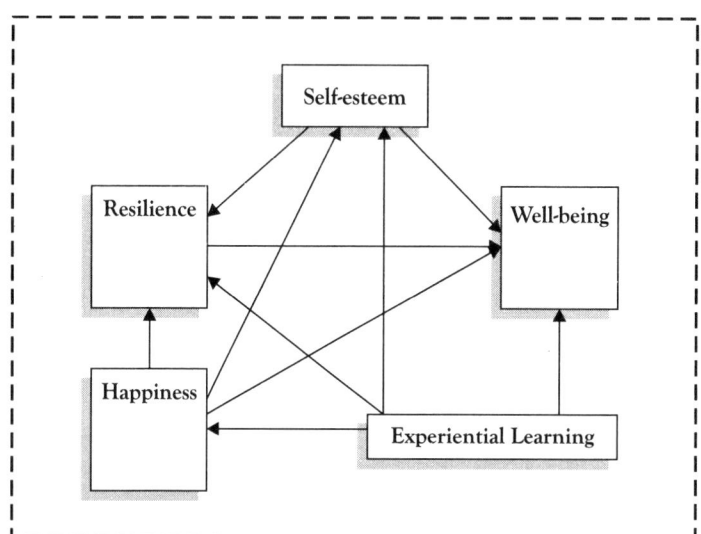

Figure 16.2: Showing the Revised Model of Relationship among Variables Based on Obtained Results

Source: Authors.
Note: The solid lines show positive association and the broken lines show negative association between the variables.

APPENDIX 16A

Table 16A.1: Basic Statistics Pertaining to Time Point One

Variables	F1se	F2se	F2wb	F5wb	F6wb	F11wb	F12wb	F15wb	F1hpp	F1res	F2res	F4res
F1se	(0.78)	0.37	-0.16	-0.33	-0.26	-0.22	-0.66	-0.25	-0.44	-0.51	-0.34	-0.63
F2se		(0.75)	-0.22	-0.32	-0.39	-0.49	-0.24	-0.49	-0.39	-0.51	-0.39	-0.52
F2wb			(0.85)	0.42	0.50	0.18	0.28	0.24	0.40	0.36	0.59	0.33
F4wb				0.15	0.30	0.30	0.23	0.50	0.51	0.56	0.41	0.44
F5wb				(0.75)	0.34	0.12	0.35	0.26	0.43	0.36	0.36	0.37
F6wb					(0.87)	0.38	0.17	0.20	0.32	0.70	0.50	0.69
F11wb						(0.70)	0.30	0.59	0.37	0.57	0.27	0.45
F12wb							(0.82)	0.40	0.30	0.17	0.20	0.47
F15wb								(0.70)	0.21	0.40	0.21	0.38
F1hpp									(NA)	0.58	0.57	0.64
F1res										(0.87)	0.51	0.66

	F2res	F4res
F2res	(0.78)	
F4res	0.50	(0.82)
M	8.7	8.27	8.4	11.97	7.53	9.13	14.17	9.10	5.2	18.9	10.33	10.73
S.D.	2.51	2.29	2.93	3.49	3.19	2.62	3.19	2.28	1.10	4.6	3.09	2.65
No of items	4	4	2	3	2	2	3	2	1	5	3	3

Source: Authors

Notes:
F1se = Positive Self-esteem
F2se = Feeling of Worth
F2wb = Close Relation with Others
F5wb = Autonomy
F6wb = Planned Accomplishment
F11wb = Purpose in Life
F12wb = Positive Relation with Others
F15wb = Environmental Mastery
F1hpp = Happiness
F1res = Tenacity and Self-assurance
F2res = Public Self-confidence
F4res = Happy Outlook

Coefficients appearing on the diagonal in parentheses are Cronbach's alpha Reliability Coefficients for the respective sub-scales.

NA = Not available, due to single item measure.

References

Andrews, F. M. and Withey, S. B. (1976). *Social indicators of well-being: America's perception of quality life*. New York: Plenum.
Beasley, M., Thompson, T. and Davidson, J. (2003). Resilience in response to life stress: The effects of coping style and cognitive hardiness. *Personality and Individual Differences*, 34, 77-95.
Bradburn, N. M. (1969). *The structure of psychological well-being*. Chicago: Aldine.
Bradburn, N. M. and Coplovitz, D. (1965). *Reports on happiness*. Chicago: Aldine.
Braithwaite, J. and Law, H. (1985). Structure of human values: Testing the adequacy of the Rokeach Value Survey. *Journal of Personality and Social Psychology*, 49, 250-63.
Brockner, J. (1988). *Self-esteem at work*. Lexington, MA: Lexington Books.
Cacioppo, J. T. and Berntson, G. G. (1999). The affect system: Architecture and operating characteristics. *Current Directions in Psychological Science*, 8, 133-37.
Cacioppo, J. T., Gardner, W. L. and Berntson, G. G. (1999). The affect system has parallel and integrative processing components: Form follows function. *Journal of Personality and Social Psychology*, 76, 839-55.
Campbell, A., Converse, P. E. and Rodgers, W. L. (1976). *The quality of American life*. Beverly Hills, CA: Sage.
Coopersmith, S. (1967). *The antecedents of self-esteem*. San Francisco: Freeman.
Davidson, R. J. (1993). The neuropsychology of emotion and affective style. In M. Lewis and J. M. Haviland (Eds), *Handbook of emotions* (pp. 143-54). New York: Guildford Press.
DeNeve, K. and Cooper, H. (1998). The happy personality: a meta-analysis of 137 personality traits and subjective well-being. *Psychological Bulletin*, 124, 197-229.
Diener, E. (1984). Subjective well-being. *Psychological Bulletin*, 95, 542-75.
Diener, E. and Diener, M. (1995). Cross-cultural correlates of life satisfaction and self-esteem. *Journal of Personality and Social Psychology*, 68, 653-63.
Judge, T. A. and Bono, J. E. (2001). A rose by any other name: Are self-esteem, generalized self-efficacy, neuroticism, and locus of control indicators of a common construct? In: B. W. Roberts and R. Hogan (Eds), *Personality psychology in the workplace* (pp. 93-118). Washington, DC: American Psychological Association.
Keyes, C. L. M., Ryff, C. and Shmotkin, D. (2002). Optimizing well-being: The empirical encounter of two traditions. *Journal of Personality and Social Psychology*, 82, 1007-22.
Kling, K. C., Hyde, J. S., Showers, C. J. and Buswell, B. N. (1999). Gender differences in self-esteem: A meta-analysis. *Psychological Bulletin*, 125, 470-500.
Klohnen, E. (1996). Conceptual analysis and measurement of the construct of ego-resiliency. *Journal of Personality and Social Psychology*, 70, 1067-79.
Kobasa, S. C. (1979) Stressful life events, personality, and health: An inquiry into hardiness. *Journal of Personality and Social Psychology*, 37, 1-11.
Luft, J. (1969). *Of human interaction*. Palo Alto, CA: National Press.

Major, B., Cooper, M. L., Cozzarelli, C., Richards, C. and Zubek, J. (1998). Personal resilience, cognitive appraisals, and coping: An integrative model of adjustment to abortion. *Journal of Personality and Social Psychology*, 74, 735-52.

Rosenberg, M. (1985). Self-concept and psychological well-being in adolescence. In: R. L. Leahy (Ed.), *The development of the self* (pp. 205-46). Orlando, FL: Academic Press.

Rosenberg, M. and Pearlin, L. I. (1978). Social class and self-esteem among children and adults. *American Journal of Sociology*, 84, 53-77.

Ryff, C. (1989a). Happiness is everything, or is it? Explorations on the meaning of psychological well-being. *Journal of Personality and Social Psychology*, 57, 1069-81.

——. (1989b). In the eye of the beholder: Views of psychological well-being among middle and old age adults. *Psychology and Aging*, 4, 195-210.

Schwarz, N. and Clore, G. L. (1983). Mood, misattribution, and judgments of well-being: Informative and directive functions of affective states. *Journal of Personality and Social Psychology*, 45, 513-23.

Seligman, M. and Csikszentmihalyi, M. (2000). Positive psychology: An Introduction. *American Psychologist*, 55, 5-14.

Tugade, M. M. and Fredrickson, B. L. (2004). Resilient individuals use positive emotions to bounce back from negative emotional experiences. *Journal of Personality and Social Psychology*, 86, 320-33.

Watson, D., Wiese, D., Vaidya, J. and Tellegen, A. (1999). The two general activation systems of affect: Structural findings, evolutionary considerations, and psychobiological evidence. *Journal of Personality and Social Psychology*, 76, 820-38.

Wessman, A. E. and Ricks, D. F. (1996). *Mood and personality*. New York: Holt, Rinehart & Winston.

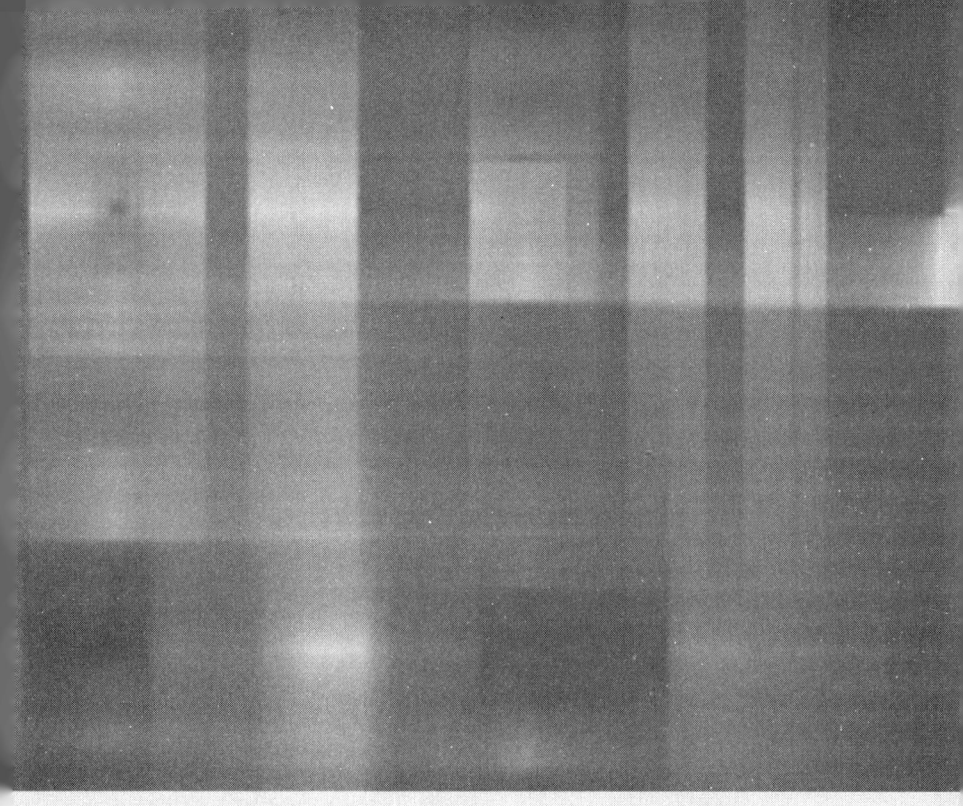

Part V

CHALLENGES AHEAD

Introduction

In the current social scenario, we need to attend to many aspects of health that have a social dimension. Since the issues are multi-disciplinary, they are being dealt with by different groups of scholars coming from diverse disciplines such as sociology, anthropology and preventive and social medicine. Therefore, to have a glimpse of the complexity of the issues, mention of some such issues seems to be in order.

1. The role of changing social structure, particularly the changes in the family structure in which there is a clear move from joint or extended to nuclear family, in determining health status by decreasing social support and depriving from the traditional folk knowledge.
2. The social determination of access to health care. The likelihood of health provisions and facilities for the poor, women and children is low. The problem is increasing with decreasing the safety net for them with decreasing focus on public sector and increase in privatization.
3. Changing nature of 'work' that makes stress and burnout as inevitable components of professional careers leading to risk for health.
4. Emerging worldview and the idea of 'good life' of people that equates it with consumerism and results in faulty lifestyle, leading to health hazards.
5. Deteriorating condition of environment and its adverse impact on health. Particularly the harmful impact of toxic elements introduced by pesticides, increasing pollution of air, water and soil, introduction of toxic metals and other substances in eatables, drinking water and air.
6. Allowing people, particularly children, to work under hazardous conditions.
7. Migration of the people from village to urban centres and increase in the number of slum dwellers.
8. Rise in the diseases of poverty (mal- and under-nutrition related diseases, tuberculosis (TB), etc.) and affluence (hyper tension, CHD, diabetes, etc.).

9. Health problems emerging from use of spurious drugs and unnecessary use of diagnostic procedures and drugs for moneymaking.
10. Protection of the rights of patients as consumers.

The contributions in this section try to examine some of the above challenges that need our attention. The first contribution is on health modernity by Amar Kumar Singh. Modernity is a concept that has been treated in many ways and conveys diverse shades of meaning and diverse images to different people. In fact, there is considerable degree of ambivalence about it. By exploring in the context of various discourses, Singh argues that in the social science scholarship, modernity relates to economic, social and political development. He points out that a democratic political system needs a democratic personality in its citizens. After providing an account of related studies on social change and modernity, Singh concludes that modernity is committed to individual dignity, equality and freedom. It believes in secularism and prefers democratic and socialistic forms of socio-political organization. It combines individual growth with social responsibility. Rationality and humanism are the core underlying foundations of modernity. As a syndrome of personality cum attitudinal traits, it comprises traits such as rationality, internal locus of control, openness to change, work commitment and aspirations. The attitudes include social equality, women's rights, family planning, civic rights, democracy, secularism and political participation. It facilitates personal growth and social responsibility.

Unfortunately, health has been missed in the past formulations of modernity although well-being of the common man is unquestioningly the main pursuit of modernity. Health and well-being decisively influence the efficacy and well-being of the individual. Singh, therefore, proposes the concept of health modernity, which is related to other aspects of modernity, i.e., political, personality and socio-cultural. He recognizes that all the dimensions of modernity are interlinked and affect each other. Singh developed a measure of modernity dealing with health, personality, sociocultural and the political. The present chapter reports the study of health modernity defined as scientific knowledge of attitudes to health and disease leading to behaviour conducive to better physical and mental well-being. He carried out surveys of health modernity in south Bihar. The results showed that the extent of health modernity was very low in the low socio-economic status (SES) group ranging from 0 to 20 per cent in rural and 3 to 23 per cent in urban areas. The tribal and Muslims had the lowest, about 2 per cent. Singh recommends health education, particularly for mothers. Such a step is important to ensure the cherished goal of health for all. While the chapter reports an old empirical data, but the scene has not changed much. The chapter also shows the significance of inter or multi-disciplinary dialogue while working on any societal problem. Rich in drawing the work from sociology, anthropology, as well as use of policy documents and secondary data, to advance the argument is an important learning from this piece of work. In a recent work, Halyal (2000) also indicates wide gaps in health modernity among women.

Sagar Sharma has drawn attention to the problem of hypertension—a serious health hazard for the urban Indians engaged in the blue colour jobs and struggling to make their fortune in the competitive and demanding life that tends to move increasingly on a faster pace. He particularly relates to the psychosocial factors and emotional markers associated with high blood pressure. The problem is becoming alarming as hypertension is identified as a key risk factor for cardiovascular diseases. It has been reported that while positive life conditions work as buffers, the perceived impact of life stress having negative affectivity have negative consequences. Sharma extends the current research on emotional vital signs among the clinically diagnosed hypertensive patient group. His findings clearly establish that the hypertensive male patients are marked by greater negative impact of life events stress, trait anger, anger suppression and trait anxiety but lower outward expression and control of angry feelings as compared to the normotensive control group. The discriminant function analysis revealed that trait anger was the most potent discriminator. It was followed by two modes of anger coping, i.e., anger-out and anger-in, and then negative impact of life events stress. The message of the study is that suppressed anger is more dangerous than expressed anger.

In the third contribution, Shalini Bharat has shared how Acquired Immune Deficiency Syndrome (AIDS) is perceived and interpreted within a particular cultural setting, in the context of local beliefs and norms of gender relations. Using focused group discussions with young and adult men and women in lower and lower middle income groups in Mumbai, the study revealed the following themes about AIDS: (*a*) it is an alien disease, 'imported' to India by people from abroad; (*b*) it is dreadful and incurable; (*c*) it is a shameful disease contracted through sex with 'others' such as prostitutes and 'loose character' women; (*d*) it is a disease of the promiscuous, those indulging in multi-partner sex, entertaining clients and engaging in sexual perversity; (*e*) it is an invited disease, because people get it due to their own irresponsible behaviour and unrestrained indulgence in sexual pleasures; (f) it is God's punishment for one's sin; (g) it is a disease of 'others', those who indulge in behaviour such as promiscuous lifestyle, including drinking, visiting prostitutes, overspending and having black money; (h) it is a contagious and polluting disease, caused by germs; (i) it is associated with uncertainty as one never knows who may be an AIDS patient in one's neighbourhood; and (j) it is a men's disease, as it was the male sexual behaviour that lead them to seducing women and multiple sex partners, due to which they contracted AIDS. A key finding was that AIDS was generally not personalized as a problem for own community members, and there was a tendency to deny the possibility of risk. The implication of the study is that much needs to be done by way of communication of accurate information about AIDS to encourage people to voluntarily seek information. This may be done by dovetailing AIDS education programmes with ongoing reproductive health programmes, to facilitate community members' access to them without anxiety and fear. Voluntary counselling and testing centres for HIV would also help in this effort.

Damodar Suar reports a study of health problems faced by people under the impact of a disaster. The super cyclone that hit the coastal state of Orissa in 1999 resulted in destruction of a very large magnitude. The available knowledge generally comes from Western countries that are characterized by an individualistic ethos and rich infrastructure. The Indian society largely subscribes to a vertical collectivist culture and presents a different scenario. The study showed that the affected people who were close to the epicentre of the cyclone and lost their loved ones and property experienced greater degree of stress than the unaffected ones who were away and did not experience any loss. The Post Traumatic Stress Disorder (PTSD) was evident among the survivors. The provision of external support reduced anxiety and depression and the amount of loss experienced by the survivors significantly increased the degree of external locus of control and anxiety. It is argued that there is need to manage psychological crisis at the same footing as it is normally done to manage material crisis, failing which, a substantial proportion of survivors may continue with certain health problems of a relatively enduring nature.

REFERENCE

Halyal, P. S. (2000). Health modernity a way to overcome the areas of ignorance and misconceptions of health in women. *Indian Psychological Review, 54-55,* 125-32.

17

Health Modernity: Concept and Correlates

AMAR KUMAR SINGH

POPULAR USAGES OF MODERNITY

Modernity has varied connotations. It refers to latest miracles of science, such as space-satellites, test-tube babies, nuclear reactors and less spectacular ones which have become commonplace things of developed societies like air conditioning, long-distance telephone calls and open-heart surgery. Modernity also refers to latest gadgets used by the affluent section of the society for comfort, and more for status, such as refrigerator, television, video and movie camera.

Modernity is also supposed to be Westernized styles and manners of dress, food, language and customs. Thus, jeans is modern and *saree* or *dhoti* is traditional; cake is modern and *rasgulla* is traditional; *kulfi* is traditional, Kwality ice-cream modern; pastry modern and *sewai* traditional; long hair is traditional and bobbed hair modern; English modern and Hindi, Bengali, Tamil, and more definitely Sanskrit, traditional. The blind imitation of Western ways takes such ridiculous forms as the bridegroom, clad in woollen three-piece suit, on the back of a mare, sweating in humid heat, marching in procession to the bride's house to marry her with the traditional seven rounds of the fire and Sanskrit *slokas* chanted by the Brahmin priest. A lipstick-smeared, pot-smoking, discotheque-swinging, pill-consuming girl is the ultimate symbol of *modernity*.

Modernity is also used in relation to time. The present is modern, past is traditional. Anything new is modern, and everything old is traditional. Taj Mahal is traditional, whereas multi-storeyed skyscraper is modern.

Turmeric paste is traditional, whereas AVON cosmetics are modern. Nail polish and eyeshadow are modern and *mehendi* is traditional. A party given in a hotel is modern, whereas at home it is traditional. A picnic is modern and a community feast is traditional. A toothbrush is modern, and a *datwan* is traditional. Hooka-smoking, though less harmful, is traditional and cigar or pipe-smoking, particularly with a tilt, is modern.

Above all, modernity is antonym of tradition. Anything opposed to *tradition* ipso facto becomes *modern*. The list of such themes is long. It includes abandonment of traditions, good as well as bad, and acceptance of new ways, some of which are good, while others worse than the abandoned traditional ways.

Modernity, therefore, is a much used and abused word. It is used in a positive as well as in a negative sense. There is fascination and admiration for it and also derision and ridicule. It refers to glorious human achievements. It also includes perverse and debased values and behaviour.

Not surprisingly, therefore, there is a great deal of ambivalence about modernity. The tug of war between tradition and modernity continues. The parties involved are often not clear about the ideals for which they are fighting. They are intoxicated by slogans of modernity and tradition, the contents and implications of which are left undefined and vague, embedded in such emotion-laden phrases as 'the Indian Way of Life'.

Modernity involves acceptance of scientific rationalism against religious faith and adoption of new innovations and methods of doing things, which challenge and compete with the old ones. At both levels, modernity has been resisted. Copernicus was asked, under threat to his life, to deny his discovery that the earth revolved round the sun and not vice versa. This he did to save his life, but coming out of the court he announced that despite his denial the earth still revolved round the sun!

If such a secular discovery displeased the Traditionalists to the extent of demanding the head of Copernicus, the shock created by Darwin's atheistic theory of evolution is not surprising. It was bitterly opposed as it shook the very foundation of religion and demolished the religious concept of man and his divine origin. In early days of industrial revolution, the Luddites, in Britain, went amuck breaking the factory machines. In India, the opposition to modernity has been stronger because of the association of some aspects of modernity with Westernization and British colonialism. The satirical poems of Akbar Allahabadi (1846-1920) expressed the sentiment of opposition to Westernization and modernization: 'Mr. Darwin is far from truth I will not accept that his ancestors were apes ...' and '... we have to drink the tap-water and to read the printed letters causing stomach upset and sore-eye; blessed be the Emperor Edward'.

Though many popular images of modernity are false and represent ridiculous caricatures and superficial aspects of modernity, it is possible to discern and identify some popular images which correlate with the essence of modernity. Inkeles and Singh (1983) picked up some uniquely Indian popular images of modernity in relation to religiosity, social customs and habits, which had significant positive correlations with Overall Modernity (OM) scale used in six different countries. An Indian who scored high on the OM scale was the one who preferred tap water against well water, toothbrush against *datwan*, allopathic medicine against indigenous ones, disapproved of dowry, wearing of ornaments by women, better food for the husband than that of his wife, the school teacher punishing the son of an ordinary farmer for not doing the home task but not the son of the rich landlord and believed that the *Sadhu/Fakir* (the holy men) produced sweets from a seemingly empty bag by trick and not by supernatural power.

CORRELATES OF MODERNITY

Modernity is often used as synonym of urbanization, industrialization, education and income. Individuals and societies with higher degrees of these are considered to be blessed with modernity compared to those who are unfortunate to have lesser degree of these. Thus, a person in Bombay or Delhi is believed to be more modern than one in a village. A factory worker is more modern than a farmer, an educated person more modern than an illiterate, a rich more modern than a poor. Modernity is influenced by these factors, and there is a positive correlation between these and modernity. They tend to increase the level of modernity. However, these per se are not modernity. Not all urban, industrial, educated and rich persons are modern, and not all rural, agricultural, uneducated and poor persons are traditional. On the contrary, a particular rural person may be more modern than a particular urban person, and similarly, a farmer may be more modern than an industrial worker, an uneducated compared with an educated one, and a poor may be more modern than a rich. Modernity is not an economic, demographic and a sociological concept. These are correlates of modernity rather than modernity itself, Modernity is a psychological concept. It relates to certain attitudes and values. A person having these values and attitudes will be modern irrespective of his sociological classification or his external appearance. Thus, Gandhi with his traditional, even primitive, dress of loincloth was more modern in his thinking than Paris-tailored three-piece suit doners.

Gandhi was more modern because of his adherence to time punctuality, despite his old-fashioned watch hanging from his loincloth than the wearers of ultra-modern electronic quartz watches. A Middle East Sheikh, despite his abundant wealth, is less modern than a poor Indian who believes in the equality of the sexes.

SOCIAL SCIENCE USAGES OF MODERNITY

In social science literature, modernity has been used in relation to economic, social and political development. It has been argued that the third world countries, including India, have remained economically backward and democracy has not taken roots in their soils because of the absence of certain psychological qualities which are prerequisites of development.

Max Weber (1958a), a German sociologist, in his seminal essay entitled *The Protestant Ethic and the Spirit of Capitalism*, originally published in German in 1904-1905, had argued that the relatively higher economic development of Protestant countries, compared with the Catholic ones, was due to reinterpretation of Christianity by Calvinist theology which gave religious sanctity to pursuit of wealth but withheld it from consumption; thus creating the psychological trait of 'This-worldly Asceticism' as opposed to 'Other-worldly Spiritualism'. Work became worship. The Protestant Ethic was inspired by such preaching as 'You may labour to be rich for God, though not for the flesh and sin' (Weber, 1958a, p. 176). Thus, psychological attitudes and motivations became the mainspring of economic development. The failure of political development on the third world countries, including India, has also been explained by the psychological prerequisites. A democratic political system needs democratic personality in its citizens. Most of the third world countries borrowed the British democratic system with adult franchise and independent judiciary. But the democratic institutions did not find nourishment from the native soil because the values continued to be feudal and non-egalitarian. Most third world countries have lapsed into military, theological or ideological dictatorships. In India, democracy has dragged on limping, with strong remnants of feudalism, social inequality, corruption and sycophancy.

The psychological prerequisites of socio-economic and political development have been labelled as modernity. A vast literature has mushroomed on this theme in the Western social science (Almond and Verba, 1965;

Apter, 1965; Black, 1967; Eisenstadt, 1966, 1973; Inkeles, 1983; Inkeles and Smith, 1974; Lerner, 1958; Marrion, 1966; Myrdal, 1968; Smith, 1965; Weiner, 1966).

MODERNITY AND THE INDIAN SOCIETY

The concept of modernity has been used to explain the development and the non-development of countries in almost all parts of the world. It has also been used to explain the non-development of India. Max Weber (1958b) himself, in his book *The religion of India*, argued that Hinduism, like Catholicism, was other-worldly and lacked the essence of 'Protestant Ethic'. Max Weber has found many disciples, non-Indian as well as Indian (Kapp, 1963; Loomis and Loomis, 1969; McClelland, 1961; Mishra, 1962; Myrdal, 1968; Rosen 1966). However, the Max Weber thesis on India has not found support in several empirical studies. McClelland (1961), who had taken the Max Weberian stand in his book *The Achieving Society*, did not find that orthodox Hindu religious beliefs were a barrier to economic entrepreneurship (McClelland and Winter, 1969). There was no difference between 'active' and 'inactive' businessmen in relation to their attitudes towards fatalism, respect for tradition, conformity to caste rules and religious behaviour (Winter and McClelland, 1975). Milton Singer (1975) found that 'traditional Hindu institution and beliefs are compatible with modern industrial organization and that they are being adopted by the successful industrial leaders in Madras city to supply the motivations and a positive social ethic for an ongoing industrialisation' (p. 41). Inkeles and Smith (1974) found that industrial experience and education were effective agents of change and modernization. Singh (1967; 1975) has reviewed the literature on Hindu culture and modernization in India and has refuted the Max Weberian thesis. He has argued that the lack of modernization in India can be explained by secular factors such as education, industrialization and urbanization. The data of Harvard University study of modernization in India has persuasive empirical evidence that secular factors are relatively more important than the religious ones in shaping modern attitudes.

The concept of modernity has emerged as a crucial one in the study of social change and development in India. Several studies have examined the relationship between tradition and modernity, the factors influencing modernity and the process of modernization (Damle, 1955; Desai, 1971;

Kuthiala, 1973; Mulay and Ray, 1973; Raghuvanshi, 1984; Rogers, 1969; Rudolph and Rudolph, 1967; Sharma, 1979; Shils, 1961; Singer, 1959, 1972, 1975; Singh, A. K., 1968; Singh, S. N., 1979; Singh, Y., 1973; Srinivas, 1972; Srivastava, 1976).

SANSKRITIZATION, WESTERNIZATION AND MODERNIZATION

Social change in modern India has been explained with three main concepts: Sanskritization, Westernization and Modernization. Srinivas (1972), the author of the concept, has described sanskritization as:

> ... the process by which a 'low' Hindu caste, or tribal or other group, changes its customs, rituals, ideology, and way of life in the direction of a high, and frequently 'twice-born' caste. Generally, such changes are followed by a claim to a higher position in the caste hierarchy than that traditionally conceded to the claimant caste by the local community (p. 6).

The caste-bound closed Indian society did not permit individual social mobility. Sanskritization provided group social mobility of the entire caste, by acquiring wealth, adopting high caste surnames, vegetarianism and even *purdah* for women, donning of sacred thread and tracing their origin of the caste to an ancient holy saint. Interestingly, the high castes, aspiring to Westernize themselves, were abandoning the very social customs and values the low castes were adopting. For the low castes, the high and dominant castes were the reference group, whereas for the high castes it was the British. Sanskritization implied two ladders of social mobility; sanskritization was the first, and it was the necessary precondition for the second, i.e., Westernization. Sanskritization explained social change in rural India, but proved inadequate to explain change in urban industrial India. For many individuals, and some social groups, the road to Westernization was direct and did not pass via sanskritization. With the increasing decline in the respectability of the values inherent in sanskritization as correlates of social status, sanskritization is becoming an ineffective explanation of social change in contemporary India.

Westernization implies science and technology and the values of democracy and social equality. Srinivas has considered Humanitarianism as the core value of Westernization, which means 'an active concern for the welfare of all human beings irrespective of caste, economic position, religion, age and sex. Equalitarianism and secularisation are both included in Humanitarianism' (1972, p. 48). It is true that science and technology have developed more in Western countries in the modern era of human civilization. However, the ancient civilizations also have contributed significantly to the development of science. The numerals, the placing of digits and the concept of zero were invented in India and these have been the basic bricks of scientific development. The first printing press was invented in China. The Babylonian civilization of Egypt had the technology to preserve mummies for thousands of years. Admittedly, the Western countries in modern era have made dominant contributions to science and technology. However, the contributions of non-Western civilization cannot be ignored. Science is a continuous development, and no civilization can claim exclusive share in its development. Similarly, the democratic policy was known and practised in ancient India. Lichchwi dynasty was an example of democracy. So also is the *panchayati* system which still is prevalent and often more effective than the formal legal system. Despite its commitment to social equality, the Western countries have practised imperialism and colonialism and many democratic Western nations are still supporting apartheid in South Africa. The humanitarian values of democracy and social equality are not exclusive in origin to the Western countries; nor have these values been fully adhered to by the Western countries. The concept of Westernization, therefore, becomes very difficult to define.

The concept of modernization refers to the process of social change in which the individual imbibes certain attitudinal-cum-personality traits conducive to socio-economic and political development as well as individual self-actualization. These traits have been labelled as modernity.

These traits are neither Western nor Eastern; neither ancient nor contemporary. These traits are related to individual and socio-economic development by a priori logic and by empirical evidence. Modernity is the bridge between change and development, and is the mediating and intervening factor between them. Sanskritization looks backward, modernity is futuristic. Westernization is parochial, modernity is universal. Modernity, too, has its own value preferences. It is committed to individual dignity, equality and freedom. It believes in secularism. It prefers democratic and socialistic forms of socio-political organization. It combines individual growth with social responsibility.

Modernity, by comparison, emerges as a more useful concept than sanskritization and Westernization for the analysis of contemporary Indian society. It is also a more relevant model for future development.

CHARACTERISTICS OF MODERNITY

Modernity, as discussed earlier, consists of psychological qualities necessary for socio-economic and political development. Before we attempt a definition of modernity, let us first list its main characteristics. The most important of these are:

1. Modernity is a psychological concept. It is a mentality. It is an inner quality and lies in the individual. It is part of the personality system.
2. Modernity is not external. It is not related to one's dress, appearance and material possessions. Modernity is not synonymous with certain indices of development such as, income, industrialization, urbanization and education.
3. Modernity is not Westernized urban lifestyle of the rich upper strata of the society. Therefore, Western dress and cosmetics, manners and speech, food and eating styles, do not guarantee modernity. Neither the imported gadgets, nor the Western university education, ensure modernity.
4. Modernity consists of a syndrome of personality-cum-attitudinal traits. The personality traits include rationality, internal locus of control, openness to change, work commitment and aspirations. The important socio-cultural and political attitudes include social equality, women's rights family planning, civic rights, democracy, secularism and political participation.
5. Two important themes underlie the various components of modernity: Rationality and Humanism. Rationality covers such issues as internal locus of control, openness to change and family planning. Humanism covers the issues of social equality, women's rights, civic rights, democracy and secularism.
6. Modernity facilitates personal growth and development as well as social responsibility. The traits of rationality, openness to change, internal locus of control, work commitment, aspirations and family planning help the individual in his personal growth and development. Similarly, the favourable attitudes to social equality, women's right, democracy, civic rights and secularism make him socially responsible and humane.
7. Modernity makes the individual an effective agent of socio-economic and political change and development.
8. Modernity is a multi-faceted concept. It has many dimensions. It views the individual in totality. It embraces his entire personality.

9. Modernity enriches the quality of life by enabling a person to live more meaningfully, intelligently and effectively.
10. Modernity helps the individual in adjustment to a plural democratic and scientific society.

DEFINITION OF MODERNITY

Modernity is an aggregate of certain personality-cum-attitudinal traits which facilitate individual growth and development with social responsibility and make the individual an effective agent of socio-economic and political development.

THE CONCEPT OF HEALTH MODERNITY

Omission of Health Modernity

The omission of health, as a component of modernity, is perhaps a consequence of concern, at times bordering to obsession, with economic and political development. In most scales measuring modernity, health has been completely ignored or there is only marginal inclusion of health. Some scales of modernity have a few items on health. But these are to measure rationality in relation to health with such items as whether one believes that illness can be cured by prayers and saints. Health is not an independent dimension of modernity.

The omission of health as a component of modernity is because of the fact that the main concern was Economy and Polity and not Man. It is now increasingly realized that concern for economic and political development is because of the concern for Man. The well-being of the common man is the main pursuit of modernity. The importance of economic development lies in the fact that it helps and facilitates human development. With Man as the centrepiece of development, health assumes a key status as a component of modernity. Health and disease very decisively influence the efficacy and well-being of the individual.

Importance of Health Modernity

The omission of health attitudes, as a component of modernity, is rather unfortunate. The health attitudes are as important as other components included in the concept of modernity.

In fact, it can be argued that they are even more important than some other components. The health attitudes are the pillars on which the structure of the personality is constructed. Health attitudes of parents, particularly of the mothers, influence the child even before he is born in the prenatal stage of development. The knowledge and attitudes of the mother about dos and don'ts during pregnancy and early years of childhood about diet and nutrition, immunization, breast feeding, supplementary food, common diseases of infants and children and their simple domestic treatment such as oral re-hydration, monitoring of development with the growth chart, developmental milestones of physical and language development, etc., have very crucial and decisive influence on human development. Therefore, the concern for health modernity comes before the concern for other dimensions of modernity. Health modernity is more directly associated with life than other dimensions of modernity.

The importance of health modernity is demonstrated by the tragic consequences of its absence for human development. The lack of health modernity results in enormous loss of young children. The painful loss is entirely avoidable as Grant, Director General United Nation's Children's Fund (UNICEF), has pointed out: 'The cost of immunising all the third world's infants works out at approximately five dollars per child. The cost of not doing so works out at approximately five million deaths a year' (1981, p. 9). The tragedy of Indian children and how they are the victims of lack of health facilities and modernity has been graphically described by Gopalan:

> ... of the nearly 23 million children who will be born in our country in 1983 nearly 3 million may be expected to die before they reach the first year, another one million more will drop by the way side before they complete their childhood, of the remaining 19 million nearly 9 million will emerge into adulthood with impaired physical stamina, low productivity and poor mental abilities because of serious under nutrition and ill-health during their childhood, yet another 7 million who will suffer milder forms of malnutrition may reach adulthood with less striking physical and mental impairment. Only less than 3 million of the 23 million to be born in 1983 will become truly health, physically fit, productive and intellectually capable citizens of this country. Thus, the full genetic potential for growth, physical and mental development, would have been achieved by less than 19 % of the children born; and even this may perhaps be an over-estimate. (Gopalan, 1983, pp. 17–20)

The importance of health modernity is also because of its practical usefulness. It is easier to intervene with and improve health modernity than with other dimensions of modernity, particularly in a short span of time. It is easier to inform and educate people about nutrition, immunization, family planning and other health habits than to inculcate or change personality and socio-political modernity. The results of intervention in the area of health are more concrete, more visible and more easily measurable.

If modernity is a prerequisite for social, economic and political development, health modernity is the prerequisite for human development, which undoubtedly is the summum bonum of all development. The individual must be alive and cognitively competent to be economically productive, socially liberal and politically democratic. Admittedly, health modernity does not ensure and guarantee social, economic and political modernity, but, nonetheless, it is the fundamental precondition of all development.

Linkage between Health and Other Dimensions of Modernity

To emphasize the importance of health modernity is not meant to undermine the importance of socio-cultural, political and personality modernity. Heath modernity does not ensure social and political modernity, and the latter are important determinants of the quality of civilized life. In fact, health modernity itself is, in large measure, determined by political modernity. The access to health and nutritional facilities are determined by political power, which also determines the important sociological correlates of health modernity, such as, education and income.

Werner and Bower (1983) have prefaced their book entitled *Helping health workers learn* by a section labelled 'Why this book is so political?' Werner states that when he wrote his earlier book *Where there is no doctor* (1982), he saw disease in physical terms.

> Little by little, I became aware that many of their losses—of children, of land, of hope—not only have immediate physical causes, but also underlying social causes. That is to say, they result from the way people treat or affect the lives of others.

Health modernity cannot be developed in isolation. In fact, it is not a choice between health modernity and other dimensions of modernity. The dimensions of modernity are interlinked affecting each other. The different dimensions of modernity are not dichotomous concepts. The dimensions are sub-concepts of the total concept of modernity. The different dimensions are positively inter-correlated. If a person has openness to change, he is also more willing to accept family planning and new methods of treatment of diseases. Grant (1984) has indicated the linkage of different dimensions and totality of one's worldview in relation to family planning: 'To expect adults who cannot control or plan any other major aspect of their lives to suddenly start planning their families is to misunderstand what powerlessness means' (p. 30).

The importance of health modernity lies in the fact that it can be the starting point of inculcation of personality modernity, which is a general predisposition reflecting itself in all dimensions, i.e., health, socio-cultural and political. In this sense, personality modernity is the core of modernity. The components of personality modernity such as rationality, locus of control and openness to change can be developed in relation to health. Health modernity may be the means to develop personality modernity.

MODERNITY: DIMENSIONS AND THEMES

Singh (1984) has included four main dimensions in his Modernity Scale, namely, Personality, Socio-cultural, Political and Health. Each of the four dimensions has five themes and each theme has five items, thus yielding a total of 100 items on a five-point Likert Scale. The dimensions and themes of the Modernity Scale are given in Table 17.1.

Profile of Modernity

A modern person has certain personality-cum-attitudinal traits which distinguish him from a non-modern person. These traits cover different aspects of life and society. A modern person is rational, is open to change, is committed to work and has aspirations. He is not fatalistic, and he believes that hard work and ability, not luck, determine success. He is willing to give up old and sacred religious customs as they have become economic strains. He is willing to work even if he can live comfortably without doing any work. A modern person is liberal in his socio-cultural attitudes. He supports women's rights, social equality and family planning.

Table 17.1: Dimensions and Themes of Modernity

Dimensions	Themes	Items
Health	Scientific versus Superstitious Belief Scientific Understanding Diet and Nutrition Child Care Family Planning	25
Personality	Rationality Aspirations Locus of Control Openness to Change Work Ethics	25
Socio-cultural	Religious Attitudes Social Equality Caste System Social Customs Attitude to Women	25
Political	Democracy Secularism Civic Rights Political Identification Political Participation	25

Source: Author.

He opposes casteism and orthodox social customs. He disapproves of the customary practice of wife giving better food to her husband than what she takes herself. He supports widow remarriage and birth control. The social liberalism of a modern person is matched by his political liberalism. He supports democracy, civic rights and secularism. He believes that every citizen should have full freedom to criticize the government. He realizes the political usefulness of opposition parties. He is not limited within the narrow boundaries of family, caste and religion; he is conscious of his wider socio-political responsibilities. He is rational and has scientific attitudes towards health and disease, and diet and nutrition. He does not believe that the cure of illness depends on the mercy of God, nor does he believe that mental illness is caused by evil spirits. He is against overeating because he knows that it is as harmful as inadequate eating. He believes that women, like men, also need physical exercise. These are only a few illustrations of the mental makeup of a modern person. He is scientific, rational, liberal, humane and effective.

HEALTH MODERNITY SCALE

The Modernity Scale, described above, includes health as one of its four dimensions. This Modernity Scale can be used for socio-psychological studies of social change and development. Singh (1984) has argued the necessity of an independent and comprehensive Health Modernity Scale (HMS), which can be used for measuring health modernity and health status of a population and to obtain benchmark data for informed intervention programme. This enlarged independent HMS consists of 10 dimensions, namely: (a) Scientific versus Superstitious Belief; (b) Scientific Understanding; (c) Diet and Nutrition; (d) Breast Feeding; (e) Family Planning; (f) Child Care; (g) Attitude to Females; (h) Health Information; (i) Health Habits; and (j) Health Indicators. Thus, the HMS covers attitudes and knowledge, as well as behavioural habits and environmental conditions. Each dimension from I to VII has been measured by 10 items on a five-point scale with scores of 1–5, the latter indicating highest health modernity. Other dimensions have been measured by pre-coded closed questions. The HMS is available in English and Hindi. Examples of items are given in Table 17.2. The health modernity is individual as well as societal. The former consists of attitudes, information and behaviour; and the latter is reflected in social and demographic indicators.

Table 17.2: Health Modernity Scale (HMS): Dimensions and Illustrative Items

Dimension	Illustrative Item
I. Scientific versus Superstitious Belief (SS)	1. Great saints can cure such diseases which cannot be cured by doctors (1–5)
	2. Insanity is caused by evil spirits (1–5)
II. Scientific Understanding (SU)	1. Women also need physical exercise as much as men do (5–1)
	2. Once insane, one can never a completely normal person (1–5)
III. Diet and Nutrition (DN)	1. It is better to take an injection for getting vitamins than taking milk, egg or other foods (1–5)
	2. Overeating makes a man ill as does inadequate food (5–1)
IV. Breast Feeding (BF)	1. The first breast milk after child's birth is harmful to the new born infant (1–5)

(Table 17.2 continued)

(*Table 17.2 continued*)

Dimension	Illustrative Item
	2. Breast feeding spoils the figure of the mother (1–5)
V. Family Planning (FP)	1. Children born after 3–4 years of interval have much better chances of survival than those born within one or two years (5–1)
	2. Vasectomy makes a man impotent.
VI. Child Care (CC)	1. Child is likely to be mentally retarded if he/she does not talk by two years (5–1)
	2. During diarrhea, the child should not be allowed to eat and drink; fasting is the best medicine for it (1–5)
VII. Attitude to Women (AW)	1. The wife should give her husband better food than she has herself (1–5)
	2. God has made women such that they can never be equal to men (1–5)
VIII. Health Information (HINF)	1. What is the exact proper weight of a healthy normal child at birth, at six months, at one year, at two years and at three years (Correct 2, Incorrect 1)
	2. At what exact age the child should be immunized against TB, diphtheria/whooping cough/tetanus/polio, measles (Correct 2, Incorrect 1)
IX. Health Habits (HH)	1. How often do you take bath, (Daily/bi-weekly/tri-weekly/weekly/occasionally (5–1)
	2. How often do you do physical exercise: daily/often/occasionally/seldom/never (5–1)
X. Health Indicators (HIND)	1. Whether the children in the family have been immunized against TB/Diphtheria/whooping cough/tetanus/polio/measles? (Yes 2, No 1)
	2. Whether there is incidence in the family of: infant and child mortality, blindness/defective eye-sight, physical handicap, mental retardation, mental illness, abortion, premature birth, etc. (No 2, Yes 1)

Source: Author.
Note: There are 10 dimensions of health modernity. Two examples of items of each dimension are listed below by way of illustration.

Profile of Health Modernity

A person with health modernity has scientific and rational attitudes to and knowledge of health and disease which are also reflected in his/her behaviour and environmental conditions. He/she does not believe that saints can cure incurable diseases, nor does he/she believe that insanity is caused by evil spirits or sins of past lives. He/she does not rely on amulets and prayers for the cure of illness. The person has scientific understanding of physical and mental health. He/she knows that women need physical exercise as much as men do. He/she knows that serious diseases like TB, typhoid and polio can be prevented by immunization. He/She knows that mental illness is curable and a mentally ill person can regain normalcy and can then be trusted with responsibility. The person is against smoking, drinking alcohol and overeating. The person knows the nutritional value of different kinds of food and nutritional requirements of different age groups and pregnant women. Breast feeding is favoured against bottle feeding. It is known that the first breast milk is beneficial to the baby and breast feeding, contrary to fashionable belief, does not spoil the figure of the mother. The person believes in small family size and is willing to use birth control methods including abortion, contraception and vasectomy, not believing in the rumour that the last causes impotency. It is believed that spacing of children is beneficial to them. The person is aware of the important milestones of development and growth of children. He/she knows home care for common diseases of children such as oral re-hydration for dehydration caused by diarrhea. He/she also knows that the body weight is a good indicator of child's health and what the expected weight in different ages is. The person with health modernity has a favourable and positive attitude towards women, believes in equality of sexes and respects the dignity of women. Health modernity means being informed of health- and growth-related issues such as the minimum weight of a healthy baby at birth and at various ages; ages when important developmental behaviours occur such as sitting, crawling, walking and speaking, and ages at which immunization against various diseases are given.

The health habits are important indicators of health modernity. The person abstains from smoking, drinking alcohol and using intoxicating drugs. He/she observes cleanliness of body, clothes and house. The children are immunized. The married couple use birth control methods. And finally, health modernity reflects itself in actual observable facts, in the physical and environmental conditions, in sanitation, family size, incidence of illness and death.

HEALTH MODERNITY SURVEY

Using the concept of health modernity and the scale discussed above, an ICMR-sponsored survey of the extent of health modernity in south Bihar was conducted (Singh, 1984). The sample consisted of 1,280 cases taken from Chotanagapur region. There were 320 cases from each of the four main ethnic-religious groups, namely, Hindus, Muslims, Tribal Christians and Tribal Hindus/Sarnas. The sample in each ethnic group was stratified on the basis of: (a) SES (a combination of education, occupation, income and caste/tribe): Low and High; (b) Residence: Rural-Urban; (c) Sex: Female and Male; and (d) Age: 20–30 yrs, and 31–40 yrs. An additional sample of 160 cases was taken from rural Santhal Parganas to include the Santhal tribe, the largest in Bihar. Thus, the total sample consisted of 1,440 cases. Only 23 per cent had health modernity, i.e., had correct scientific attitudes to and knowledge of health and disease. It may be noted that this was when half of the sample belonged to high socio-economic status, having an educational level of BA or more in urban and Intermediate in rural, an income of rupees 1,000 or more in urban and 700 or more in rural areas, and they belonged to high castes and had occupations with high prestige. The extent of health modernity was very low in the Low SES groups, ranging from 0 to 2 per cent in rural and 3 to 23 per cent in urban areas in different sample groups. The tribal Hindu/Sarnas and Muslims had the lowest, about 2 per cent. The SES was the most powerful correlate of health modernity. The F value in each of the four ethnic-religious groups, as well as in the total sample, was statistically significant at 0.01 level. In each sample group comparison, the high SES had, without exception, higher health modernity than the low SES counterpart group (Figures 17.1 and 17.2).

HEALTH STATUS AND ITS CORRELATES IN INDIA

Singh (1983a), in his paper 'Health modernity education in India', has surveyed the health status in India in relations to such health indicators as infant and child mortality, birth weight, premature birth, malnutrition, fertility rate and life expectancy. He has concluded that:

> ... the dismal and depressing health status in India is reflected in numerous health-related statistics, particularly in relation to children and women, the two most important population groups ... not merely because of their

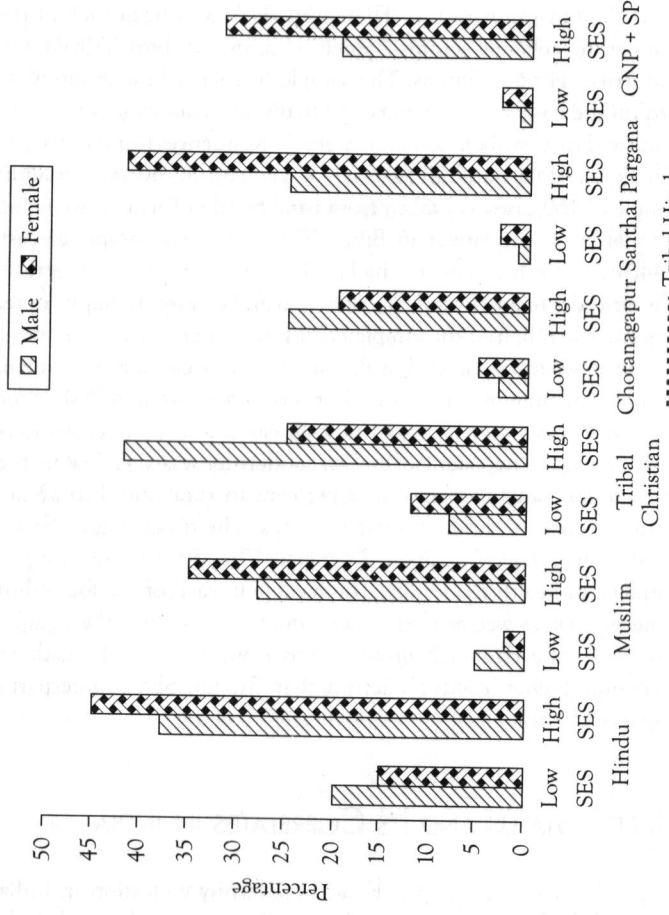

Figure 17.1: Extent of Health Modernity

Percentage of 'Modern' (4–5) Scorers on Five Point Scale (Rural)

Source: Author.

Figure 17.2: Extent of Health Modernity
Percentage of 'Modern' (4–5) Scorers on Five Point Scale (Urban)

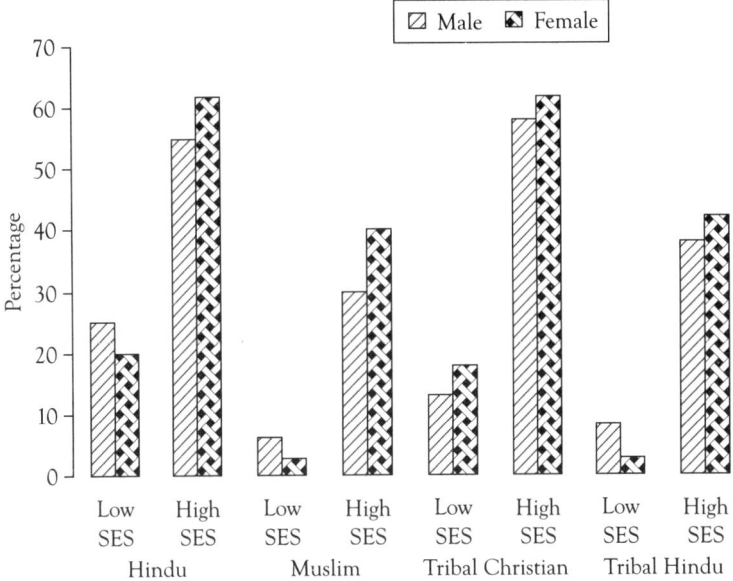

Source: Author.

numbers ... but also because of the fact that they are the most crucial segments of the population which determine the quality of the health of the community and, therefore, any intervention for improving the health status of the community must necessarily concentrate substantially on these two main target groups. (p. 28)

The facts about several important health indicators have been summarized in Table 17.3, which gives an overall picture of health status in India at a glance. As can be seen, India lags behind not only developed countries like Sweden and Japan, but also Sri Lanka in relation to important health indicators such as, infant mortality, child mortality, crude birth/death rate, total fertility rate, birth weight, life expectancy, adult literacy and GNP per capita income. Almost one-third of the babies are below the minimum required weight of 2,500 g. Almost 90 per cent of the children are not immunized; even in Delhi, with better health facilities, only one-third of the children are immunized. Majority of the population is malnourished; in the lowest group the percentage is as high as 95. According to one

Table 17.3: Health Status and Its Correlates in India

Health Indicator	Fact	Source
Infant Mortality (0–1 year)	120 in India per 1,000 live births, compared to 43 in Sri Lanka and seven each in Japan and Sweden (1981 data) IMR is higher in rural and female populations compared with urban and male. 1978 IMR for Rural Males, Rural Females, Urban Males, Urban Females were 130, 142, 69 and 71, respectively.	Grant, 1982 Ghosh, 1980, p. 75
Child Mortality (Less than five years)	17 in India, per 1,000 live births, compared to five in Sri Lanka and less than one percent in Japan and Sweden (1980 data) 16% of the Indian population is under five; it contributes 50% of the total deaths.	
Crude Birth/Death Rate	35/13 in India compared to 27/6 in Sri Lanka, 13/6 in Japan and 11/11 in Sweden (1981 data)	Grant, 1984, pp. 40–41
Total Fertility Rate	5.3 in India compared to 3.4 in Sri Lanka and 1.8 in Japan and 1.6 in Sweden	Grant, 1982, pp. 152–53
Birth Weight	About 33% of the babies are below 2,500 g and about 10% below 2,000 g. In India, 30% of infants are born with low birth weight compared to 21% in Sri Lanka, 5% in Japan and 4% in Sweden (1979 data)	Ghosh,1980, p. 75 Grant, 1984, pp. 40–49 Quoted by Grant, 1984, p. 28

Premature Birth	New Delhi figures for 1969–1974 show that IMR is related to birth weight. For birth weights under 1,000 g, between 1,001–1,500 g, 1,501–2,000, 2,001–2,500, 2,501–3,000 and over 3,000, the IMR were 1,000, 615, 238, 59, 21 and 18, respectively.	Chhabra and Pettersson, 1979, p. 23
	About 17% of all births in India are premature because of maternal malnutrition; about one-third of premature infants die.	
Immunization	Rural infants below age one year: percentage of immunized with polio vaccine, triple vaccine and BCG: less then one, about four and about 12, respectively. Corresponding figures for urban population: 11, about 24 and 40 (1979 data).	Register General of India, 1981, p. 37 Ghosh, 1980, p. 76, Hooja et al., 1976
	Not more than 10% of children are immunized. Even in Delhi with comparatively better facilities only about 33% children are immunized.	
Weaning	For 36% of all infants in villages and 40% among urban poor mothers breast milk is the only food.	Grant, 1984–7, p. 34
	Delayed weaning is first unintentional push down the slope of malnutrition.	
Malnutrition	Percentages of malnourished populations: Rural, 57; Lowest income group, 95; Highest income group, 19; Children 1–5 years, 86.	Grant, 1984, pp. 40–41, Premi, 1982, p. 74

(Table 17.3 continued)

(Table 17.3 continued)

Health Indicator	Fact	Source
	Malnutrition is underlying cause in 7% of deaths in 0–5 years and is an associated cause in 46%. About 6,600 children in 0–5 years die every day because of malnutrition.	UNICEF, 1981, pp. 32–33, Berg, 1970
Anaemia	In India, around half the number of preschool children and pregnant mothers have been reckoned to suffer from anaemia.	Haxton, 1983
Mental Retardation	2.5% of the total population is mentally retarded. Total number = approximately 15 millions. A large portion of this is due to malnutrition.	Kulkarni, 1983
Blindness	12,000 children in 1–5 years become blind every year due to vitamin A deficiency.	Gupta, 1980, p. 96
Goitre	One mentally retarded child is born every two hours in goitre-prone Tarai regions of Bihar and UP.	AIIMS, *The Times of India*, 11 July 1983
Leprosy	Estimated cases: 3.2 millions, approximately 20% of these are infections and 25–30% are deformed.	UNICEF, 1981, p. 27 UNICEF, 1984, p. 34
Malaria	There were over two million cases in 1982.	UNICEF, 1984, pp. 34–40
Tuberculosis	About 10 million suffer annually and about 500,000 die.	UNICEF, 1984
Poliomyelitis	About 200,000 children are affected yearly and about 2,000 die.	UNICEF, 1984
Tetanus	Nearly 230,000–280,000 thousand infants die within the first month of life due to neo-natal tetanus.	UNICEF, 1984

Measles	200,000 children die annually due to measles-related complications	UNICEF, 1984
Diarrhea	Causes 4.4 of deaths in the first year and 30.5% in 1–4 years. Incidence is 500 per 1,000 children; 1.5 million annually die.	UNICEF, 1984
Medical Attention	Nearly 58% of rural and 29% of urban infant deaths are not attended by trained medical practitioners.	UNICEF, 1984, p. 29
Life Expectancy	52 years in India compared with 69 in Sri Lanka and 77 in Japan and Sweden (1981 data)	Grant, 1984, pp. 40–41
Adult Literacy Rate Male/Female	55/29 in India compared with 87/76 in Sri Lanka, 99/99 in Japan and 99 (Male + Female combined) in Sweden (1980 data). Indian national average literacy rate in 1981 was 36% for male and 25% for female.	Grant, 1984, pp. 40–41 Census of India, 1981
GNP Per Capita US Dollar	India 260, Sri Lanka 300, Japan 100,800, Sweden 14,870 (1981 data).	Grant, 1984, pp. 40–41
Physical Quality of Life Index (PQLI)	PQLI = combination of literacy rate of age 15 or more, Life Expectancy at age one year, and IMR. Range of scores is 0–100. National average is 34.3, Kerala 100 (highest) and UP 5.3 (lowest).	UNICEF, 1981, pp. 30–31
Health Modernity	The extent of health modernity in low SES Tribal Hindu/Sarna and Muslims in south Bihar was only 2%. The corresponding percentages in Tribal Christian and Hindus were eight and 18. About two-thirds in rural High SES Muslims, and Tribals did not have health modernity.	Singh, 1984, p. 102

estimate, about 6,600 children in the age range of 0-5 years die everyday because of malnutrition. In the same age range, about 12,000 children become blind every year due to vitamin A deficiency. The Physical Quality of Life Index—a combination of literacy rate, life expectancy and infant mortality rate—is an important health indicator. The scores on this index have a range of 0-100. The national average is only 34.3, which means that the country has just about one-third of what is required. Uttar Pradesh, the biggest state with the largest population, has a score of only 5.3. These are some of the grim statistics about the health status of India. We have picked up only a few important references, but numerous studies repeat and reconfirm the same story.

The poor health status in India is largely a consequence of its poor socio-economic conditions. Illiteracy and poverty, with their numerous manifestations, adversely influence the health status. About 51 per cent of the rural and 38 per cent of the urban populations exist below the poverty line, making an enormous total of 317 millions (Singh, T.N., 1983, p. 10). Three out of four women (75 per cent) and more than half (53 per cent) of the male population are illiterate; only 36 per cent Indians are literate. The IMR, an important indicator of health status, is closely associated with socio-economic factors (Table 17.4). The IMR in urban population is lower than the rural. Higher the level of education of the women, lower is the IMR in both rural and urban groups. The IMR is lower in working women than in non-working ones. Higher the age of women at marriage, lower is the IMR. Families having electric light and tap water have lower IMR compared to those using oil lamp and well water. The availability of social amenities such as water supply, motorable road, bus stand, railway station, primary school and medical facilities lower IMR.

How socio-economic conditions affect health status is demonstrated by the comparison of Bihar, having the highest IMR, and Kerala, with the lowest. Kerala, compared with Bihar, has higher per capita income, high literacy rate, higher per capita expenditure on medical and public health, higher doctor-population ratio and higher number of beds per 1,000 population.

Poverty and illiteracy make it impossible to improve the health status. The situation is made worse by lack of dissemination of scientific information about health and disease and the persistence of superstitious beliefs and incorrect information.

The health status and modernity of the poor and the illiterate are understandably low. But on several issues of health modernity, even higher levels of education and income have little impact. A study of 400 educated

Table 17.4: Infant Mortality Differentials in India (1979)

	Rural	Urban
Infant Mortality Rates		
India	136	71
Level of Education of Women		
Illiterate	145	88
Literates Below Primary	101	57
Primary and above	71	47
Work Status of Women		
Workers	142	98
Non-workers	134	64
Age at Marriage of Women		
Below 18 years	156	88
18–20 years	132	67
21 years and over	90	46
Source of Lighting		
Electric Light	90	55
Oil Lamp	157	114
Source of Drinking Water		
Tap	112	66
Well	143	84
Presence/Absence of Social Amenities		
Water Supply: with/without	113/140	
Motorable Road:	116/145	
Bus Stand:	114/144	
Railway Station:	91/136	
Primary School:	133/148	
Medical Facilities:	117/141	

Sources: Registrar General of India. (1981). *Survey of Infant and Child Mortality.* 1979–A Preliminary Report, pp. 26–33. New Delhi: Ministry of Home Affairs.

women, with a minimum of a Bachelors degree, in Ranchi town, revealed that majority of them believed that 'the first breast-milk after child's birth was harmful to the new born infant', that 'the mother should not breast-feed her child when she is ill as it may harm the child', that 'breast-feeding spoils the figure of the mother' and that 'fasting was the best medicine for diarrhoea'. Most of them did not know the correct age when the child should be immunized against common diseases; nor did they know the minimum weight expected of an average healthy baby at birth and at different ages. They were ignorant of the major development milestones about speech and motor activities. Though there was acceptance of small family size norm and adoption of birth control measures, only a few had correct information about reproductive system and birth control methods. Singh (1983b) has concluded that:

> The near-absence of scientific knowledge of and attitude to health and disease, diet and nutrition, childcare, breast-feeding, family planning and health habits make these educated women, some with brilliant academic careers and a few with even Ph.D. degrees, no more than educated illiterates so far as health modernity is concerned.

HEALTH MODERNITY EDUCATION

The facts about the health status and health modernity of India logically lead to the inescapable necessity of health education. Mahler, Director General of WHO, has underlined this point:

> It is not accidental that health education was given the pride of place in the Alma-Ata Declaration; nor is it accidental that the global strategy constantly refers to educational interventions as the means par excellence for enlisting the involvement of people in all walks of life and making them true artisans of health and development. (1983, p. 4)

Ramalingaswami, Director General of ICMR, also confirms this statement:

> There is perhaps no greater priority in the entire health field than that of education and communication to induce a way of thinking and behaving in the people that would be conducive to early disease recognition, disease prevention and health promoting. (1984, p. 353)

The health of the child is the crux of the issue. Health education for children obviously has to be done mainly through the mothers, a vast majority of whom are illiterate and poor. Health education, therefore, has to be outside the formal educational system. The mother has to be the main focus of health education because 'for almost all children, the most important primary health care worker is the mother' (Grant, 1984, p. 30). Health education is perhaps the most important means and hope for achieving the goal of Health For All by the year 2000. The enormous loss of human life, pervasive ill health and consequently low quality of human efficiency can be substantially prevented by health modernity education. The scientific and technological know-how has provided low cost preventive methods for the most common disease of children, which take the heaviest toll. Indeed, it is a humiliating indictment on our civilization that so many children are allowed to die or be crippled and maimed, when they could have been healthy and economically and socially useful citizens. Grant, writing about the health, or more appropriately ill health, of the children of the developing countries had painfully pointed out that:

> ... It is neither socially nor economically acceptable to have 500,000 children a year being affected by poliomyelitis when 20,000 shots of vaccine cost less than dollars 1000. Nor, is it either humane or sensible to have allowed over 500 children to lose their eye-sight everyday during 1981 when vitamin A tablets costing only a few cents could have prevented it. (1982, p. 22)

The situation continues to be equally agonizing in 1984 as Grant describes it in his report on *The state of world's children, 1984*:

> These children do not die from exotic causes requiring sophisticated cures. Five million of them die in the stupor of dehydration caused by simple diarrhoea. More than three million die with the high fevers of pneumonia. Two million die marked by the rash of measles. A million and half die racked by the spasms of whooping cough. Another million die with convulsions of tetanus. And for every child who dies, many more live on in hunger and ill-health. There has to be a better way forward, and there is. (1984, p. 8)

And, yes, indeed, there is a better way. Millions of lives can be saved, and their health protected, by simple and economical preventive methods.

> The oral rehydration therapy, universal child immunization, the promotion of breast-feeding, and the use of child growth charts are all low-cost, low-risk, low-resistance people's health actions which do not depend on the economic and political changes which are necessary in the longer term if poverty itself is to be eradicated. They are, therefore, available now. (Grant, 1983, p. 21)

Ramalingaswami, Director General, ICMR, agrees with this statement: 'We possess almost all the knowledge we need to be able to make the dream of "Health For All" a reality. The dream is not a shibboleth, but is realisable' (1983, p. 13). Grant, Executive Director UNICEF, researches this point in his latest report on *The state of the world's xhildren, 1984*:

> Any government which now decides to make a serious commitment to saving the lives and protecting the health and growth of its children can now move towards that goal ... The evidence leaves no room for doubt that low cost techniques are available ... The Challenge is now primarily political rather than technical or financial. (1984, p. 3)

CONTENT OF HEALTH MODERNITY EDUCATION

Six themes for health education were suggested by the UNICEF mnemonic GOBI-FF to mean Growth Chart, Oral Re-hydration, Breast Feeding, Immunization, Food Supplement and Family Planning (Grant, 1983, p. 38). To these six themes, Singh, A.K. (1983a, p. 31) had added one more F to represent attitude to females, because, he argued, that 'women can be made agents and means of health improvement of the community only in the context of their own status and dignity'. Coincidentally, an extra F has been added to the UNICEF mnemonic to represent Female Education (Grant, 1984, p. 5), which, though not exactly the same as dignity and respect for women suggested by Singh, is a related and overlapping theme. Female education is easier to define, promote and monitor than female status and dignity, and generally female education and female status are positively correlated, but not always. Therefore, the attitude to female, incorporating dignity of and respect for women, may remain a separate theme. In addition to these eight important themes, the health modernity education may also include the other dimensions of HMS, namely: (*a*) Scientific versus Superstitious Belief; (*b*) Scientific Understanding; and (*c*) Health Habits.

The goal of 'Health for All' remains distant and elusive for most Indians, but it can be achieved by political will and commitment. Health modernity education can contribute significantly to the realization of this goal. The Planning Commission, Government of India, has emphasized the importance of health education in its document 'The Approach to the Seventh Five Year Plan 1985–80': 'Achieving active community participation and involvement in health and health related programme should also be part of the strategy. In particular, active community participation and involvement of non-governmental organisations in a massive health education effort is urgently needed ...' (1984, pp. 22–23).

ACKNOWLEDGEMENTS

The concept of health modernity reported in this chapter has been developed in an ICMR Project conducted by this author jointly with Professor Eswara Reddy, Head, Department of Adult and Continuing Education, Osmania University, Hyderabad. Professor D. Sinha, Director, A.N.S. Institute of Social Studies, Patna, and Professor G. G. Prabhu, Head, Department of Clinical Psychology, NIMHANS, Bangalore had served as consultants. In the formulation and crystallization of the concept of health modernity, the active contribution of Professor Usha K. Luthra, Senior Deputy Director, ICMR, and Dr D. K. Menon, Director, National Institute of Mentally Handicapped, Secunderabad, is gratefully acknowledged.

REFERENCES

Almond, G. A. and Verba, S. (1965). *The civic culture*. Boston: Little Brown and Co.

Apter, D. E. (1965). *The politics of modernisation*. Chicago: The University of Chicago Press.

Berg, A. D. (1970). Nutrition as a national priority: Lessons from the Indian experiment. *The American Journal of Clinical Nutrition*, 23(7), 1396-408.

Black, C. E. (1967). *The dynamics of modernisation*. New York: Harper Torch Booke.

Chhabra, R. and Pettersson, W. (1979). *The situation of children in India*. Stockholm, Sweden: SIDA, Information Division.

Damle, Y. B. (1955). *Communication of modern ideas and knowledge in Indian villages*. MIT, Cambridge, Massachusetts.

Desai, A. R. (Ed.). (1971). *Essays on modernisation of underdeveloped societies*. Bombay: Thacker & Co. Limited.

Eisenstadt, S. N. (1966). *Modernisation: Protest and change*. Englewood Cliffs, NJ: Prentice-Hall, Inc.

———. (1973). *Tradition, change and modernity*. New York: John Wiley and Sons.

Ghosh, S. (1980). Priorities in child health. In *Profile of child in India*. Ministry of Social Welfare, pp. 74-88. New Delhi: Government of India.

Gopalan, C. (1983). Nutrition at the base. *Seminar*, February, 282, 19-24.

Grant, J. P. (1982). *The state of the world's children (1981-82)*. New York: UNICEF.

———. (1983). *The state of the world's children (1982-83). New Hope in Dark Times*. New York: UNICEF.

———. (1984). *The state of the world's children, 1984*. New Delhi: UNICEF.

Gupta, Satya. (1980). Health and nutrition education of mothers child care, in *Profile of the child in India*. Report submitted to Ministry of Social Welfare, Government of India, New Delhi, pp. 89-100.

Haxton, D. P. (1983). *Against anaemia.* New Delhi: UNICEF.
Hooja, V., Ghosh, S., Mittal, S. K. and Verma, R. K. (1976). Immunisation status in the urban community. *Indian Pediatrics,* 13(10), 747-50.
Inkeles, A. (1983). *Exploring individual modernity.* New York: Columbia University Press.
Inkeles, A. and Singh, A. K. (1983). Indian image of modernity in cross-cultural perspective. In A. Inkeles (Ed.), *Exploring individual modernity* (pp. 129-37). New York: Columbia University Press.
Inkeles A. and Smith, D. H. (1974). *Becoming modern: Individual changes in six developing countries.* Cambridge: Harvard University Press.
Kapp, K. W. (1963). *Hindu culture, economic development and social planning in India.* Bombay: Asia Publishing House.
Kuthiala, S. K. (1973). *From tradition to modernity.* New Delhi: Abhinav Publications.
Kulkarni, J. L. (1983). Retrieval from retardation. *Future,* 6, 39-42 (New Delhi: UNICEF).
Lerner, D. (1958). *The passing away of traditional society: Modernising the Middle East.* Glencoe, IL: Free Press.
Loomis, C. P. and Loomis, Z. K. (1969). *Socio-economic change and the religious factor in India: An Indian symposium of views on Max Weber.* New Delhi: Affiliated East-West Press Pvt. Ltd.
Mahler, H. (1983). Health for all: Every one's concern. *World health,* April-May, 2-4.
Marrion, J. Jr. (1966). *Modernisation and the structure of societies.* New Jersey: Princeton University Press.
McClelland, D. C. (1961). *The achieving society.* Princeton M.I., Van Nostrand.
McClelland, D. C. and Winter, L. G. (1969). *Motivating economic achievement.* New York: The Free Press.
Mishra, V. (1962). *Hinduism and economic growth.* Bombay: The Oxford University Press.
Mulay, S. and Ray, G. L. (1973). *Towards modernisation: A study of peasantry in rural Delhi.* Delhi: National.
Myrdal, G. (1968). *The Asian drama: An inquiry into poverty of nations.* New York: Pantheon.
Planning Commission. (1984). *The approach to the seventh five year plan 1985-90.* New Delhi: Planning Commission, Government of India.
Premi, M. K. (1982). *The demographic situation in India.* Paper No. 80, February. Honolulu, Hawaii: East-West Centre.
Raghuvanshi, M. S. (1984). *Modernising rural youth: The role of formal education.* Delhi: Ajanta Book International.
Ramalingaswami, V. (1983). The Greatest Health for the Greatest Number. *Future* (New Delhi: UNICEF).
———. (1984). Science and public health. *India International Centre Quarterly,* 11(3), 346-54.

Registrar General of India. (1981). *Survey on infant and child mortality, 1979.* New Delhi: Office of the Registrar General, India, Ministry of Home Affairs.

Rogers, E. M. (1969). *Modernisation among peasants: The impact of communication.* New York: Holt Rinehert and Winston, Inc.

Rosen, G. (1966). *Democracy and economic change in India.* Chicago: Aldin Publishing Co.

Rudolph, L. I. and Rudolph, S. H. (1967). *The modernity of tradition.* Chicago: The University of Chicago Press.

Sharma, S. L. (1979). *Modernising effects of university education.* New Delhi: Allied Publishers Pvt. Ltd.

Shils, E. (1961). The intellectuals between tradition and modernity: The Indian situation. *Comparative Studies in Society and History,* Supplement I. The Hague, Mounton & Co.

Singer, M. (Ed.). (1959). *Traditional India: Structure and change.* American Folklore Society: Philadelphia.

———. (1972). *When a great tradition modernises.* New Delhi: Vikas Publishing House Pvt. Ltd.

———. (1975). Industrial leadership, the Hindu ethic and the spirit of socialism. In A. K. Singh (Ed.), *Hindu culture and modernisation* (pp. 19-44). Psychology Department, Ranchi University.

Singh, Amar Kumar. (1967). Hindu culture and economic development in India. *Conspectus, Quarterly Journal of India International Centre,* 1, 9-32.

———. (1968). What cities and factories do to rural migrants: Dehumanisation or modernisation. Harvard University, centre International Affairs, Mimeo.

———. (1975). *Hindu culture and modernisation.* Post Graduate Department of Psychology, Ranchi University.

———. (1983a). Health modernity education in India. *Social Change,* 13(2), 27-34.

———. (1983b). *Health modernity in educated women.* Department of Psychology, Ranchi University.

———. (1984). *Health and modernity and its correlates in South Bihar.* ICMR, Report, Department of Psychology, Ranchi University.

Singh, S. N. (1979). *Industrialisation in modern perspective.* New Delhi: Classical Publications.

Singh, Tarlok. (1983). A decade for ending rural poverty. *Seminar,* 282, 14-19.

Singh, Yogendra. (1973). *Modernisation of Indian tradition.* Delhi: Thomson Press (India) Limited.

Smith, C. (1965). *Modernisation and traditional society.* Bombay: Asia Publishing House.

Srinivas, M. N. (1972). *Social change in modern India* (Indian education). New Delhi: Orient Longman.

Srivastava, S. K. (Ed.). (1976). *Tradition and modernisation.* Allahabad: Indian International Publications.

UNICEF. (1981). *Child atlas of India.* New Delhi: UNICEF.

UNICEF. (1984). *An analysis of the situation of children in India.* New Delhi: UNICEF.

Weber, Max. (1958a). *The protestant ethic and the spirit of capitalism* (trans. Talcott Parsons). New York: Charles Scribbner's Sons.

———. (1958b). *The religion of India* (trans. H. H. Gerth and Martindale Don). The Free Press, Glencoe.

Weiner, Myron. (Ed.). (1966). *Modernisation: The dynamics of growth.* Voice of America Forum Lectures.

Werner, D. (1982). *Where there is no doctor,* Indian Edition. New Delhi: Voluntary Health Association of India.

Werner, D. and Bower, B. (1983), *Helping health workers learn.* New Delhi: Indian education, Voluntary Health Association of India.

Winter, D. G. and McClelland, D. C. (1975). Need for achievement and Hindu culture. In A. K. Singh (Ed.), *Hindu culture and modernisation* (pp. 109-28). Ranchi: Psychology Department, Ranchi University.

18

Life Events Stress, Emotional Vital Signs and Hypertension

SAGAR SHARMA

Hypertension (HT) has been a major focus of biomedical and psychosomatic research for decades since it is the largest risk factor for cardiovascular disorders (CVDs), and is also known as a 'silent killer' as people go on for years without knowing its presence. There is a continuum of cardiovascular risk associated with the level of elevated blood pressure (BP) or HT; the higher the BP, the greater the risk for both coronary events and stroke (see Bittner, 2002; Brezinka and Kittel, 1996; Carrol, Smith and Sheffield, 1997; Gupta, 1997a, 1997b; Kop, 1997).

One area of inquiry and dispute has been the link of psychosocial factors and emotional markers (for example, stress, negative emotions/affectivity) to the pathophysiology of HT, and in turn to CVD (see Jorgenson, Johnson and Koloziej, 1996; Markovitz, Jonas and Davidson, 2001; Kranz and McCeney, 2002; Pickering, 2001). Studies that examined the role of stress (stressful life events or job/occupational stress) along with the indicators of negative affectivity in the onset and exacerbation of HT and related cardiac illness include those by Peter, Alfredson and Knutson (1999), Samova, Diarra and Jacobs (1995), Siegrist (1997) and Uchino and Garvey (1997). The related research has also shown that specific life events related to some kind of 'loss' are a greater risk factor for Essential Hypertension (EH). For instance, Levenstein, Smith and Kaplan (2001), in a prospective study of treated HT in general population, showed that the reality of unemployment or lowered occupational status increased the likelihood of developing HT. Most recently, a mild real-life condition (university examination) has been seen to increase arterial pressure and impair cardiovascular homeostasis (Lucini, Nabiato and Clerici, 2002). Such changes contribute to the link between psychological stress and increased cardiovascular risk of HT. However, another group of studies observed life events or work stress per se to be unrelated to EH (for example, Curtis, James and Raghunathan, 1997; Lazaro, Valdes and Marcos, 1993; Lindquist, Beilin and Knuiman, 1997; Pawar, 1994). Moreover, the prevailing pattern of such inconclusive evidence is further highlighted by Caputo, Rudolph and Morgan (1998). They argued that those experiencing positive life events are more likely to have high diastolic BPs, while Hobfoll and Spielberger (1992) suggest that positive life events indeed may act as stress buffers, thus alleviating BP levels. It seems that it is not the number/frequency of negative or positive life events per se that is important. What appears to be significant is their perceived impact as a psychological distress and other negative consequences.

The emotional vital signs (EVS) that are most critical to an individual's well-being are anger, anxiety and depression (Spielberger, Ritterband and Sydeman, 1995; Spielberger, Sydeman and Owen, 1999). A common link for all these negative emotions or markers of negative affectivity is a perceived loss of control over one's environment. Thus, it might be important to examine these emotional configurations as precursors or concomitants of HT (Sharma, Krishna and Spielberger, 1996). Out of these three EVS, anger and anxiety are the ones most often implicated as being associated with HT.

Trait anger (T-anger), or anger proneness, is a relatively stable personality trait that is manifested in the frequency, intensity and duration of anger experience. It is argued that persons with high T-anger, by virtue of their propensity towards anger and their long-term exposure to its pathophysiological sequelae, might be particularly susceptible to HT/CVD. However, T-anger has been studied less extensively and the findings to date are equivocal. Meta-analysis of the studies dealing with the relationship of T-anger and cardiovascular reactivity/elevated BP demonstrate small and variable relations (Suls, Wan and Costa, 1995). Also, Friedman, Schwartz and Schnall (2001) observed no significant differences on T-anger between mild hypertensives and those with normal BP. In a more recent review, however, Pickering (2001) found T-anger to be generally related to HT (see also Ghosh and Sharma, 1998). Given the inconsistent nature of the findings based on a rather limited research, further investigations are warranted on the role of T-anger in the onset and aggravation of cardiac illness/events such as HT.

Likewise, there is also a considerable variation across studies regarding the association of modes or styles of anger expression and EH/elevated BP. Anger suppression (anger-in [AX/In]) rather than anger proneness is seen as a critical factor in the development of HT (for example, Ghosh and Sharma, 1998; Helmers, Baker and O'Kelly, 2000; Samova et al., 1995; Sharma et al., 1996), but not in all (for example, Mueller, Grunbaum and Labarthe, 2001; Ohira, Tanigawa and Leo, 2000; Ohira, Iso and Tanigawa, 2002; Porter, Stone and Schwartz, 1999; Vandervoort, Ragland and Syme, 2001). Another set of studies indicate that outward expression of anger (anger-out [AX/Out]) is associated with HT status/greater BP than the suppressed anger (see Schwenkmezger and Hank, 1996; Seigman, 1994; Vogele, Jarvis and Cheesman, 1997), whereas some others showed that either expressed anger is inversely related to BP levels (for example, Ohira et al., 2002; Sharma et al., 1996) or extreme expressions of anger (AX/In or AX/Out) in either direction have adverse cardiovascular consequences (Everson, Goldberg and Kaplan, 1998). Further, with respect to control of anger (anger-control [AX/Con]), hypertensive patients tend to be lower on control of anger expression than the normotensives (Ghosh and Sharma, 1998; Sharma et al., 1996). In a recent study, Davidson, MacGregor and Stuhr (2000) further suggest that constructive anger expression (a form of anger control) may have an independent beneficial association with BP.

Like T-anger and the modes of anger expression, the data linking T-anxiety to HT/elevated BP also remains ambiguous. In a group of cross-sectional studies, hypertensive patients reported higher T-anxiety than the normotensives (for example, Chaudhry, Singh and Bhardwaj, 1994; Ghosh and Sharma, 1998; Sharma et al., 1996), whereas no such differences were observed in another group of studies (for example, Friedman et al., 2001). In a review by Jonas, Franks and Ingram (1997), four prospective studies failed to show an association, while three prospective studies supported the etiological significance of anxiety in HT (see also Jonas and Lando, 2000). Increased cardiovascular reactivity has been proposed to be a critical mediator in the development of HT and CVD. Contrary to this expectation, Young, Nesse and Weder (1998) demonstrated that individuals with high T-anxiety demonstrated reduced cardiovascular reactivity. Despite its longevity, the debate over whether a relationship exists between psychological variables (for example, stress, EVS) and HT remains unsettled. Most of the preceding research often favoured single factor, univariate analysis disregarding possible interaction of situational (contextual) and dispositional (personality) variables. A combination of socio-cultural and/or psychological stressors and EVS might synergistically induce greater psycho-physiological activities related to HT than either factor alone. In fact, there is some evidence suggesting that chronic/acute stressors interact with EVS in frequent triggering of the physiological stress reactions to contribute to the development of HT (see Anderson, McNeily and Myers, 1992; Jorgenson et al., 1996; Myers and McClure, 1993; Samova et al., 1995; Schwenkmezger and Hank, 1996; Thomas, 1997).

In view of the preceding overview, the present attempt in respect of patients with diagnosed HT determines the (*a*) negative and positive impacts of life events stress (LES); (*b*) levels of T-anger and T-anxiety (EVS); (*c*) dominant modes of coping with anger, i.e, AX/In, AX/Out, AX/Con and (*d*) the optimum set of variables (LES and EVS) which in combination or synergistically separate/discriminate these hypertensive patients from their normotensive–control counterparts.

METHOD

Participants

Hypertensives

Eighty married males diagnosed as hypertensives consented to participate in this study. The Diagnostic Protocol included structured medical history, BP readings that fulfilled WHO/ISH (1993) criteria for Systolic Blood Pressure (SBP) and Diastolic Blood Pressure (DBP) or both which had to be exceeded on three different occasions, laboratory tests such as total serum cholesterol with direct enzymatic level, albuminuria, electro-cardiogram recordings, etc. The diagnosis had been conducted by cardiologists at the Outpatient Clinic of Cardiology Unit of a state-administered medical college/hospital. All the patients were under medication/treatment, and thus aware of their hypertensive status. The M ± ISD values of five BP readings for these patients were 153.60 + 8.82 (SBP) and 105.59 + 7.83 (DBP), respectively. These patients thus continued to be mildly hypertensive despite being on regular medication ever since their diagnosis. Their Mean vs. ISD age in years was 56.46 + 10.63 (with 40 each in 40 + and 55 + years ranges). All of them were educated (12th grade +), either in job or retired and belonged to middle socio-economic status (SES) background. These patients had no previous history of MI, angina pectoris, intermittent claudication, and no current non-CHD illness including diabetes mellitus or secondary complication.

Normotensive controls

Eighty married males attending the Surgical/Orthopaedic Outpatient Clinic of the same Hospital were identified to willingly serve as normotensive controls. The M+1SD values of five BP readings in respect of this group were 132.45 + 5.28 (SBP) and 78.33 + 4.22 (DBP), respectively. Their corresponding mean ± ISD age in years was 55.76 + 10.62 (with 40 each in 40 + and 55 + years ranges). These controls were well-matched for age distribution, educational and SES status. None of these patient-controls had a history of HT or any other CHD or non-CHD illness including diabetes mellitus.

Measures

Life events stress scale (LESS)

The Hindi language version of the LESS (Ghosh, 1999) has 49 culturally relevant stressful life events. The LESS requires the respondents to identify the life events experienced during last two years, rate their desirability as well as their impact. The impact ratings are made on a 7-point scale ranging in terms of severity/intensity from extremely negative (-3) to extremely positive (+3). This procedure records not only the number/frequency of life events/stresses in the last two years, but also the degree of their perceived impact. In this study, two indicators were considered, *negative impact* (total impact of stressful events perceived as negative) and *positive impact* (total impact of events perceived as positive). Such standard measures of life events can be used cross-culturally with a degree of confidence (McAndrew, Akanda and Turner, 1998).

State-trait anger expression inventory (STAXI)

The Hindi adaptation of Spielberger's (1988) STAXI (see Sharma et al., 1996; 2003) was utilized to assess the emotional vital sign characterized by T-anger and modes of anger coping, i.e., AX/In, AX/Out and AX/Con. Only 34 out of 44 STAXI items were used since the rest pertain to state-anger (S-anger). While 10 items assess T-anger (anger proneness), the three STAXI subscales (8 items each) assess the frequency with which anger is held in or suppressed (AX/In), outwardly expressed (AX/Out) or covertly controlled (AX/Con).

State-trait anxiety inventory (STAI)

T-anxiety, the other EVS, was measured with the 20-item Hindi form of the T-scale of the STAI (Spielberger, Sharma and Singh, 1973; Spielberger and Sharma, 1976) of the English STAI (Spielberger, Gorsuch and Lushene, 1970).

Both the STAI and STAXI are excellent tools for use across cultures. The STAI has been translated and adapted into more than 50 languages and dialects. In addition to its English and Hindi versions, the STAXI is also available in the Dutch, German, Italian, Norwegian, Finnish and Chinese language versions. The cross-language equivalence, internal consistency, test-retest reliability and concurrent/construct validity of these measures of EVS have been consistently demonstrated (see also Spielberger et al., 1995, 1999).

Procedure

All the measures were administered individually to the patients with HT (treated) and also to their surgical/orthopaedic normotensive controls in the following order, LESS, STAXI and STAI. The respondents were assured of confidentiality and the likely use of their responses in treatment/recovery. Two impact ratings of life events were arrived at by a separate summing of (a) the life events perceived/experienced as negative, and (b) the life events perceived/experienced as positive. Thus, two separate indices of LES were obtained. Further, standardized scoring procedures were employed for the STAXI and STAI.

The data were first analysed for between-groups comparisons with independent t-tests in respect of LES—negative and positive impact. T-anger, modes of anger coping (AX/In, AX/Out, AX' Con and T-anxiety). Thereafter, the data on these seven measures were submitted to stepwise discriminant function analysis. By identifying the significance of selected variables in linear combination, this analysis permits (a) the understanding of synergistic role of identified discriminators in the separation of the two groups (hypertensives vs. normotensives), and (b) their classification accuracy, which is an additional indicator of the effectiveness of the discriminant function. This stepwise discriminant analysis was done on Pentium-based machine using SPSS-PC + (Statistical Package for Social Sciences) Software with procedure 'DISCRIMINANT' (see Nie, Hull and Jenkins, 1975; Klecka, 1985).

RESULTS

Hypertensive Patients vs. Normotensive Controls, Group Comparisons

The means and standard deviations for LES (negative and positive impacts), T-anger, modes of anger-coping (AX/In, AX/Out, AX/Con) and T-anxiety are shown in Table 18.1.

Table 18.1: Life Events Stress (Negative and Positive Impacts), Trait Anger, Modes of Anger Expression and Trait Anxiety in Hypertensives and Normotensives

Variables	Hypertensives (N = 80)		Mormotensives (N = 80)		t
	Mean	SD	Mean	SD	
Life Events Stress, (Negative Impact)	5.07	4.81	1.75	2.64	5.35**
Life Events Stress, (Positive Impact)	1.85	2.77	1.90	2.09	0.13
T-Anger	18.84	5.13	13.21	2.99	8.47**
Anger-In	21.37	3.49	17.26	3.07	7.91**
Anger-Out	13.17	3.29	14.42	2.17	2.83*
Anger-Con	24.S	I 4.82	27.18	2.94	3.76*
T-Anxiety	35.41	7.73	28.17	5.75	6.72**

Source: Author.
Notes: * $p \pm 0.01$
** $p \pm 0.001$

When compared to the normotensive controls, the hypertensives scored significantly higher on the negative impact of LES (t = 5.35; p < 0.001), but no such a significant difference was observed on the positive impact of LES. With respect to the EVS of T-anger and the modes of anger coping, the hypertensives were significantly higher on T-anger or anger proneness (t = 8.47; p < 0.001), AX/In (t = 7.91; p < 0.001), but significantly lower on AX/Out and AX/Con (t = 2.83 and 3.76, respectively; p < 01) than their normotensive counterparts. Consistent with the direction of group-contrasts observed with either negative impact of LES or T-anger, the patients with HT also reported higher score on the second EVS, i.e.,

T-anxiety or anxiety proneness (t = 6.72; p < 0.001) than the normotensive controls. When considered together, the composite profile of hypertensive patients, when compared to normotensive controls, comprised greater negative impact of LES, higher T-anger as well as suppression of anger and T-anxiety, but a lesser outward expression and control of anger. Given these findings, the issue of which of these measures in combination differentiated the hypertensive patients from their normotensive-patient controls appeared salient.

Hypertensive Patients vs. Normotensive Controls, Discriminant Analysis

Table 18.2 provides a summary of the outcome of stepwise discriminant analysis.

Table 18.2: Stepwise Discriminant Analysis with Respect to Patients with Hypertension vs. Normotensive Controls (N = 80 in each group)

Variables	F-to-remove	Wilk's Lambda	Wilk's Lambda Decrement	Standardized Discriminant Function Coefficient
T-Anger	52.44	0.687	0.313	0.789
Anger-Out	39.87	0.541	0.146	−0.700
Anger-In	20.34	0.468	0.073	0.467
Negative Impact of Life Events	6.96	0.448	0.020	0.291

Source: Author.

As can been seen, a set of four discriminators (i.e., T-anger, AX/Out, AX/In, and the negative impact of LES formed the discriminant function (Eigen value = 1.22). T-anxiety and AX/Con, however, did not comprise this function. Based on F-to-remove values, the selected set of four discriminators were arranged in the rank order of their relative importance for discrimination/separation between groups of hypertensives and the normotensives. As is evident in Table 18.2, T-anger, with the largest F-to-remove value (F = 52.44), made the highest contribution to the overall discrimination above and beyond the contribution made by other selected variables, i.e., AX/Out (F = 39.87), AX/In (F = 20.34) and negative impact of LES (F = 6.96). The values of Wilk's Lambda corroborated the observed group differences over the same set of four discriminating variables. Since T-anger increased maximum within-groups cohesiveness, this EVS was the first to be selected, followed by AX/Out, AX/In and the negative impact of LES, in that order. The values of Wilk's Lambda decrement further supplement/confirm the relative and unique contribution of each variable to the discriminant equation above and beyond the contribution of the preceding variable. While developing the discriminant function equations, standardized discriminant function (SDF) coefficients are also created. The magnitude of these SDFs, regardless of signs, also depict the relative and unique contribution of each variable to the discriminant function (see Table 18.2). These SDFs provided an additional confirmation to the conclusions derived on the basis of F-to-remove and Wilk's Lambda/decrement values. Specifically, the SDF values also documented that T-anger contributed the highest to the discrimination/separation of the hypertensives from their normotensive controls (SDF = 0.789), followed by AX/Out (SDF = –0.70), AX/In (SDF = 0.467) and negative impact of LES (SDF = 0.291). The direction of significant differences in respect of these discriminators was generally consistent with the signs of SDF loadings.

In respect of discriminant analysis, another crucial question is the classification accuracy based on identified set of discriminators. Klecka (1985) suggested that classification accuracy can be used along with F-to-remove, Lambda and SDF coefficients to indicate the amount of discrimination contained in selected variables. However, he pointed out that if chance accuracy is 50 per cent (as in the case of two-groups of equal sizes), the classification accuracy should be at least 62.5 per cent (25 per cent greater than that is achieved by chance). Based on discriminant function (comprising T-anger, AX/Out, AX/In and negative impact of LES), the correct classification rate for the patients with HT was 66 (82.5 per cent). The corresponding classification for the normotensive controls was 75 (93.5 per cent). Thus, 14 (17.5 per cent) of the 80 cases of hypertensive group were misclassified, whereas, in respect of the normotensives, only 5 (6.5 per cent) out of 80 were not correctly classified. This combination of discriminators was more accurate in correct identification of normotensives than the hypertensives. Nevertheless, the overall classification accuracy of known cases turned out to be 88 per cent (which is higher than 62.5 per cent). An additional confirmation thus emerged regarding the degree of group discrimination/separation, i.e., between hypertensive and normotensive groups.

Discussion

The findings that characterized patients with HT vis-à-vis their normotensive controls, document a relatively (a) greater negative impact of LES; (b) higher T-anger and anger suppression (AX/In); lower outward expression (AX/Out) and control of anger and (c) a higher T-anxiety.

With respect to the role of LES in HT and the related CVD, the evidence so far is mixed. While some studies support the role of stressful life events in the onset and progression of HT (for example, Fisher, 1996; Uchino and Garvey, 1997), others found no significant differences in the frequency of experienced stressful life events (for example, Lazaro et al., 1993; Pawar, 1994). As indicated earlier, the number/frequency of life or job events per se does not seem to be important. What appears to be significant is their perceived negative impact either directly or through a maladaptive coping with negative consequences such as HT and related risks (for example, Curtis et al., 1997; Lau, Huis and Lam, 1996; Lindquist et al., 1997). Additionally, O'Brien, Haynes and Mumby (1998) and Seibt, Brucsein and Schcuch (1998) highlighted the role of recovery process, and not stress per se, in the development of HT. Recent studies are now more concerned with specific life events/stresses involving some kind of 'loss' such as bereavement, divorce, unemployment, anticipated or actual job loss, effort-reward imbalance on job, etc. Such specific life events with their inherent negative impact are increasingly seen as stronger risk factors for HT (for example, Blumenthal, Thyrum and Siegal, 1995; Levenstein et al., 2001; Lucini et al., 2002; Peter et al., 1999; Schnall et al., 1992; Schnall, Landsbergis and Baker, 1994; Siegrist, 1997). While in the present study, the positive impact of LES turned out to be a non-significant variable, the possibility of positive life events impacting as stress buffers vis-à-vis HT/elevated BP, needs to be further explored (for example, Caputo et al., 1998; Fredrickson and Levenson, 1998).

Another finding related to T-anger (anger proneness), which was higher in patients with HT. When operationally defined, the hypertensives having high T-anger are likely to have (a) stronger propensity to experience and express anger indiscriminately and (b) greater disposition to express anger when criticized or treated unfavourably by others. Some earlier studies of HT tend to support this finding (for example, Ghosh and Sharma, 1998; Madigan, Dale and Cross, 1997; Pickering, 2001). However, a meta-analysis by Suls et al. (1995) showed little support for a connection between T-anger and chronically elevated BP. Nonetheless, it is possible that this conclusion of Suls et al. relates, in part, to their focus on T-anger self-report scores derived by averaging across items, varying in their linkages to or specification of an interpersonal context. It is quite possible that methods with stronger interpersonal foci or contexts (for example, structural interviews or a recall of life events just prior to responding to anger-scale items) may affect the strength of the association between T-anger and HT.

With respect to the modes of anger expression/coping, this study revealed that patients with HT resorted to higher anger suppression, lower outward expression as well as control over their angry feelings. Holding anger in appears to be a critical factor in the development of HT (see Ghosh and Sharma, 1998; Helmers et al., 2000; Samova et al., 1997). Moreover, the support for suppressed anger–HT hypothesis is seen in a meta-analytic review by Jorgenson et al. (1996). This meta-analysis of 295 relevant effect sizes confirmed the expectation that HT/chronically elevated BP would be associated with lower affect-expression or higher anger suppression (see also Ohira et al., 2002). Further, Jorgenson et al. (1996) argued that the prediction of HT can be maximized if anger-suppression measures are used that are linked to specific social contexts. Moreover, suppressed anger has been observed to be associated with avoidance coping style (Sharma and Acharya, 1989). It seems that a significant psychological process meditating between suppressed anger and HT could be the more frequent use of avoidance coping (see also Ohira et al., 2002; Spielberger, 1988). The more frequent and dominant use of suppression of anger by the hypertensives can also be attributed to their fear of retaliation as well as loss of social approval and desirability. There is also evidence to show that the inhibition of anger causes heightened autonomic arousal, which eventually leads to HT. Though it is not clear how it might happen, but the underlying premise usually is that inhibiting emotions leads to acute increase in physiological response parameters that may in the long run do damage. Further, studies may examine the interaction of anger proneness (T-anger) and anger-coping styles (especially anger suppression) in jointly determining the HT status/chronically elevated BP and consequential ill-health outcomes. Besides higher anger suppression, the hypertensives resorted not only to a lower AX/Out but also to a lesser control of the outward expression of their angry feelings. The findings are consistent with some of the earlier studies (for example Davidson et al., 2000; Ghosh and Sharma, 1998; Otten, 1993; Sharma et al., 1996). The research in this area has repeatedly revealed a relation among cardiovascular reactivity, anger and anger expression, with a larger body supporting suppressed anger–HT hypothesis. Yet the strength and direction of this relation is not yet fully clear.

It is still uncertain whether it is suppressed or openly exhibited anger that relates to cardiovascular reactivity. Moreover, there is a little related research on AX/Con mode of coping. It is now argued that the suppression or control reflect two distinct ways of dealing with anger (Spielberger, 1988). As indicated earlier, AX/In is associated with many negative (avoidance) copying styles (Sharma and Acharya, 1989), while AX/Con is significantly associated with several positive personality features. Persons relying on AX/Con rather than AX/In have more stable personalities with better psychosocial resources. This appears to be an important reason why AX/Con seems to be a healthier way of dealing with angry feelings, whereas AX/In would pose a major health risk (Julkunen, 1996).

The finding of higher T-anxiety (anxiety proneness) in patients with HT are supportive of earlier work by Chaudhry et al. (1994), Ghosh and Sharma (1998), Greenglass (1996), Jonas and Lando (2000), Markovitz et al. (2001), Pickering (2001), Pogotto et al. (1992), Sharma et al. (1996) and Vogele et al. (1997). In an earlier review, Jonas et al. (1997) reported that out of seven prospective studies, three tended to support the etiological significance of anxiety in HT. On the basis of the findings of this study, it can be speculated that individual differences in anxiety and anger proneness (T-anxiety and T-anger), contribute to the etiology of HT by enhancing anger suppression. Nonetheless, the observed differences in this study on the negative impact of life events and EVS are specific to the HT-normotension dichotomy.

A special feature of this study is the identification of a set of four discriminators and their relative power on the basis of simultaneous consideration of multiple indices of discrimination such as F-to-remove, Wilk's Lambda/decrement and SDF coefficients. The discriminant function that synergistically separated individuals with HT from the normotensives comprised T-anger (which emerged as the most potent discriminator), followed by two modes of anger expression (AX/Out, AX/In), and then negative impact of LES. The high degree of classification accuracy further confirmed the effectiveness of this discriminant function. The third emotional vital sign of trait depression (T-depression) was not considered in this study. The inclusion of T-depression could possibly lead to an almost perfect classification accuracy since this emotional vital sign is now being increasingly seen as a strong independent risk factor in cardiovascular disease (see Pickering, 2001; Sheps and Sheffield, 2001). Contrary to expectations, T-anxiety did not emerge as a significant discriminator. It is important to recognize that the outcome of discriminant analysis is also influenced by the inter-correlations between measures. For the hypertensive and normotensive groups, the correlations between anger and anxiety measures ranged from 0.48 to 0.78 ($p \leq 0.001$). This indicated a considerable overlap in these two constructs in respect of the samples under consideration. Being a relatively stronger and consistent factor in cardiac illness, T-anger could have been preferred as the most potent variable in the discriminant function at the cost of T-anxiety.

The special finding of this study is the identification of T-anger as the most potent discriminator along with modes of anger coping, and in combination with a situational variable (perceived negative impact of LES). The co-occurrence of a situational variable (LES) as an outcome I, in interaction with dispositional variable of T-anger and its coping as an outcome 2, vis-à-vis HT, suggests that psychological stressors and EVS and corresponding behavioural tendencies can synergistically influence the pathophysiology and etiology of HT and related cardiac illness (see Anderson et al., 1992; Everson and Salonen, 1997; Jorgenson et al., 1986; Myers and McClure, 1993; Thomas, 1997). It is suggested that future research needs to determine the role of chronic socio-cultural/psychological stressors (for example, crowding, chronically unequal and insecure neighbourhood, environmental degradation) in interaction with psychological risk factors (for example, the indicators of negative affectivity) in the frequent triggering of the physiological stress reactions (for example, Sympathetic Nervous System [SNS]-mediated Sodium retention and vasoconstriction) that are thought to contribute to the development of HT and related cardiac illness.

While this study delineated the powerful role of T-anger in HT, relatively little attention has been devoted to the study of this emotional vital sign, especially in India. Nevertheless, in a series of prospective studies, the significant causal role of T-anger as a risk factor has now been determined vis-à-vis acute and/or silent MI, cardiac revascularization procedure, premature cardiovascular disease and ischemic stroke (see Chang, Ford and Meoni, 2002; Kawachi, Sparrow and Spiro, 1996; Mittleman et al., 1995; Williams, Paton and Seigler, 2000; Williams, Nieto and Sanford, 2001; Williams, Nieto and Sanford, 2002). Such studies showed that higher proneness to anger places normotensive persons at significant risk of CHD morbidity and mortality or stroke, independent of biological risk factors. In most of such studies, including the present study, Spielberger's STAXI was employed to assess overall T-anger score. However, Spielberger's concept of proneness to anger is composed of two distinct components—angry temperament and anger-reaction. In a recent prospective study, Williams et al. (2001) showed that a strong angry temperament rather than anger in reaction to criticism, frustration or unfair treatment places normotensive middle-aged persons at increased risk for cardiac events and may confer a CHD risk similar to that of HT. Future research needs to take into account this distinction within the concept of T-anger. Moreover, T-anger–HT/CHD relationship could be directly causal or a proxy for another truly causal factor.

The strengths this study include the use of (a) culturally sensitive and carefully adapted measures of LES, STAXI and STAI, (b) clinical normotensive controls; (c) identification of a set of discriminators based on the simultaneous consideration of different indices of discriminant analysis and (iv) its situation × dispositional (interactional) perspective. Despite meaningful findings, there are some study limitations. A cross-sectional design was employed for treated/medicated individuals with HT. Therefore, the observed findings might not be causal, and also the over-reporting of events/symptoms cannot be ruled out. Illness itself can be a source of distress. Thus, relatively higher levels of LES and EVS observed in patients with HT may not be an exclusive etiological association but in part a consequence of diagnosis (see Rostrup and Ekeberg, 1992). Moreover, this study could not control for confounders/covariates of obesity, family history, smoking, alcohol abuse and other related factors. A longitudinal research with necessary controls for such confounders, though a difficult course, is required to demonstrate the prospective and synergistic links between stress, EVS and subsequent impairment of cardiovascular homeostasis resulting in CVD.

Notwithstanding these limitations, this study at least confirmed the association of LES and EVS as concomitants of HT status. This implies that either cognitive–behavioural techniques for management of stress, anger and anxiety (negative affectivity) require to be incorporated in the overall interventional package for hypertensive patients or at least these techniques, alongwith the cultivation of positive emotions, could be utilized as adjuncts to medication (see Deffenbacher, 1999; Fredrickson and Levenson, 1998; Kondwani and Lollis, 2001; Pandya, 1999; Sheu, Irvin and Lin, 2003).

REFERENCES

Anderson, N. B., McNeily, M. and Myers, H. F. (1992). A contextual model for research of race differences in autonomic reactivity. In E. H. Johnson, W. D. Gentry and S. Julius (Eds), *Personality, elevated blood pressure and essential hypertension* (pp. 197-216). Washington, DC: Hemisphere.

Bittner, V. (2002). Women and coronary heart disease factors. *Cardiovascular Risk, 9*, 315-22.

Blumenthal, J. A., Thyrum, E. T. and Siegal, W. C. (1995). Contribution of job strains, job status and marital status to laboratory and ambulatory BP in patients with mild hypertension. *Journal of Psychosomatic Research, 39*, 133-44.

Brezinka, V. and Kittel, F. (1996). Psychosocial factors of coronary heart disease in women: A review. *Social Science and Medicine, 42*, 1351-65.

Caputo, J. L. Rudolph, D. L. and Morgan, M. (1998). Influence of positive life events on blood pressure in adolescents. *Journal of Behavioral Medicine, 21*, 115-29.

Carrol, D., Smith, G. D. and Sheffield, D. (1997). The relationship between socioeconomic status, hostility and blood pressure reactions to mental stress in men: Data from the Whitehall II study. *Health Psychology, 16*, 131-36.

Chang, P. P., Ford, D. E. and Meoni, L. A. (2002). Anger in young men and subsequent premature cardiovascular disease: The precursors study. *Archives of Internal Medicine, 162*, 901-06.

Chaudhry, S., Singh, M. and Bhardwaj, P. (1994). Anxiety and depression in idiopathic hypertension. *Indian Journal of Clinical Psychology, 21*, 18-21.

Curtis, A. B., James, S. A. and Raghunathan, T. E. (1997). Job strain and blood pressure in African Americans: The Pitt County Study. *American Journal of Public Health, 87*, 1297-1302.

Davidson, K., MacGregor, M. W. and Stuhr, J. (2000). Constructive anger verbal behaviour predicts blood pressure in population-based sample. *Health Psychology, 19*, 55-64.

Deffenbacher, J. L. (1999). Cognitive-behavioral conceptualization and treatment of anger. *Journal of Clinical Psychology, 52*, 295-309.

Everson, S. A. and Salonen, J. T. (1997). Interaction of workplace demands and cardiovascular reactivity in hypertension of carotid atherosclerosis: Population-based study. *British Medical Journal, 314*, 553.

Everson, S. A., Goldberg, D. E. and Kaplan, G. A. (1998). Anger expression and incident hypertension. *Psychosomatic Medicine, 60*, 730-35.

Fisher, S. (1996). Life change, personal control and disease. *South Africa Journal of Psychology, 26*, 16-22.

Fredrickson, B. L. and Levenson, R. W. (1998). Positive emotions speed recovery from the cardiovascular sequelae of negative emotions. *Cognition and Emotion, 12*, 191-220.

Friedman, R., Schwartz, J. E. and Schnall, P. L. (2001). Psychological variables in hypertension: Relationship to casual ambulatory blood pressure in men. *Psychosomatic Medicine*, 63, 19-31.

Ghosh, S. N. (1999). Life events stress in patients with bronchial asthma and peptic ulcer. In D. M. Pestonjee, U. Pareek and R. Agrawal (Eds), *Studies in stress and its management* (pp. 219-26). New Delhi: Oxford and IBH.

Ghosh, S. N. and Sharma, S. (1998). Trait anxiety and anger expression in patients with essential hypertension. *Journal of the Indian Academy of Applied Psychology*, 24, 9-14.

Greenglass, E. R. (1996). Anger suppression, cynical distrust and hostility: Implications for coronary heart disease. In C. D. Spielberger and I. G. Sarason (Eds), *Stress and emotions* (Vol. 16) (pp. 205-25). Washington DC: Taylor and Francis.

Gupta, R. (1997a). Epidemiological evolution and rise of coronary heart disease in India. *South Asian Journal of Preventive Cardiology*, 1, 14-20.

—— (1997b). Meta-analysis of hypertension epidemiology in India. *Indian Heart Journal*, 49, 43-48.

Helmers, K. F., Baker, B. and O'Kelly, B. (2000). Anger expression, gender and ambulatory blood pressure in mild unmedicated adults with hypertension. *Annals of Behavioral Medicine*, 22, 60-64.

Hobfoll, S. E. and Spielberger C. D. (1992). Family stress. Integration of theory and measurement. *Journal of Family Psychology*, 6, 99-112.

Jonas, B. S. and Lando, J. F. (2000). Negative affect as a prospective risk factor for hypertension. *Psychosomatic Medicine*, 62, 188-96.

Jonas, B. S., Franks, P. and Ingram, D. D. (1997). Are symptoms of anxiety and depression risk factors for hypertension? *Archives of Family Medicine*, 6, 43-49.

Jorgenson, R. S., Johnson, B. T. and Koloziej, M. E. (1986). Elevated blood pressure and personality: A meta-analytic review. *Psychological Bulletin*, 120, 293-320.

Julkunen, J. (1996). Suppressing your anger: Good manners or bad health? In C. D. Spielberger and I. G. Sarason (Eds), *Stress and emotion* (Vol. 16) (pp. 227-40). Washington, DC: Taylor & Francis.

Kawachi, I., Sparrow, D. and Spiro, A. (1996). A prospective study of anger and coronary heart disease. *Circulation*, 94, 2090-95.

Klecka, W. R. (1985). *Discriminant analysis*. London: Sage.

Kondwani, K. A. and Lollis, C. M. (2001). Is there a role for stress management in reducing hypertension among African Americans. *Ethnicity and Disease*, 11, 788-92.

Kop, W. J. (1997). Acute and chronic psychological risk factors for coronary syndrome: Moderating effect of coronary artery disease severity. *Journal of Psychosomatic Research*, 43, 167-81.

Kranz, D. S. and McCeney, M. K. (2002). Effects of psychological and social factors on organic disease: A critical assessment on coronary heart disease. *Annual Review of Psychology*, 53, 341-69.

Lau, G. K., Huis, W. H. and Lam, S. K. (1996). Life events and daily hassles in patients with atypical chest pain. *American Journal of Gastroenterology*, 91, 2157-62.

Lazaro, M. L. Valdes, M. and Marcos, J. (1993). Borderline hypertension, daily stress and physiological variables. *Stress Medicine*, 19, 215-20.

Levenstein, S., Smith, M. W. and Kaplan, G. A. (2001). Psychosocial predictors of hypertension in men and women. *Archives of Internal Medicine*, 61, 1341-46.

Lindquist, T. L., Beilin, L. J. and Knuiman, W. (1997). Influence of life style, coping, and job stress on blood pressure in men and women. *Hypertension*, 29, 1-7.

Lucini, D., Nabiato, G. and Clerici, M. (2002). Hemodynamic and autonomic adjustments to real life stress conditions in humans. *Hypertension*, 39, 184-88.

Madigan, M. F. Jr., Dale, J. A. and Cross, J. D. (1997). No respite during sleep: Heart-rate reactivity to rapid eye movement sleep in angry men classified as Type A. *Perceptual and Motor Skills*, 85, 1451-54.

Markovitz, J. H., Jonas, B. S. and Davidson, K. (2001). Psychological factors as precursors to hypertension. *Current Hypertension Reports*, 3, 25-32.

McAndrew, F. T., Akanda, A. and Turner, S. (1998). A cross-cultural ranking of stressful life events in Germany, India, South Africa and the United States. *Journal of Cross-cultural Psychology*, 29, 717-27.

Mittleman, M. A., Maclure, M., Sherwood, J. B., Mulry, R. P., Tofler, G. H., Jacobs, S. C., Friedman, R., Bensen, H. and Muller, J. E. (1995). Triggering of acute myocardial infraction onset by episodes of anger. *Circulation*, 92, 1720-25.

Mueller, W. H., Grunbaum, J. A. and Labarthe, D. R. (2001). Anger expression, body fat, and blood pressure in adolescents: Project Heart Beat. *American Journal of Human Biology*, 13, 531-38.

Myers, H. F. and McClure, R. E. (1993). Psychological factors in hypertension in blacks: The case of an interactional perspective. In J. C. S. Fray and J. G. Douglas (Eds.), *Psychophysiology of hypertension in Blacks* (pp. 69-89). New York: Oxford University Press.

Nie, N. H., Hull, C. H. and Jenkins, K. (1975). *SPSS, statistical package for social sciences*. New York: McGraw Hill.

O'Brien, W. H. Haynes, S. N. and Mumby, P. E. (1998). Differences in cardiovascular recovery among healthy young adults with or without a family history of hypertension. *Journal of Psychophysiology*, 12, 17-28.

Ohira, T., Iso, H. and Tanigawa, T. (2002). The relation of anger expression with blood pressure levels and hypertension in rural and urban Japanese communities. *Journal of Hypertension*, 20, 21-27.

Ohira, T., Tanigawa, T. and Leo, H. (2000). The impact of anger suppression on blood pressure levels in white-collar workers with low coping behaviour. *Environmental Health and Preventive Medicine*, 5, 37-42.

Otten, H. (1993). Relationships of anger expression to cardiovascular reactivity and blood pressure in men. In V. Hodapp and Schwenkmezger (Eds), *Arger and Argerausdruck* (pp. 193-215). Bern: Huber.

Pandya, R. (1999). Stress management through exploring the inner space. In D. M. Pestonjee, U. Pareek and R. Agrawal (Eds), *Studies in stress and its management* (pp. 281-90). New Delhi: Oxford & IBH Publishing.

Pawar, N. B. (1994). A study of stress and personality factors of the patients of some psychophysiological disorders (i.e., asthma, peptic ulcer and essential hypertension. Unpublished doctoral thesis, University of Pune, Pune.

Peter, R., Alfredson, L. and Knutson, A. (1999). Does a stressful psychosocial environment mediate the effects of shift work on cardiovascular risk factor. *Scandinavian Journal of Work Environment*, 25, 376-81.

Pickering, T. G. (2001). Mental stress as a causal factor in the development of hypertension and cardiovascular disease. *Current Hypertension Reports*, 3, 249-54.

Pogotto, V., Fallo, F. and Fava, G. A. (1992). Anxiety sensitivity in essential hypertension. *Stress Medicine*, 8, 113-15.

Porter, I. S., Stone, A. A., Schwartz, J. E. (1999). Anger expression and ambulatory blood pressure: A comparison of state and trait measures. *Psychosomatic Medicine*, 61, 454-63.

Rostrup, M. and Ekeberg, O. (1992). Awareness of high blood pressure influence on psychological and sympathetic response. *Journal of Psychosomatic Research*, 36, 117-23.

Samova, L. I., Diarra, K. and Jacobs, T. Q. (1997). Psychophysiological study of hypertension in blacks, Indian and white African students. *Stress medicine*, 11, 105-11.

Schnall, P. L., Landsbergis, P. A., Pieper, C. F., Dietz, D., Gerin, W., Schlussel, Y., Warren, K. and Pickering, T. G. (1992). The impact of anticipation of job loss on psychological distress and worksite blood pressure. *American Journal of Industrial Medicine*, 21, 417-32.

Schnall, P. L., Landsbergis, P. A. and Baker, D. (1994). Job strain and cardiovascular disease. *Annual Review of Public Health*, 15, 381-411.

Schwenkmezger, P. and Hank, P. (1996). Anger expression and blood pressure. In C. D. Spielberger and I. G. Sarason (Eds), *Stress and emotion* (Vol. 16) (pp. 241-59). Washington, DC: Taylor & Francis.

Seibt, R., Brucsein, W. and Schcuch, K. (1998). Effects of different stress settings on cardiovascular parameters and their relationship to daily life BP in normotensive and bordeline hypertensives. *Ergonomics*, 41, 634-48.

Seigman, A.W. (1994). From Type A to hostility to anger: Reflections on the history of coronary-prone behaviour. In A. W. Seigman and T. W. Smith (Eds), *Anger, hostility and heart* (pp. 1-21). Hillsdale, NJ: Erlbaum.

Sharma, S. and Acharya, T. (1989). Coping strategies and anger expression. *Journal of Personality and Clinical Studies*, 5, 15-18.

Sharma, S., Krishna, A. and Spielberger, C. D. (1996). Anger and anxiety in hypertensive patients in India. In C. D. Spielberger and I. G. Sarason (Eds), *Stress and emotion* (Vol. 16) (pp. 261-68). Washington, DC: Taylor & Francis.

Sharma, S., Krishna, A. and Spielberger, C. D. (2003). The Hindi anger expression scale: Construction and validation. In C. D. Spielberger and I. G. Sarason (Eds), *Stress and emotion* (Vol. 17) (pp. 197-206). Washington, DC: Taylor & Francis.

Sheps, D. S. and Sheffield, D. (2001). Depression, anxiety, and the cardiovascular system: The cardiologist's perspective. *Journal of Clinical Psychiatry*, 8, 12-16.

Sheu, S., Irvin, B. L. and Lin, H. S. (2003). Effects of progressive muscle relaxation on blood pressure and psychosocial status for clients with essential hypertension in Taiwan. *Holistic Nursing Practice*, 17, 4147.

Siegrist, P. R. (1997). Chronic work stress, sickness absence and hypertension in middle managers: General and specific sociological explanation. *Social Science Medicine*, 45, 1111-20.

Spielberger, C. D. (1988). *State-trait anger expression inventory: Professional manual*. Odessa: Psychological Assessment Resources.

Spielberger, C. D. and Sharma, S. (1976). Cross-cultural measurement of anxiety. In C. D. Spielberger and R. Diaz-Gurrero (Eds), *Cross-cultural anxiety* (pp. 13-25). Washington, D. C: Hemisphere/Wiley.

Spielberger, C. D., Gorsuch, R. L. and Lushene, R. E. (1970). *Manual for state-trait anxiety inventory*. Palo Alto, California: Consulting Psychologists Press.

Spielberger, C. D., Ritterband, L. M. and Sydeman, S. J. (1995). Assessment of emotional states and personality traits: Measuring psychological vital signs. In J. N. Butcher (Ed.), *Clinical personality assessment, practical approaches* (pp. 41-58). New York: Oxford University Press.

Spielberger, C. D., Sharma, S. and Singh, M. (1973). Development of Hindi edition of the state-trait anxiety inventory. *Indian Journal of Psychology*, 48, 11-20.

Spielberger, C. D., Sydeman, S. J. and Owen, A. E., (1999). Measuring anxiety and anger with state-trait anxiety inventory (STAI) and the state-trait anger expression inventory (STAXI). In M. E. Maruish (Ed.), *The use of psychological testing for treatment planning and outcome assessment* (2nd ed.) (pp. 993-1021). Mahwah: Lawrence Erlbaum Associates.

Suls, J., Wan, C. K. and Costa, P. T. Jr. (1995). Relationship of trait anger to resting blood pressure: A meta-analysis. *Health Psychology*, 14, 444-56.

Thomas, S. P. (1997). Women's anger: Relationship of suppression to blood pressure. *International Congress of Behavioral Medicine*, 20, 15-27.

Uchino, B. N. and Garvey, T. S. (1997). The availability of social support reduces cardiovascular reactivity to psychological stress. *Journal of Behavioural Medicine*, 20, 15-27.

Vandervoort, D. J., Ragland, D. R. and Syme, S. L. (2001). Anger expression and hypertension in transit workers. *Ethnicity and Disease*, 11, 80-89.

Vogele, C., Jarvis, A. and Cheesman, K. (1997). Anger suppression, reactivity and hypertension risk: Gender makes a difference. *Annals of Behavioral Medicine*, 19, 61-69.

WHO/ISH Mild Hypertension Liasion Committee (1993). Summary of 1993 World Health Organization-International Society of Hypertension guidelines for the management of mild hypertension. *British Medical journal*, 311, 1541-46.

Williams, J. E., Nieto, F. J. and Sanford, C. P. (2001). Effects of an angry temperament on coronary heart disease risk: The atherosclerosis risk in communities (ARIC) study. *American Journal of Epidemiology*, 154, 230-35.

———. (2002). The association between trait anger and incident stroke risk: The atherosclerosis risk in communities (ARIC) study. *Stroke*, 33, 13-20.

Williams, J. E., Paton, C. C. and Seigler, I. C. (2000). Anger proneness predicts coronary heart disease. Prospective analysis from the atherosclerosis risk in communities (ARIC) study. *Circulation*, 101, 2034-39.

Young, E. A., Nesse, R. M. and Weder, A. (1998). Anxiety and cardiovascular reactivity in the Tecumseh population. *Journal of Hypertension*, 16, 1727-33.

19

Perception of AIDS in Mumbai: A Study of Low Income Communities

SHALINI BHARAT

... I sometimes feel it will not be any illness but this name—AIDS—that will kill me... (Male, HIV positive, 42 years)

INTRODUCTION

The understanding that AIDS (Acquired Immune Deficiency Syndrome) is not only a biomedical problem but also a social one was acknowledged early on in the epidemic, given its socio-economic and psychological impact on individuals, families and society in general. As a result, there have been a number of research attempts to understand the social dimensions of the problem. Currently available Indian researches have been limited mainly to assessing knowledge and awareness about AIDS, patterns of high-risk behaviour and the impact of AIDS education programme (see Aggarwal, Sharma and Indrayan, 1997 for a compilation of research work on AIDS). The social context in which HIV is transmitted, experienced and managed, and the socio-cultural meanings attached to HIV and AIDS, have been the subject matter of only a few studies thus far (see Bharat, 1996; Bharat and Aggleton, 1999; Bharat, Singhanetra-Renard and Aggleton, 1998).

In most developing countries, illnesses are experienced and managed within the household and communities (Ankrah, 1993). In this sense, illnesses are not just individual concerns, but they are the 'concerns' of the household and the community as well. However, even as households and communities assume significant roles in the care and support of their sick members, their responses, supportive or discriminatory, are shaped by their perceptions and meanings associated with illnesses. These perceptions and meanings are in turn shaped by the social construction of illnesses. Evidence from medical anthropology suggests that illnesses have various characteristics that lend themselves to figurative thinking about health problems: signs and symptoms, etiology and social characteristics of those who have an illness or are perceived to be particularly at risk (Lieban, 1992).

In her outstanding work on illness metaphors, Sontag (1989; 1991) explained that every disease has certain associated myths, ideologies and metaphors. These may be positive or negative, may change over time, may be based on incomplete knowledge and may have a powerful impact on sick persons and their caregivers. For example, beliefs and perceptions about how an illness is acquired may influence attributions to causality; sickness may be attributed to the person or to factors in his or her environment or to a combination of both. Further, causality attributed to a health condition may influence the ways in which care is provided—with compassion and understanding or with anger and resentment. Social perceptions of a disease also affect the people's efforts to prevent the disease, their sense of control over the disease and, more importantly, their social interactions with sick individuals. Research on disease explanatory models (Kleinman, 1980) revealed that people everywhere make attempts to perceive and attribute meanings to various diseases, infer signs and symptoms, grade diseases according to intensity, and label and categorize them as curable/incurable and contagious/non-contagious. Such perceptions generally differ from those held by medical professionals and often are dismissed as lay persons' beliefs and misconceptions.

Diseases such as leprosy, syphilis, TB and cancer in particular have been attributed with various meanings and symbols with consequences, generally discriminating in nature, for the sick individuals (Douglas, 1970; Gussow, 1989; Sontag, 1989). Taking the example of leprosy, Gussow (1989) noted that as leprosy disappeared from Europe and America and became endemic in some of the colonies, it began to be perceived as a disease of the 'inferior peoples'. Consequently, early Chinese immigration into America was seen as a potential source for the spread of leprosy in that country, condensing the perception of leprosy into a powerful symbol of danger and defilement. Sontag (1989) illustrated the use of the language of warfare in descriptions of cancer. According to her, '... cancer cells do not simply multiply; they are invasive'. Indeed, in common language, the word cancer is used to convey invasion as in colonization or Westernization. For instance, Nichter (1981) reported that in most parts of South Asia, the word cancer is used as a metaphor for the invasive activities of Western capitalism and the ill-effects of a Western lifestyle. While symptoms and disease progression help in characterizing illnesses such as cancer and TB, certain other diseases are more inherently associated with their etiology than symptomatology. For instance, the perceived etiology of syphilis carries with it a stigma for those who are infected with it (Lieban, 1992). It is commonly perceived as afflicting those who have low moral worth and sinful behaviour. AIDS is yet another disease that closely follows such negatively perceived diseases as syphilis due to its etiology. AIDS has been strongly associated with moral denigration and lifestyles involving deviant and perverse sex, intravenous drug use and promiscuity. According to Sontag (1989), 'The drug usage behavior, which produces AIDS, is judged to be more than just weakness. It is indulgence, delinquency ... addiction to chemicals that are illegal and to sex regarded as deviant ... a disease not just of sexual excess but of perversity.' The metaphoric use of language in AIDS is a powerful indication of the stigma attached to it (Sontag, 1989). At least seven metaphors have been used in interpreting the meaning of AIDS (Gilmore and Somerville, 1994).

1. AIDS as death—not only biological but social and sexual as well, and depicted often by images of skulls and bones.
2. AIDS as punishment—for immoral and sinful behaviour such as homosexuality and commercial sex.
3. AIDS as crime—the HIV-infected are perceived as criminals and 'guilty' of harming their 'innocent' victims (their sexual partners, for example).
4. AIDS as war—it is interpreted as an enemy or an invader to be fought with warlike zeal and preparedness.
5. AIDS as otherness—it is seen as a problem of 'them' and not 'us' and a distinction is made between the 'infected' and the 'uninfected', the 'sick' and the 'well'.
6. AIDS as horror—HIV infection is interpreted as an abject, terrorizing invader or demon and those infected are demonized.
7. AIDS as villain—the infected are perceived as villains for creating the epidemic and those not infected are seen as heroes.

Several studies provide evidence of the usage of such metaphors in other places. In Thailand, for example, AIDS is seen as a dirty disease associated with promiscuity, homosexuality and prostitution (Songwathana and Manderson, 1998). In some developing countries, AIDS is also seen as a 'woman's disease' because of its perception as a sexually transmitted disease and its association with prostitutes who are regarded as the reservoir of Sexually Transmitted Disease (STD) and HIV infection (Songwathana and Manderson, 1998). Shame and social disgrace are other meanings associated with AIDS where those infected are seen as bringing ignominy to society (Bharat, 1996; Omangi, 1997). Paying for their sins as part of their *karma* is how Buddhist countries such as Thailand perceive AIDS (Songwathana and Manderson, 1998).

The routes of transmission of the AIDS virus, and its impact on the social economic and personal lives of the infected and affected people have led to the conception that AIDS is not just a biomedical problem. The social dimensions of AIDS are far too serious and complicated; this means that its prevention requires an understanding of its cultural context, both at the micro level (individual's household, community) and at the macro level (poverty, urbanization, gender relations).

This paper seeks to understand how AIDS is perceived and interpreted within a cultural setting. It investigates the level of knowledge related to the transmission of the AIDS virus, its causes, prevention methods and the meanings attached to AIDS as an illness. Data reported here are drawn from a larger qualitative research that examined the household and community responses and coping patterns to HIV/AIDS in Mumbai (Bharat, 1996; Bharat and Aggleton, 1999; Bharat et al., 1998). The more specific objectives of the study are: (*a*) to examine the nature and dynamics of household and community responses to HIV/AIDS; (*b*) to investigate the cultural, social, economic and demographic correlates of the household and community responses and to study the inter-relationships at the household and community levels and (*c*) to suggest intervention strategies for the prevention of AIDS.

AIDS Scenario in India

Estimates made by the Joint United Nations Programme on HIV/AIDS (UNAIDS/WHO, 1998) suggest that at the beginning of 1998, over 30 million people globally were infected with the HIV that causes AIDS and that nearly 11.7 million people had already succumbed to the disease.

The heaviest burden of the HIV epidemic was reported in the developing countries of sub-Saharan Africa and Asia, the latter with nearly 4 million infected with HIV. Among the Asian countries, India reportedly has the largest number of individuals with AIDS after Thailand (the two countries together account for an estimated 95 per cent of reported AIDS cases in the region). The first case of AIDS in India was detected in 1986 in Chennai in a female sex worker. The early phase of the epidemic elicited a general denial of the problem from all quarters. It was considered the problem of a highly selective group of people—those with high-risk behaviour, namely, sex workers, injecting drug users and professional blood donors. The general masses were thought to lead a 'morally pure' life and, hence, not likely to acquire the dreaded virus. However, by the early 1990s, 'denial' had given way to a 'reluctant acceptance' of the epidemic as a real public health problem. The government established the National AIDS Control Organisation (NACO) in 1992 as an executive body of the Ministry of Health and Family Welfare to address the problem. A strategic plan for the prevention and control of AIDS in India for a five-year period, 1992–97, was prepared with support from the World Bank, the WHO and other international bodies. Sero surveillance data reported by the NACO over the last one decade showed increasing HIV incidence. Data collected in February–March 1998, for example, revealed that HIV infection was prevalent in all parts of the country (NACO, 1997–98). Almost 75 per cent of all currently reported infections are through the sexual transmission route, 8 per cent through blood and 8 per cent through injecting drug use. Over 90 per cent of the reported cases were from the sexually active and economically productive age groups of 15–59 years (NACO, 1997–98). A disturbing trend of increasing HIV prevalence, among women attending an antenatal clinic and those who are married and monogamous, has shifted the exclusive focus of the AIDS programme from high-risk behaviour groups to the general population with low risk of infection (Gangakhedkar et al., 1997; NACO, 1997–98).

THE RESEARCH SETTING AND ITS SOCIO-CULTURAL CONTEXT

This paper draws from a study conducted in Mumbai between 1994 and 1995 (Bharat, 1996). Mumbai, with a population of nearly 10 million people (Census of India, 1991), is India's second largest city. A combination of social, demographic, political and economic factors have transformed this city into an overpopulated, congested and polluted one with increasing space demands made on a land mass that has natural limitation to its geographic expansion. Inmigration of job seekers, primarily males, has resulted in an adverse sex ratio (820 females per 1,000 males; Census of India, 1991). Migration has also produced large squatter settlements with little access to safe drinking water, choked drainage system and extreme squalor. Despite its urban and civic problems, Mumbai remains the dream city for people in search of economic affluence and prosperity. In socio-cultural terms, it mirrors the rest of Indian society with perhaps only some evidence of a cosmopolitan, progressive society. While the facade is of a metropolitan city offering anonymity and a fast-paced work culture, the city is not entirely rid of traditional norms of gender relations and attitudes. Thus, just as elsewhere in India, male sexuality is acknowledged and accepted, and sexual needs of men are understood and justified in more liberal terms. Norms governing women's sexual lives are extremely rigid in comparison. Virginity and marital fidelity remain the normative ideals for the general population of women in the city (Bhende, 1995; George and Jaswal, 1995).

METHODOLOGY

Findings reported here pertain to the community-based data of the larger study on household and community responses to HIV/AIDS (Bharat, 1996). For the purpose of this study, a community was understood in terms of neighbourhood or cluster of households within a geographical boundary. Participants were drawn from two lower income (slum) and three lower middle class (*chawls*[1]) communities to explore their responses to HIV and AIDS. The two slum communities were located in the eastern and western suburbs, and the three lower middle-class communities were located in the central part of the city.

A qualitative research approach was adopted to situate the perception of AIDS within the social-cultural context of the participants (Boulton, 1994). Since the purpose was to explore the community

---

[1] *Chawls* are one-room tenement buildings housing mainly the working-class population.

members' understanding and perception of AIDS, the focused group discussion (FGD) method was chosen which allows such explorations at group levels (Morgan, 1988). A total of 18 FGDs were held with young and adult men and women in their communities. This was done to ensure representation of both genders as well as generations. The distribution was: 10 FGDs with men (6 with older men aged 30-45 years and 4 with younger men aged 18-25 years) and 8 FGDs with women (5 with older women aged 30-45 years and 3 with younger women aged 18-22 years).

The specific topics covered were level of awareness and understanding about HIV/AIDS, perception of causes, patterns of sexual behaviour, perception of the risk of HIV infection in the community and their ways of coping with the epidemic. In this paper the focus is on (a) the understanding of HIV/AIDS—its nature, causes, transmission routes, ways of prevention; (b) meanings attributed to HIV/AIDS and (c) risk perception of infection with HIV.

The entry points for the communities were the local youth clubs or libraries that characterize many such communities in Mumbai. In one slum community, however, the point of entry was the household of an HIV-infected person. The common features of these communities were poor hygienic conditions, ill-ventilated rooms, lack of space, overcrowding and a concomitant lack of privacy. A majority of the male *chawl* residents worked as low-ranked professionals (technicians, junior engineers) in factories and private firms. The women were mainly housewives, although some of them were school teachers, nurses or community health workers. Men in the slum communities worked as low-skilled workers and their wives as domestic servants or as maids in hospitals.

A question guideline was developed in the local language for the purpose of FGDs (Bharat, 1996). Male and female moderators and recorders were employed to conduct FGDs with their respective gender groups. However, in two cases, female staff conducted FGDs with young men after they had spent sufficient time in the community discussing health issues in general. Each focus group comprised 5-10 participants and the discussion lasted approximately two hours.

THE FINDINGS

The findings reported here are thematically arranged with a number of verbatim quotes to accurately present the people's own voices. People's perceptions are grouped under single-idea domains.

While most respondents were familiar with the word AIDS, they did not know the full form of the acronym, and very few people knew about HIV. Those who did, referred to HIV as the *jeevanu* (micro-organism) that causes AIDS. But, their conception of *jeevanu* was nothing like that of an invisible virus as in biomedical terms.

In general, men had greater knowledge and awareness, but more misconceptions as well about AIDS. The group of younger girls was least communicative on AIDS-related issues as their awareness was at a very preliminary level. FGDs with this group explored sexual health issues such as experiences at first menstruation, and their attitudes and beliefs regarding gender relations.

AIDS is an Alien Disease. A majority of the participants, both men and women, had heard about AIDS, 'the new disease', which was 'imported' to India by people from abroad.

> .... It is a new disease ... it was not there before, I never heard about it ... these people who come from other countries, bring such problems ... and our government allows them to come (younger men).
>
> ... the foreigners (*videshi*) have no morals, they (do) free sex, they bring AIDS ... (older men).
>
> ... this new disease has no cure. So many people come to this city from other states and other countries. Who can control people's behaviour ... the foreigners bring all such problems ... (older men).

Many similar statements indicate that for the average members of a community, AIDS is the latest entrant in their lives. By treating it as a new disease, they seem to distance it from themselves in time and by associating it with foreigners, they distance themselves at a cultural level too. Clearly the onus for spreading AIDS in the city is on the non-natives who are sometimes referred to as *videshis* but may also include people from other states.

AIDS is Dreaded. AIDS is commonly perceived as a dreadful (*bhayanak*), incurable (*la-ilaaj rog; iska ilaaj nahin*) and a dirty disease (*gandi bimari*). Its very name spells doom. During a discussion one woman did not want to verbalize the word AIDS. She said, '.... Don't even take its name, it's a bad disease (*kharab bimari*)'.

Like the earlier conception of TB, it was seen as a *maharog* (big disease) that is lethal.

> ... Once a person has AIDS all is over (*sab khatam samjho*), no chance of living after that (older men).

A person with AIDS knows that he will not live longer ... generally he dies in 6–8 months (older men).

Indeed, the lethality and certainty of death in AIDS was powerfully conveyed by advertisements in the early 1990s carrying images of skulls and bones. These images seem to have stayed on with the people even as they have been replaced by those of demons and devils. The older men opined, '... It [AIDS] is like the Ravana we burn on *Dushera*' (younger men). 'Last year we burnt the AIDS Ravana[2] ...'. AIDS conjures up horrifying images of dying early, dying without support and care, of being hated and ridiculed. According to the older men, ' ....In AIDS people suffer—nobody takes care, even family members, I have heard, leave them, and they generally die very young.' The horror that AIDS creates makes people wish they have nothing to do with it. The younger men said, 'We hope there is no one with AIDS here ...'

AIDS is a Shameful Disease. During discussions AIDS was most strongly associated with its sexual mode of transmission. Almost all the participants across different communities mentioned that AIDS was contracted through sex with 'others' such as prostitutes and other 'loose character' women (*charitraheen auratein*). It was, therefore, considered shameful (*sharmnak*) and a dirty, disgusting disease (*gandi bimari*). It was said to reveal the dark side of those injected. The older men believed, '... you get to know of the dirty face (*gandi soorat*) of people'. It was not just that AIDS was a shameful disease (*sharmnak bimari*), but also that it brought shame upon the infected and their families.

> ... people will not like if somebody has AIDS. Certainly it brings shame to the family ... how will they face others ... everybody will look down upon them (older women).
>
> ... if a boy has this dreaded disease then everybody will know that he was 'going out' and every one will comment about his family, their character. You know how people are, they just want an opportunity ... it will be such a shameful thing (older men).

Shame and horror were the most enduring images which emerged during the discussion on AIDS as participants dwelt at length on morals and values.

---

[2] The reference here is to the burning of the effigy of Ravana, the demon king by a local AIDS NGO which sought to personify AIDS as the modern day Ravana.

AIDS is a Disease of the Promiscuous. When questioned as to how one may get AIDS, most participants said it resulted from having sex with prostitutes.

> ... prostitutes are the agents ... they give it to men who are in the habit of going to them (younger men).
> ... prostitutes are the spreading medium ... (younger women).
> ... one gets AIDS by going to the outside women (*bahar ki aurtein*) (older men).
> ... if you keep relations with several women [you get AIDS] (older men).

People indulging in multi-partner sex, entertaining clients, engaging in sexual perversity (*yon vikrati*) and those without morals were particularly at risk to contract the infection. These included men who go 'out' (to prostitutes for sex), homosexuals (*samlingi vyakhti*), beer bar girls, bad women and one who stepped aside (from the right path).

Even as other risk behaviours were mentioned, such as homosexuality and injecting drug use, heterosexual transmission of AIDS was the focal issue during all FGDs. It centred around promiscuous, illicit, multi-partner sexual behaviour of both married and unmarried men. Men commonly talked about those who indulged in 'outline' behaviour, that is, those who strayed from the (right) path.

> ... Those who go 'outline', visit the prostitute (*vaishya*), keep relations with several women, they get AIDS (older men).
> .... Those who cannot be satisfied with their wife alone, they seek sex in the market (*bazar*)... they can get AIDS (younger men).
> Some men here indulge in several relations, they go 'out' to those bad women, ... it is possible that they have AIDS (older women).

AIDS was thus seen as a disease of sexual excesses and sexual misadventures. Prostitutes figured prominently in all discussions, although there was mention of 'other women' too who granted sexual favours without seeking any payment. According to the older women, 'One may not go to the prostitute (*dhandewali*) ... it is possible for some men to seek it with other women without payment'.

AIDS is an Invited Disease. Some respondents, mainly from the lower middle income group (*chawl* residents), believed that the people themselves were to be blamed for AIDS. For example, the older men asserted, '.... You get it because of your own irresponsible (*gairjimmedar*) behavior, nobody told you to get it ... you had fun and *mazza*, now pay for that'.

Personal weakness giving in to sexual pleasures and all-round erosion of culture in society were cited as reasons for people to contract diseases such as AIDS. Most of the older men echoed these observations: '... where are morals today? ... there is no self-control (within people) ... so there is AIDS and other such diseases. These people themselves bring it home ... what can be done now'.

The underlying views were that AIDS was 'knowingly' inflicted upon the self by infected persons who were mainly seen as belonging to the slums. Consequently, there was little sympathy or supportive attitude towards those infected with the virus, and hatred towards them was justified. The older women forcefully asserted, '.... If you do something wrong, then be ready to face its results also ...'.

AIDS is God's Punishment. Those who perceived AIDS to be self-inflicted, believed that AIDS was a punishment for one's sinful behaviour, and sinful behaviour was mainly interpreted as promiscuous behaviour.

> ... when these people have the time and money to spend on such things, visit outside women (*bahar ki auratein*) then surely God will punish ... (older women).
>
> ... when you have a wife at home, why do you go 'outline', away from the good/moral path ... then one has to pay for all this ... (younger men).

AIDS implies a strong moral judgement. It is seen as a disease of the less virtuous. Sexual excesses and adventures are not sanctioned by society. Such behaviours are considered sinful and the message is that they will surely not go unpunished.

AIDS is a Disease of 'Others'. The respondents' perceptions tended to associate AIDS with 'other people'—those who indulged in 'such' behaviour, that is, promiscuous lifestyle, including drinking, visiting prostitutes, overspending, having black money.

> ... it [AIDS] will mainly happen to people who go to the sex worker (*dhandewali aurat/bai*), who drink too much, gamble ... of course they should have black money (*do number ka paisa*) to spend for all this ... it will not happen to just anybody ... there has to be some reason, isn't it? (older men)
>
> ... there is no AIDS in this community. Why will it be? We are all householders (*grihastha*, that is, family people) here (older women).

The key point here is that AIDS was generally not personalized or perceived as a problem for their own community members. There was a tendency to deny the possibility of risk. This was in spite of the fact that the FGDs on sexual patterns highlighted the presence of risk behaviour in slum communities. For instance, the age of initiation into sexual activities was reported to be as low as 13–14 years for males, often in the company of older boys or under peer pressure to visit red-light areas. Paying for sex was reported to be common among men in the age group of 18–40 years with independent sources of income, and among school dropouts doing odd jobs. While most women tended to deny that their husbands visited prostitutes, they acknowledged that it was in the nature of men to indulge in sex outside even when there was a 'good' wife at home. Men often compared the habit of seeking 'outside' sex with eating in a restaurant despite food being available at home. Some of the older men said, '.... Even if food (at home) is good, you feel like eating out at a hotel.' Others added, '.... The "hen" at home is like grain (*ghar ki murgi daal barabar*) .'

Within the communities, age and income class served to create the 'us' and 'them' divide in relation to AIDS. For example, AIDS was perceived by older men in slums as a possible problem for the younger age groups— today's youth—but not for themselves.

> ... I can't say anything about the (sexual) behavior of young boys in our community ... but some of them are clearly going 'outline' ... who knows some of them may have it (AIDS) but it can't be a problem with other household men (those who have families) (older men).

Among the younger age groups, the discussion generally focused on the risk of AIDS to 'those' who have 'such' lifestyles, especially people in the neighbouring communities. For those living in *chawls*, the slum population constituted 'the others', while for the slum residents, 'others' were those living across the road in apartment buildings (housing mainly middle-class people). The younger men said, '.... Why explore (this problem) with us ... just find out what happens there, in those buildings, I am sure there is AIDS there ...' Middle-aged married men living in a *chawl*, who were comparatively better educated, believed that AIDS was a problem of the poorer groups.

> ... those who are educated possess TV and newspapers for information and therefore can take precautions ... it is the illiterate people living in the slums who lack such sources of information and need to be told ... (older men).

The findings of the study, however, revealed that personalization of AIDS was beginning to occur among younger age groups following greater awareness such as that generated due to participation in focus group discussions on AIDS. This was confirmed by the increased demand for AIDS literature among young boys in the slum community in the wake of an AIDS awareness camp. In short, the group discussions revealed the people's difficulty in acknowledging AIDS-related risk behaviour in their own communities, especially among their own age and class members. Consequently, low AIDS-risk perception was observed among the respondents.

Marital status was also identified as an important variable. Male married householders were perceived to have lower risk of infection than unmarried males. In one of the slums, older married men expressed, '... men like us who have sexual relations with our wife any number of time will not get AIDS'. They added, '... the unmarried people are really at risk ... you can't say about their behavior (sexual).'

Female sex workers were uniformly identified as the 'others' who could get AIDS, while housewives tended to see themselves as less vulnerable. Some of them were even offended by the question: 'What AIDS! ... are we those kind of women ... as if we will get it (AIDS).' Their attitude was further reinforced by health workers. At an AIDS awareness camp for women, the health worker began by saying, '... we are all family women here ... so there is no question of relations outside ...'. Here the assumption was that AIDS is contracted only through the sexual mode of transmission. Infected blood and needles were not considered as other sources of infection.

AIDS is a Contagious and Polluting Disease. Some participants pointed to the role of micro-organisms or germs as causative factors in AIDS, although not all of them were able to name it correctly as HIV. 'I don't know the name, but I know it is caused by germs (*jeevanu*).'

Some respondents, mostly men, of both age groups, had some conception of the AIDS micro-organisms but they had little knowledge of its nature and functioning from a biomedical perspective. Some thought it was an 'insect' (*jantu/kida*) that could fly and is in the air. These views were based on their belief in causal contagion of the AIDS virus. Some of their responses are indicative of this belief.

> ... if one in the family has (AIDS), every body can get it...
> ... micro-organisms (of AIDS) fall through air...
> ... Its virus can spread by talking to the infected person ... so we must maintain distance ....
> ... We must keep clothes and vessels of the AIDS person separate—if we touch his things we can get AIDS.
> ... Upon contact with our body it (germs) can immediately cause AIDS ...

Other beliefs about causal contagion were revealed through their views that AIDS is caused by mosquitoes. Toilets were seen as sources of possible spread of the disease. These beliefs were accompanied by a fear of common toilets in communities. The older men in a slum said, '... the gases from the urinals ... when our urine falls on `others' urine ... the gases that flow out can cause the disease.'

Belief in causal contagion conveys the notion of easy and imminent transmissibility of the virus. At the same time, such beliefs carry the notion of pollution and contamination as well. The older women believed, '... even the air around such persons is dangerous, one should not touch them ... why take chance'.

Underlying the perceptions of AIDS as a defiling and polluting disease are the popular cultural conceptions of pure/impure and hygiene and cleanliness. Normally, things associated with an ill person are considered to be impure and unhygienic, more so if there is fear and dread associated with a health status. Body products such as fluids, odour and breath are thought to carry illness-producing germs and, hence, to be avoided. AIDS, with its association with 'immoral' sex, is doubly polluting because such sex means 'unnatural desires' that adversely affect health and are the cause of cultural decay. The younger men said, '... there are some people who enjoy perverse sex, it is not natural, their health goes down quickly ...'. The older women, on the other hand, argued, 'AIDS shows how our culture (*sanskriti*) is decaying.'

AIDS is Associated with Uncertainty. Most illnesses are understood in terms of some visible bodily signs and symptoms. Physically healthy-looking individuals are usually not 'suspected' of harbouring any illness. The response to an illness is usually in relation to its symptoms such as skin colour, disfigurement, weight loss, and hair thinning. A person with AIDS is generally described as one who loses body resistance, grows weak and thin.

> ... His bones become powdery and useless like in paralysis. AIDS viruses go into the marrow of the bones and grow there, so they become weak ...
> ... body turns black ...
> ... the blood solidifies.
> ... instead of urine they pass red water and develop red and yellow spots on eyes and their body turns yellow ...

In AIDS, the viral infection may not be manifested in physical symptoms for a long time. This makes the people uncertain, including those infected with HIV. The respondents mentioned thinness, dark skin, sudden ill health, especially among young men, as the diagnostic symptoms of AIDS. Even in the case of those who had some idea about viral causation, the concept of HIV infecting the body and not being manifested in body symptoms was not convincing enough till some signs were visible; for example, the younger men believed, 'We don't know any AIDS cases— no body looks like having AIDS.'

'Looking like AIDS', that is, thin and emaciated, was important for people to give any response. In the absence of recognizable AIDS cases, the response was one of uncertainty, suspicion and fear of accidental contagion. The younger men opined, '... actually one never knows who may be an AIDS patient in your neighbourhood ... it is better to keep to oneself'.

AIDS is a Disease that Isolates People. Closely related to the contagious and polluting perception of AIDS is the perception that it demands isolation of the infected individual. Responses of medical professionals and instructions issued to family members of the HIV-infected individual are frequently the basis for such perceptions.

> ... advertisements say that (it) is not a contagious disease then why do doctors and nurses not touch them (the patients with AIDS) ... (younger men).
> ... why was ... (somebody's) wife asked to wear gloves and mask when entering his room ... (older women).

Even when the respondents had not actually interacted with persons infected with AIDS, it symbolized danger with a signal to keep distance from them.

AIDS is a Men's Disease. In nearly all FGDs, it was the male sexual behaviour that was the focal point of discussions in relation to AIDS. Men were perceived as having sexual needs that propelled them towards those seducing women (*woh auratein jo lubhati hain*) or to multiple sex partners as a consequence of which they contracted AIDS.

> ... these men who go to the 'outside' (*bahari*) women ... they have a high chance of getting AIDS ... (younger men)
> ... see, men have their needs [*yeh* (sex) *unki jaroorat hai*]... they will go wherever they get it... why doesn't somebody chuck out these women doing this business (*dhandewali*–sex worker) ... (older women).

The underlying perception was that men were victims of AIDS because of their (just) sexual needs. Even when they were blamed and held guilty of moral transgressions, they were still portrayed as 'those who get AIDS', 'those who face the consequences (in the form of AIDS) for their sinful (sexual) behavior'. In contrast, descriptions of women mainly centred around their role of causative agents. They made men suffer by transmitting the AIDS virus. While most discussions centred around prostitutes as causative agents, other women (housewives mainly) were also held responsible. This view was held by both older men and women. According to the older men, ' ... Housewives can also give (AIDS) ... some housewives have relations with ten-ten men'. The older women believed, '... Some women (other than prostitutes) are also bad ... not only men'.

Responses such as these are suggestive of the non-commercial context of sex in communities where it is the housewives who are-alleged to be involved with men other than their married partners. While discussions on the sexual excesses of men made them out to be the innocent/guilty victims of their sexual escapades, women in a similar situation were seen as agents who transmitted the AIDS virus and not as the likely victims of AIDS. It is significant to note that FGDs did not focus on how married women may be vulnerable to infection through sex with their husbands who visited sex workers. AIDS is, indeed, a man's disease in popular perception.

Discussion

Throughout human history, illnesses that are contagious, incurable and those related to sexual organs have given rise to feelings of fear, dread and shame in society. They have served to stigmatize the infected and created labels and categories for them (Gilmore and Somerville, 1994). Like leprosy, TB and syphilis, AIDS has also joined the ranks of such dreaded diseases (Sontag, 1989; 1991).

Literature on social symbolism of illnesses informs how social perceptions are important in understanding people's response to illnesses and their illness-coping mechanisms. These may then be incorporated in disease prevention and stigma-reduction strategies.

The findings presented here are a reconfirmation of the several AIDS metaphors and symbols described by Sontag (1991), and Gilmore and Somerville (1994). These include the perceptions of AIDS as a dreaded, shameful, invited and 'othered' disease. In addition, AIDS perceptions in Mumbai underscore its alienness, its sexual connotation and the commercial sex context, its highly 'contagious' nature and its androcentric focus. These perceptions may be understood in relation to local health beliefs and norms of gender relations.

Broadly speaking, four observations may be made on the basis of people's perceptions of AIDS in Mumbai.

1. Knowledge and awareness about AIDS is at a very basic level. In addition, several misconceptions are prevalent about modes of transmission through casual contact, clothes, etc., and about who can and cannot get AIDS.
2. AIDS is highly feared and stigmatized. Because there is no cure as yet, it generates anxiety and concern for life. Further, due to its perceived close links with sex, promiscuity and prostitution, AIDS serves as a metaphor for sinful and immoral behaviour. For most respondents, AIDS belonged to the domain of 'consequences of sinful, self-willed behaviour'. This etiology of AIDS, that is, by having sexual relations with members of other risk behaviour groups such as prostitutes, makes it a stigmatized disease. In this sense, AIDS is perceived more etiologically than symptomatically. Its sex connection is highlighted more than its physical symptoms.
3. AIDS is located mainly within the context of sexual mode of HIV transmission excluding all other modes, that is, through blood, infected needles and mother to child. Further, it is the heterosexual relationship that is closely scrutinized as a risk behaviour for AIDS and not so much homosexual behaviour. This heterosexualization of AIDS in communities is done primarily within the framework of commercial sex to the exclusion of sexual relations without monetary transactions such as those between regular or married partners.
4. AIDS is generally perceived to be a man's problem. This male-centred view does not acknowledge monogamous, married women's vulnerability to AIDS due to the risk behaviour of their sexual partners.

To have a more complete understanding of the local perceptions of AIDS, it is important to discuss how these perceptions differ from those described elsewhere. One of the most striking differences is that sexual deviance and perversity symbolized by homosexuality are not closely linked with AIDS as they are in other Western countries. Thus, it is not so much sexual 'perversity' as it is the excesses of sexual indulgence and promiscuity that are associated with AIDS in Mumbai.

Another noticeable difference is the absence of criminalization of AIDS, that is, people with AIDS are not viewed as criminals (see AIDS metaphors described by Gilmore and Somerville, 1994). This probably can be explained by the perception of AIDS as a man's disease in which men are victims and sufferers, not perpetrators of a crime such as AIDS.

If, at all, there is any villainy perceived in AIDS, it is in relation to prostitutes. Slogans on AIDS indeed suggest this to be so. An analysis of health messages plastered in various sections of Mumbai as part of the AIDS-prevention campaign draws attention to the depiction of sex workers as the enemy of men (Robinson, 1998). Quoting a slogan '*Gairon ke sath sex ab nahin, Nirodh ke bina tho kabhi nahin*', Robinson has shown that the '*gairon*' is the *bahari* women (the outside women), the unclean, the not-at-home and the seducer, the commercial sex worker '... who is defined in their messages as the carrier, she becomes the enemy of the "male." Silenced here is the knowledge how AIDS actually spreads; the fact that males pass on the virus even to monogamous females and, thence, their children' (Robinson, 1998, p. 1909). There is ample evidence to show that the incidence of female-to-male HIV transmission is much lower than male-to-female transmission. Yet, both in popular perceptions and in AIDS prevention messages, the target is the commercial sex worker. In the same analysis, Robinson has also highlighted the male-centred view of AIDS prevention messages: all such messages are meant primarily for men so that they may safeguard themselves against AIDS. Men are exhorted to avoid sex workers and to use *nirodh* ('*kisi ki mohabbat bhari baton mein mat aana; nirodh ke bagair, kisi ke sath mat jana*') (Robinson, 1998, p. 1909).

The findings presented here have implications for AIDS prevention and advocacy work. First, the findings inform that people have insufficient information about AIDS that forms the basis for their misconceptions, fears and stigmatized responses towards HIV-infected people. Credible AIDS education programmes are needed to impact correct, adequate and unbiased information related to HIV AIDS. Beliefs in causal contagion of HIV through physical contact, clothing, etc., must be addressed appropriately through these programmes to eliminate segregationist tendencies. As is evident from these popular perceptions, AIDS is a stigmatized disease. People feel hesitant to even seek information on their own, lest they be suspected of being HIV positive. To encourage people to voluntarily seek information, efforts need to be made to dovetail the AIDS education programmes with the ongoing reproductive health programmes to facilitate community members' access to them without anxiety and fear. Voluntary counselling and testing centres for HIV would help in this effort.

The 'othering' of AIDS suggests that people tend to deny their vulnerability to HIV or that they live under the false belief that 'such' things happen to 'others' and not to people like them (who live in *chawls* or are educated, etc.). It is important that people be made aware of the facts so that they are capable of assessing their vulnerability to HIV and seek timely intervention.

The fear and anxiety associated with AIDS is clearly a result of the moralistic attitudes of people and their perception that prostitutes cause AIDS. Another reason for fear is the practice of equating of AIDS with death. A more balanced approach is required in AIDS-prevention slogans to avoid stigmatizing of AIDS through the targeting of sex workers and other 'women' as carriers of HIV, and to avoid fear-based messages that highlight the lethality of AIDS.

Perceptions of AIDS as an invited and shameful disease, and punishment for sinful behaviour promote prejudices and segregating tendencies in society. These need to be tackled by addressing AIDS-related discrimination through anti-discrimination law and human rights watch.

REFERENCES

Aggarwal, O. P., Sharma, A. K. and Indrayan. A (Eds). (1997). *HIV/AIDS research in India*. New Delhi: National AIDS Control Organisation.

Ankrah, E. M. (1993). The impact of HIV/AIDS on the family and other significant relationships: The African clan revisited. *AIDS Care*, 5, 5–22.

Bharat, S. (1996). *Facing the challenge. Household and community response to HIV/AIDS in Mumbai, India*. Geneva: UNAIDS/Mumbai: TISS.

Bharat, S. and Aggleton, P. (1999). Facing the challenge. Household response to AIDS in Mumbai, India. *AIDS Care*, 11(1), 31–44.

Bharat, S., Singhanetra-Renard, A. and Aggleton, P. (1998). Household and community response to HIV/AIDS in Asia: The case of Thailand and India. In J. Kaldor, T. Brown, S. Bharat and K. Zhang (Eds), *AIDS in Asia and the Pacific, second edition* (S117–S122). London: Lippincott-Raven.

Bhende, A. (1995). *Evolving a model for AIDS prevention education among underprivileged adolescent girls in urban India*. Women and AIDS Program Research Report Series. Washington, DC: International Centre for Research on Women.

Boulton, M. (Ed.). (1994). *Methodological advances in social research on HIV/AIDS: Challenge and innovation*. London: Taylor & Francis.

Census of India. (1991). *Maharashtra–Provision population totals, Paper 1 of 1991*. Series 14. Mumbai.

Douglas, M. (1970). *Natural symbols*. New York: Vintage.

Gangakhedkar, R. R., Bently, M. E., Divekar, A. D., Gadkari, D., Mehendale, S. M., Shepherd, M. E., Bollinger, R. C. and Quinn, T. C. (1997). Spread of HIV infection in married monogamous women in India. *The Journal of the American Medical Association*, 278, 2090-92.

George, A. and Jaswal, S. (1995). *Understanding sexuality: An ethnographic study of poor women in Bombay*. Women and AIDS Program Research Report Series. Washington, DC. International Center for Research on Women.

Gilmore, N. and Somerville, M. A. (1994). Stigmatisation, Scapegoating and discrimination in sexually transmitted disease: Overcoming 'them' and 'us'. *Social Science and Medicine*, 37(9), 1339-58.

Gussow, Z. (1989). *Leprosy, racism and public health*. Boulder: Westview Press.

Kleinman, A. (1980). *Patients and healers in the context of culture: An exploration of the borderland between anthropology, medicine and psychiatry*. Los Angeles: University of California Press.

Lieban, R. W. (1992). From illness to symbol and symbol to illness. *Social Science and Medicine*, 35(2), 183-88.

Morgan, D. L. (1988). *Focus groups as qualitative research*, Qualitative Research Methods Series 16. New Delhi: Sage Publications.

National AIDS Control Organisation. (1997-98). *Country scenario*. New Delhi: Ministry of Health and Family Welfare, Govt. of India, NACO.

Nichter, M. (1981). Idioms of distress. *Culture Medicine and Psychiatry*, 5, 379.

Omangi, H. G. (1997). Stigmatisation and discrimination in the context of HIV and AIDS in Kenya. *Newsletter of African Network on Ethics, Law and HIV*, 3, 4-5.

Robinson, R. (1998). Socio-logic of AIDS campaign. *Economic and Political Weekly*, 33(29 and 30), 1908-09.

Songwathana, P. and Manderson, L. (1998). Perceptions of HIV/AIDS and caring for people with terminal AIDS in southern Thailand. *AIDS Care*, 10 (suppl. 2), S155-S165.

Sontag, S. (1989). *AIDS and its metaphors*. New York: Farrer, Stratus & Giroux.

———. (1991). *Illness as metaphor, AIDS and its metaphors*. London: Penguin.

UNAIDS/WHO. (1998). *Report on the global HIV/AIDS epidemic*, Geneva.

20

Disaster and Trauma: Who Suffers and Who Recovers from Trauma, and How?

DAMODAR SUAR

The term 'disaster' is derived from the Latin word *dis astrum* meaning 'bad star'—an evil influence of a star or a planet. Words used in dictionaries like misfortune, calamity, tragedy or catastrophe for a disaster imply the sufferings of people and damage of property and infrastructure. A hazard is not a disaster unless it claims lives, inflicts sufferings, destroys property or devastates infrastructure. Often an earthquake or a flood disrupts the normal conditions within a society and causes widespread damage, destruction and human sufferings. Economic destruction, loss of human life and injury and deterioration in health and health services may warrant extraordinary responses from the state and federal administration, relief agencies and health personnel. Survivors' trauma of Orissa supercyclone (1999), Bhuj earthquake (2001) and the tsunami (2004) in India is well-reported in mass media, agency reports, few journal articles and fresh in our memory. Despite this, trauma amelioration is frequently overlooked. The techno-economic approach dominates in disaster management.

Research on post-disaster trauma poses several difficulties. First, most disasters strike suddenly and unexpectedly. There is hardly any time to devise sophisticated research strategies. Second, when individuals and communities are overwhelmed by intense fear, terror and helplessness following a disaster, ethical constraints prohibit gathering data from them. Post-disaster investigation after a year or so often entails undesirable occasions for recollection of survivors' traumatic memories when the trauma is reduced and people are already engaged in livelihood reconstruction. Third, researchers use various diagnostic and assessment procedures, diverse sampling frame and different follow-up periods that become difficult to compare findings across studies. Four, grass-root workers involving in rescue operations and providing psychosocial support are trained neither to document systematically nor publish scientifically their experiential evidence. Consequently, a rich repertoire of knowledge is lost. Five, some researchers, driven by the native knowledge, argue that while the survivors do not level their suffering as 'posttraumatic stress', why outside researchers and clinicians level the sufferings with foreign vocabulary. Moreover, researchers from developing countries fail to generate adequate knowledge on trauma because of the scarcity of funds to carry out post-disaster research. With this backdrop, this study examines about: (*a*) the disasters in India; (*b*) the post-disaster trauma; (*c*) the vulnerabilities to trauma; and (*d*) trauma amelioration.

DISASTERS: IS INDIA A POTENTIAL VICTIM?

Though varied classifications of disasters are made on the basis of consequences, administrative regions, precipitating event and cultural collapse and interaction of primary causes (natural, industrial and humanistic) with primary elements (earth, air, fire, water and people), the well-accepted taxonomy is on the basis of prime agents—nature and man—causing disasters. While natural disasters result from uncontrollable forces of nature, man-made disasters are consequences of human activities. Natural disasters can be further classified into geophysical disasters such as earthquakes, volcanic eruptions and tsunamis; hydro-meteorological disasters such as floods, cyclones, heat waves, cold waves and droughts; and pandemic waves of diseases. A natural disaster can also be a slow-onset disaster, like a drought or cold wave, and a fast-onset, like an earthquake or cyclone. Man-made disasters can be bifurcated into (non-intentional) technological disasters and (intentional) mass violence. The failure in input, process and output of technology incorporates industrial, road, rail and air accidents, mine and space explosions, shipwreck, radioactive pollution, toxic waste disposal, oil spills and building collapse. The examples are Bhopal gas tragedy, Chernobyl nuclear explosion, Three Mile Island accident, Buffalo-creak dam collapse and Exxon Valdez oil spill. Included in technological disasters are policy disasters. Those incorporate the violation of policies such as the water-logging in unplanned civic structures in desert state of Rajasthan that caused flash flood in 1996 and subsequent malarial deaths, and the inefficient public distribution system in KBK districts in Orissa that created frequent droughts. In contrast, intentional harm is a defining feature during acts of civil strife, communal riots, genocide and terrorism. Such disasters include genocide in Rwanda, 9/11 World trade centre attack, Gulf wars, Kashmir terrorist problems and Gujarat riots. Since we have control over technology and human acts, we can expect to have control over man-made disasters but not over natural disasters.

Quarantelli (2006) offers a continuum of disasters relative to the community resources, such as: (*a*) crisis: when capacity exceeds demands; (*b*) emergency: when capacity meets or somehow exceeds demands; (*c*) disaster: when demands exceed capacity; and (*d*) catastrophe: when demands overwhelm and may even destroy capacity. A disaster varies in severity depending on the scale of damage and the assistance required for meeting survivors' needs. The cumulative impact of disasters can be gauged using multiple measures of mortality, morbidity, economic loss, infrastructure damage, cultural collapse and disruption of health and health care services. Depending on damage and destruction, a severe natural disaster of rare nature in India is declared as a national calamity that can receive the assistance from central government 'calamity relief fund' up to 500 crore Indian rupees to cover up losses.

On average, a natural disaster occurs once in every 19 hours and one technological disaster once in every 25 hours (CRED, 2005) somewhere in the world. Taken together, about two disasters occur everyday. Disasters become more severe in developing countries than the developed world because of inadequate warming systems, lack of control over use of unsafe land, lack of preparedness of people and ruthless exploitation of natural resources for faster economic growth. The most vulnerable continents to disasters are Asia and Africa in terms of loss of lives, damage of property, injury and destruction of infrastructure; and the least vulnerable is Oceania. India is also a house for theatre of devastating disasters.

Extracted information for India from the database of Centre for Research on the Epidemiology of Disasters (CRED) indicates that while in the last 99 years (1908–2006), 1,083 (100 per cent) disasters strike India, in last 17 years (1990–2006), 688 (63.52 per cent) disasters and in last one decade (1997–2006), 446 (41.18 per cent) disasters hit India (Table 20.1). By and large, one disaster occurs in every nine days in agreement with the last 17 years' data, and one disaster occurs in every eight days in accordance with the last one decade data authenticating the increased occurrence of disasters in recent times (Suar, 2007). The statistics on disasters in India are also alarming.

Table 20.1: Disasters from 1997–2006

Disaster	Number[1]	Person killed	Person Injured	Homeless	Person Affected	Damage US $ 000's
Drought	4	20	0.00	0.00	390,000,000	1,498,721
	0.90	0.02	0.00	0.00	56.34	8.07
Earthquake	5	21,459	175,328	2,075,700	4,862,000	2,730,000
	1.12	25.19	84.74	53.89	0.70	14.70
Epidemic	32	2,353	0.00	0.00	319,256	0.00
	7.17	2.76	0.00	0.00	0.05	0.00
Extreme Temperature	14	7,332	0.00	0.00	0.00	0.00
	3.14	8.61	0.00	0.00	0.00	0.00
Flood	73	12,604	287	620,230	277,908,430	9,398,742
	16.37	14.80	0.14	16.10	40.15	50.60
Slides	16	997	244	2,000	212,000	0.00
	3.59	1.17	0.12	0.05	0.03	0.00

Wave/Surge	2	16,789	6,913	0.00	647,599	1,022,800
	0.45	19.71	3.34	0.00	0.09	5.51
Wind Storm	27	14,140	12,609	956,345	18,194,601	3,465,416
	6.05	16.60	6.09	24.83	2.63	18.66
Industrial Accident	26	660	1,255	0.00	100,453	429,200
	5.83	0.77	0.61	0.00	0.01	2.31
Transport Accident	202	7,039	5,368	190,000	237	28,000
	45.29	8.26	2.59	4.93	0.00	0.15
Miscellaneous Accident	45	1,786	4,894	7,750	2,000	0.00
	10.09	2.10	2.37	0.20	0.00	0.00
Total	446	85,179	206,898	3,852,025	692,246,576	18,572,879

Source: Centre for Research on the Epidemiology of Disasters (CRED), School of Public Health, Belgium.
Note: [1]The second row below the number includes percentage.

1. Indian territories are mostly disaster-prone. In India, 68 per cent of total sown area is drought-prone and 55 per cent of the area is quake-prone. The fragile Himalayan mountain ranges are extremely vulnerable to quakes, avalanches and landslides. Landslides are increasingly common in hilly regions, particularly in lower Himalayas (Himachal Pradesh and Uttarakhand), as well as Kerala and North East, and cause extensive damage to roads, bridges, human dwellings and agricultural lands regularly. Western and central India are equally unsafe. Seventy-six lakh hectares of land are flooded every year. The areas affected by flood are rapidly extending beyond the river basins of the Himalayan region to other parts. Five to six tropical cyclones form in the Bay of Bengal and the Arabian Sea every year, of which two or three lash the densely populated coastal areas. Indian is among the world's most disaster-prone areas (NDM, 2001).
2. Analysis of data from 1990–2006 from the CRED database indicates that earthquakes, waves/surges, droughts, windstorms and floods are the most devastating disasters in India (Suar, 2007). The last one decade data indicate that 45 disasters occur every year. Technological disasters of transport accident, industrial accidents and miscellaneous accidents alone account for 61 per cent of the total occurrences. These are less devastating than natural disasters (Table 20.1).
3. The consequences of natural disasters are immense in terms of loss of human life, shelter, property and livelihood. Disasters per annum claim more than 8,500 human lives, injure more than 20,500 persons, make 3.8 lakh people homeless, affect a colossal of 692 lakh people and damage property worth 18,573 lakh US dollars. The biggest killers are earthquakes, waves/surges, windstorm and floods that claim more than three-fourths (76.30 per cent) of total human lives. Droughts and floods alone affect more than 95 per cent of the total disaster-affected population. Floods alone account for more than 50 per cent of the total property damaged by disasters (Table 20. 1).
4. Devastating natural disasters are frequent visitors to India. Data from the CRED indicate that in the Orissa supercyclone on 29 October 1999, 10,000 people were killed, 126 lakh people were affected and thousands were rendered homeless. In Kutch (Gujarat) quake on 26 January 2001, more than 20,000 people died, about 44 lakhs were injured and 17 lakh people rendered homeless. On 26 December 2004, tsunami hit the coastal belt of Tamil Nadu,

Andhra Pradesh and Kerala, Andaman and Nicobar islands, UT Pondicherry, and killed more than 16,000 people, injured about 7,000 and damaged property worth (US) $10,228 lakhs. On 24 July 2005, floods took a toll of 1,200 lives and affected 200 lakh people in Gujarat, Madhya Pradesh, Goa, Orissa, Karnataka, Himachal Pradesh and Jammu and Kashmir.
5. The actual devastation greatly exceeds the documented ones. Many persons in the recent tsunami were swept in the sea without their bodies being traced, and are not counted in the list of dead persons. Most injuries such as lacerations in cyclones or fractures in earthquakes are estimated by the number admitted to hospital. But there are hundreds more who never go to a hospital, and many thousands more suffering from post-traumatic stress go completely unrecorded and untreated.
6. The long-term consequences of disasters are immense. The death/disability of a family's earning members during a disaster means a lifetime loss of income. The death of a family's livestock, loss of capital or tools of trade seize the earning capacity. During floods, salt-water contamination of land can lead to the loss of not one, but several harvests. For an already malnourished population, this would result in rise of hunger deaths.

DISASTER TRAUMA

Devastating disasters give a blow to individual and collective psyche. At the individual level, survivors experience confusion, shock, fear and anxiety immediately following the disaster. Subsequently, they report grief, anger, guilt, depression, helplessness, withdrawal, irritability, flashbacks, nightmares and somatic complaints. The intensity and duration of symptoms are directly proportional to the scale of devastation, degree of exposure, extent of survivors' resource loss and inadequate social support.

At the collective level, affected communities experience anxiety, irrational fear, social chaos and get influenced by the rapidly spreading rumour. Such fear and rumours spread following the Sarin attack on a Tokyo subway system in 1995 and the anthrax attack in the US in 2001. Long after the Marathwada earthquake in 1993, people continued to sleep in open places leaving the newly provided houses. They had the fear psychosis that there may be another quake that would collapse the houses.

Similar was the situation following devastating Bhuj (Gujarat state) earthquake in 2001 where survivors felt that the earthquake might strike again. Many preferred to sleep on the Rajkot–Bhuj highway in the chilling cold. Research on mass hysteria and panic is in infancy in India and will be not reported here. Here follows the discussion on individual-level traumas.

Trauma Victim and Symptom

Six categories of survivors suffer from trauma. Primary victims are those at the epicentre of the disaster and are most exposed. Secondary victims are the family members and friends of primary victims. Tertiary victims are the rescue, recovery and emergency personnel who experience an imbalance between the demands made on them and their abilities to cope. Fourth-level victims are members of community beyond the impact area who express their good intentions to support survivors with goods and services. Fifth-level victims are bystanders who are mentally disturbed. Sixth-level victims are researchers and clinicians who are directly affected by the intensive, prolonged and professional demands that are made on them. Though the primary and secondary victims are more affected than the others, these categories are not mutually exclusive. In some cases, the rescuers might themselves be primary victims and also be concerned about the troubles of their own families in the affected area. They might also share the concern of the immediate community and of any organization involved. Similar complicated patterns of victim-classification emerged after the radiation discharge at the Three Mile Island plant, and those most distressed were found to be the young mothers, younger (male) plant employees and those lived closest to the plant. Here follows the discussion on trauma of severely affected primary and secondary victims.

Disasters generate multiple symptoms of trauma. The general symptoms include: (*a*) grief, mourning, depression, despair; (*b*) being frightened easily, worrying; (*c*) disorientation, confusion; (*d*) obsession; (*e*) feelings of hopelessness, helplessness, feeling isolated, abandoned; (*f*) dependency, clinging or alternately social withdrawal; (*g*) suspiciousness, hyper-vigilance, fear of harm; (*h*) insomnia, nightmares; (*i*) irritability, hostility, anger; (*j*) moodiness, sudden outbursts of emotion, restlessness; (*k*) difficulty concentrating and decision-making, memory loss, slowness of thinking; (*l*) headaches, gastrointestinal symptoms, sweats, tremors, fatigue, changes in menstrual cycle, loss of sexual desire, diffuse muscular pain, suicidal ideation; (*m*) intrusive thoughts: flashbacks, feeling of 're-living' the experience; (*n*) avoidance of thoughts, places, pictures, sounds reminding the disaster; (*o*) marital conflict, drug and alcohol abuse, etc.

Some responses shown by children in post-disaster include: (a) clinging, fears about separation, fears of strangers, monsters, animals; (b) difficulty in sleeping; (c) compulsive, repetitive play which represents part of the disaster experience; (d) crying; (e) fears of specific sounds, sights or objects associated with the disaster; (f) aggressiveness; (g) suspiciousness; (h) headaches, stomach aches and pains; and (i) refusal to go to school and inability to concentrate. If their symptoms are not handled, they seem cold, insensitive and grow up with fear and anxiety. Protecting children by sending them away from their parents adds trauma of separation to the trauma of a disaster. Adolescents show more aggression, defiance of parents, delinquency, substance abuse, risk-taking behaviour and non-attendance of schools.

Reanalysis of 225 sample data from developed and developing countries including India, Norris (2005) reports the frequently studied components of disaster trauma. Those in order of priority are: post-traumatic stress disorder (PTSD), depression, non-specific distress, physical health problems and anxiety.

PTSD along with acute stress has been observed in 74 per cent (= 166) of the sample. It is an anxiety disorder. It has symptom criteria (A–F) that develop following the direct exposure to, or witnessing, or learning about a disaster (criterion A). The symptoms resulting from the exposure to the disaster include persistence re-experiencing of the traumatic event through nightmares, flashbacks or intrusive thoughts (criterion B), avoidance and numbing responses (criterion C) and increased arousal through difficulty in sleeping and hyper-vigilance (criterion D). These symptoms must be present for more than one month (criterion E) and must cause significant impairment in social, occupational or other important areas of functioning (criterion F) (American Psychiatric Association, 1994).

Investigation on PTSD in all types of disasters has observed less prevalence of avoidance and numbing symptoms (criterion C) and more of intrusion (criterion B) and hyperarousal symptoms (criterion D). This has been confirmed in the study of supercyclone in Orissa and tsunami in Tamil Nadu (Suar and Khuntia, 2004; Das, Suar and Hota, 2006). First, confirming the presence of post-traumatic stress requires a reporting of higher number of symptoms in criterion C than in criteria B and D. Second, numbing symptoms in criterion C reflect community response to a disaster and are more likely to emerge later in the course of post-traumatic stress than the symptoms in criteria B and D. Third, avoidance symptoms may not co-occur with numbing symptoms in criterion C.

Our findings (Suar and Khuntia, 2004), corroborating with the Northridge Earthquake study (McMillen, North and Smith, 2000), confirm that the avoidance and numbing symptoms serve as the 'threshold symptoms' to the diagnosis of PTSD. Only 13 per cent had PTSD in the earthquake study because all received compensation against property damage, and the sample was predominantly white, well educated and affluent. In a country like India, high proportion of survivors suffers from PTSD. Those survivors have hardly any insurance policy to receive compensation against resource loss and are poor, illiterate and having low caste status.

First, the frequency of exposure to at least one traumatic event in 5,877 respondents is found to be 61 per cent for men and 51 per cent for women (Kessler, Sonnega, Bromet, Hughes and Nelson, 1995). Though men are more exposed to traumatic events than women, women are twice as likely as men to develop PTSD. Second, high rates of PTSD are found among the survivors of technological disasters and mass violence, and low to moderate rates among the survivors of natural disasters (Norris, Friedman, Watson and Byrne, et al., 2002) suggesting that intentional/unintentional human acts intensify PTSD. Third, high rates of PTSD among disaster survivors in India (Kar et al., 2004; Mehta, Vankar and Patel, 2005; Sharan, Chaudhary, Kavathekar and Saxena, 1996; Suar, Mandal and Khuntia, 2002) suggest that the lower socio-economic status and cultural factors might have increased the incidence of PTSD.

Depression is identified in 39 per cent (= 87) samples. It is characterized by symptoms of sadness, withdrawal, pessimism, lower self-confidence, indecisiveness, concentration difficulty, anhedonia (diminished interest in life activities), guilty ruminations, loss of appetite, preoccupations with loss, etc. Related symptoms such as suicidal thoughts and remorse also increase with severity of exposure (Norris et al., 2001). In some cultures, individuals report somatic symptoms of chronic fatigue, headache, pains, gastrointestinal disturbances, problems of the heart and feelings of 'heat', rather than cognitive and affective symptoms.

Non-specific distress is observed in 35 per cent (= 78) samples. This outcome refers to the elevation of psychological and psychosomatic symptoms such as demoralization, perceived stress and negative affect.

Physical health problems are identified in 27 per cent (= 60) samples. The problems include self-reported somatic concerns, verified medical conditions of availing increased sick leave, declined immune functioning, sleep disturbances and increased consumption of alcohol, drug and tobacco.

Anxiety is found in 20 per cent (= 46) samples. It is the apprehension of danger in the environment. The individuals report tension, worry, nervousness and apprehension. Death anxiety, phobias and panic disorders are occasionally observed. In some cultures, anxiety may express through somatic symptoms of dry mouth, nausea and diarrhoea, and in others through cognitive symptoms. Children may reveal their anxiety through non-attending schools and not getting sleep easily.

First, PTSD includes anxiety and negative affect (fear, felling detached, losing interest, etc.). Hence, PTSD, depression and physical health problems can capture post-disaster trauma. Though the English word 'trauma' is derived from the Greek word 'wound', it connotes both psychological and physical impairments. In some cultures, trauma manifests more through cognitive and affective reactions, in others through physical health and behavioural problems. These symptoms can be grouped under cognitive, spiritual, affective, behavioural and physical reactions (see Table 20.2).

Table 20.2: Normal Traumatic Reactions to Disaster

Effects	Symptoms
Cognitive	Impaired concentration, decision-making and memory, intrusive thoughts, confusion, decreased self-esteem, distrust, nightmares, decreased self-efficacy, self-blame, worry, dissociation (tunnel vision, dreamlike or 'spacey' feeling)
Spiritual	Loss of faith, being punished for immoral acts, sense of world being changed, withdrawal from spiritual rituals
Affective	Shock, terror, irritability, anger, guilt, grief/sadness, fear, externalization of blame, emotional numbing, surprise, helplessness, dependency, loss of pleasure from familiar activities, anhedonia, difficulty experiencing love
Intra-personal behaviour	Suicide ideation, more tobacco consumption, alcoholism and drug abuse, sleeplessness, crying, more alertness, work alienation, decreased performance
Inter-personal behaviour	Social withdrawal, reduced relational intimacy, domestic violence, angry outbursts, remarriage, litigation, feeling rejected, over protectiveness
Physical	Fatigue, exhaustion, insomnia, cardiovascular strain, somatic complaints, reduced immune response, headache, gastrointestinal upset, decreased appetite, decreased libido

Source: Author.

Second, it is required to develop a shorter inventory of about 20 items with ecological validity to assess post-disaster trauma. This can act as a screening instrument for diagnosis and identification of traumatized and referral cases as well as an inventory for research. Third, in our country, post-disaster trauma is more widespread among those who are poor, having lower level of education and belonging to lower castes. The intergenerational trauma of social exclusion, exploitation, powerlessness, culture of poverty and devaluation of cultural practices are not recognized in assessment of trauma but those add to the trauma of a disaster. Literature on this area is growing (Danieli, 1998). Comparing the specific population vulnerable and resilient to trauma, we find out the human conditions that fuel trauma. We need to know the intergenerational and cultural factors that help to intensify trauma and the genetic factors that make some people more vulnerable to trauma.

Disaster trauma reaches the peak within the first few weeks after the disaster, continues for about one year and decreases thereafter (Norris, Friedman, Watson and Byrne, et al., 2002; Norris, Friedman and Watson, 2002; Suar and Kar, 2005). Immediately following the supercyclone in Orissa, the state hospital was overcrowded with psychiatric patients, but decreased subsequently. High-impact disasters create persistent long-term trauma. Increased anxiety, depression and post-traumatic stress persisted six years after a volcanic eruption (Howard et al., 1999), post-traumatic stress eight years after exposure to a catastrophic oil rig disaster (Holen, 1991), and such stress persisted among school children 33 years after the collapse of a coal slag heap on a mining area primary school (Morgan, Scourfield, Williams, Jasper and Lewis, 2003). In high-impact disasters with exposure to devastation, loss of lives, injuries, threat to livelihood, damage to property and community infrastructure, disaster traumas are severe, lasting and pervasive and in low-impact disasters, traumas are mild and transitory (Norris, Friedman, Watson and Byrne, et al., 2002). With every other disaster, survivors report varied degrees of trauma.

The resilience and risk of certain population are dealt in excellent reviews of literature and well-documented through programmatic research (Norris, Friedman, Watson and Byrne, et al., 2002; Norris, Friedman and Watson, 2002; Norris, 2005). Though sparse literature is available in India, here follows the discussion on the population who are more vulnerable or resilient to trauma.

Risk and Protective Factor

Exposure

Severity of exposure is operationalized in two ways: (a) the exposure to the number of stressors; and (b) the nearness of survivors' locality to the epicentre of a disaster. In tsunami, the semi-urban habitations surveyed in Nagapattnium district were nearer to the seacoast (Das, Suar and Hota, 2006). As the number of stressors increased, survivors reported more distress. In Orissa supercyclone, 87 per cent of survivors had PTSD who remained within 10 km from the epicentre compared to 11 per cent PTSD who stayed 40 km or away from the epicentre (Suar et al., 2002). More children (43.7 per cent) in high exposure areas of supercyclone are found to have PTSD than that (11.2 per cent) in low exposure areas (Kar, Mohapatra, Nayak, Pattanaik, Swain and Kar, 2007). Those nearer to the epicentre of a disaster experience more stressors.

Stressors are found to affect survivors' trauma. Those include death of family/community members, injury to self or family members, loss of property, destruction of infrastructure and (permanent or temporary) relocation. The more are the number of stressors, the more the trauma. First, all types of losses do not occur in each disaster. Physical property losses do not occur following specific natural disasters like cold wave or heat wave. Second, stressors such as death, threat to life and injury to self/family members are more potent causes of trauma. Following the Taiwan earthquake in 1999, the trauma of bereavement has found to provoke the development of psychiatric disorders including PTSD (Kuo et al., 2003). Focus group discussion with survivors of Orissa supercyclone after seven years confirm that the death of family members causes severe and lasting psychological impairment because such a loss cannot be compensated but other losses can be compensated over time (Suar, 2007).

The service providers and recovery workers clear the debris, dead bodies, interact with families of deceased victims and provide social support to the orphans, widow, widower, physically handicapped and the ravaged communities. They experience burnout being unable to meet constantly the professional demands made on them and also trauma identifying with disaster victims, their needs and sufferings.

Personal loss relates to increase in negative affect and community loss decreases positive affect (Phifer and Norris, 1989). Community devastation leads community-wide tendency for people to feel less positive about their surroundings, less optimistic, less energetic and less able to enjoy life.

Socio-demographic Characteristics

Gender

Women are at least twice as likely as men to develop PTSD. They have greater burden of symptoms and longer duration of distress in the post-disaster period (Norris, Friedman, Watson and Byrne, et al., 2002). First, in accordance with Hofstede's (1980) femininity dimension of values, and Bem's (1974a; 1974b) gender role; warmth, emotional expressiveness, compassion, nurturance and the like are feminine characteristics, and competitiveness, aggressiveness and dominance are masculine characteristics. Having the feminine characteristics, females are likely to experience greater difficulty in extinguishing emotional arousal in the aftermath of a disaster. Second, ours is a male-dominated society. Females have lower social and economic power. Females lacking power, having excessive need to be cared of and often living without permanent family and community members in the post-disaster period render them more vulnerable to distress. Moreover, in similar hazards, female trauma survivors are more likely than male trauma survivors to view the world as dangerous, are more likely to blame themselves for the trauma and to hold more negative views of themselves than male survivors (Tolin and Foa, 2002).

Roles of women also contribute to vulnerability of trauma during and after a disaster: (*a*) role of family caretakers affects their willingness to flee as disaster threatens; (*b*) less access to information after a disaster; (*c*) more susceptibility to physical insecurity, threat of violence from friends/abusers in disaster shelters; (*d*) discrimination in food and medical attention at home and disaster shelters; (*e*) lack of special attention who are pregnant or have small children; (*f*) forced remarriage after a disaster following the death of spouse; (*g*) unemployment for lack of marketable skills; and (*h*) husbands leaving wives for employment elsewhere making women isolated and more dependent on outside assistance.

In the Orissa supercyclone, women had only more anxiety than the men (Suar, Das, Hota and Prasad, 2008; Suar et al., 2002). In a vertical collectivist culture of ours where women are more confined to the house, those who show up for interviews are less likely to be traumatized. In a cross-cultural study, while more distress of women than men has been exacerbated in Mexican culture, it has been attenuated in African American culture (Norris, Perilla, Ibanez and Murphy, 2001). FGDs of men and women after seven years of supercyclone and one year of tsunami reveal that women subjectively describe the events as more devastating than that of men

(Suar, 2007). But women use the post-disaster aid to develop skills and acquire tools and take on non-traditional roles. Women after the Orissa supercyclone had formed self-help groups and earned employment and income for their families.

Age

In a cross-cultural study (Norris, Kaniasty and Conrad, et al., 2002) on effects of age in American, Mexican and Polish adults, it has been observed that for Americans, age has a curvilinear relation with post-traumatic stress revealing that the middle-aged are most distressed. Among Mexicans, age has a negative and linear relation with PTSD suggesting that the younger people are most distressed. Contrarily, in Poland, age has a positive and linear relation with PTSD signifying that the older adults are most vulnerable to disaster trauma. Differences in findings suggest that age–trauma relationship depends on the social, economic, cultural and historical context of disaster-stricken communities.

Studies revealing the middle-aged people to be worst sufferers favour the *inoculation and burden* perspective. It is argued that older people having prior experience of trauma have improved coping skills. Middle-aged people act as service-providers in a society. They suffer from trauma following a disaster which disrupts their role of providers. The *exposure and resource* perspective explains more vulnerability of older people to trauma than the younger ones. The coping capacity of older people decreases because of declining health and lower socio-economic resources. They have lesser likelihood of receiving warning, greater reluctance to evacuate, higher resistance to alter accustomed patterns of life and a severe sense of deprivation resulting from losses. They are more likely to experience disaster-related injuries, substantial economic losses and evaluate their situation as worse compared to those around them. They are also less likely to use post-disaster services of counselling and social support.

Studying the adult survivors above 18 years age, the two competing paradigms are modelled in obtained data from supercyclone in Orissa and tsunami in Tamli Nadu (Suar et al., 2008; Suar, Mishra and Khuntia, 2007). Older people are found to be suffering more from anxiety, depression and post-traumatic stress. In India, collectivistic values of interdependence, social support, cooperation and interpersonal sensitivity coexist with power distance (Triandis, 1996). Senior members are respected and obeyed. They represent the family, take care of others and provide suggestions and advices for the family and community's prosperity. First, the disasters depleted the personal (self-esteem, mastery, well-being), social, economic and work resources that survivors had built and conserved over time (Hobfoll, 2001). Elderly people, being the custodian of family and community, had greater sense of resource loss with little hope to regain the resources in the remaining years of their life. Second, the sudden crisis was painful to the elderly in our culture characterized by high uncertainty avoidance and low tolerance of ambiguity (Hofstede, 1980). Third, people in India are like prospective gardeners who expand their family tree with expectations to see all family members and relatives happy at their deathbed. Elderly people experienced separation anxiety, despair and dejection being detached from their kith and kin. Moreover, the loss of needed assistive devices, such as spectacles, hearing aids and so forth made it difficult for the elderly to approach others. All these factors may have intensified trauma of the elderly.

Effects of age on distress are found across cultures and disasters. Elderly people were more distressed after the flood in Poland (Norris, Kaniasty and Conrad, et al., 2002), the earthquake in Australia (Ticehurst et al., 1996), Turkey (Salcioglu et al., 2003), Taiwan (Yang et al., 2003) and Japan (Tanida, 1996). Individuals in the 50–59 age group were most emotionally distressed after the September 11 terrorist attack in the the US (Chen, Chung, Chen, Fang and Chen, 2003). Psychological morbidity had persisted longer in older citizens following the earthquake in Australia (Ticehurst et al., 1996) and a volcanic eruption in Japan (Ohta et al., 2003). Observations in other cultures along with ours suggest that old age is a definite risk factor for psychological sequelae in the aftermath of a disaster.

In the aftermath of a disaster, children often suffer from various water- and air-borne diseases. Analysis of the secondary data two years before and two years after the Orissa supercyclone at macro level reveals the decrease in enrolment of children in primary school up to two years after the disaster. Infant mortality suddenly has risen following the disaster (Suar and Kar, 2005). Grief of children intensifies following bereavement in family. They often regress to earlier stage of development and show thumb sucking, bedwetting and fear of sleeping alone. The traumatized parents fail to provide the required affection and care to their children. Children get more traumatized observing the trauma of their parents. Following supercyclone, 30.6 per cent of children had PTSD and an additional 13.6 per cent had sub-syndromal PTSD (Kar et al., 2007). Orphan children suffer most the trauma of losing their parents and family members. Being the lone surviving member in the family, they are vulnerable to abuse and exploitation.

Caste Status

In Western culture, psychosocial morbidity following disasters is found to be more among ethnic minorities (Norris, Friedman, Watson and Byrne, et al., 2002). In India, poor and weaker sections of the society are worst sufferers in the aftermath of disasters as they have fewer resources to cope with (Bhatt, 2001; Parasuraman and Unnikrishnan, 2001).

Studying the caste hierarchy, Srinivas (1996, p. 120) has concluded that the high castes in rural areas dominate the low castes on economic and political power, education and occupations. First, attitudes and beliefs that are mentally programmed in a vertical collectivist culture lower the abilities of low caste people to cope with the post-disaster life. It is explained by higher levels of fatalism and acculturative stress (discomfort in dealing with higher caste people). Fatalism is a global risk factor in post-disaster because it inhibits the initiation of livelihood activities. Second, low caste people live in more risk-prone areas (unstable slopes, flood plains), vulnerable homes and are likely to experience greater devastation. Third, social disarticulation occurs following a disaster. Tightly-knit social networks with neighbours and friends being vital life support sources of low caste people—emotional support, food borrowing, labour-exchange relations, child care reciprocity, etc.—are destroyed following a disaster. Social networks fail to fulfil their supportive roles. Fourth, lacking ability to influence service-providers and having restricted access to economic infrastructure, low caste survivors are not likely to receive the social support as much as the high caste survivors have. Accordingly, it has been found that supercyclone survivors belonging to low castes have experienced more post-traumatic stress, anxiety and depression compared to those belonging to high castes (Suar and Khuntia, 2004). Majority of low caste people inhabited near the epicentre of supercyclone and experienced greater devastation. They lacked social power to influence the service-provider and muster resources in the post-disaster period. Severity of exposure and lack of social power worked in tandem to induce trauma. Also, intergenerational marginalization may have also affected the trauma of low caste people.

Socio-economic Status

Socio-economic status (SES) comprises education, income and occupation. It is often difficult to assess. In our study of tsunami survivors in Nagapattinam, the affected people belonged to fisherman communities and their source livelihood was fishing. Agriculture and fishing were main occupations in costal belt for the affected communities in the Orissa supercyclone. Similarly, the affected people from the supercyclone in Orissa and tsunami in Nagapattinam had lower level of education and similar income. In the absence of wide variation on educational levels, occupations and income, it poses difficulty to assess the impact of SES on post-disaster trauma.

Education creates awareness, improves capabilities, makes people more dynamic and manipulative and helps in marshalling post-disaster services (Srinivas, 1996). The less educated survivors lack confidence and the ability to influence service-providers. They have limited access to economic infrastructure and alternative livelihood options in the post-disaster period. So also, first, people with low income live in more vulnerable places and are likely to experience greater intensity of devastation. Second, fragile resources of the poor are shattered, homes are damaged, food, cloth and health insecurity are constantly threatened in post-disaster. Their social network collapses and they become marginalized with a little hope to regain the resources in future. Third, according to the *rule of relative advantage*, victims with larger social network, better economic resources, more education and majority status receive more help than those with smaller social network, fewer economic resources, less education and minority status. Accordingly, poor people are less likely to muster post-disaster services and support. In accordance with this, we found that the illiterates in both supercyclone and tsunami survivors and low-income households in tsunami are found to suffer more from anxiety and post-traumatic stress than their counterparts (Das, Suar and Hota, 2006; Suar and Khuntia, 2004). More children and adolescents having PTSD had the lower education level and were from low-income families (Kar et al., 2007).

Physically, Mentally and Developmentally Challenged

The physically disabled, mentally ill or retarded are at risk in post-disaster period. Their needs are different from others and supportive services are disrupted. For instance, supplies of medication, assistive devices, such as wheelchairs, familiar caretakers and previous programmes of treatment may not be available anymore. Their special needs with regard to food, toilet and house are constantly threatened. Those mentally ill or developmentally delayed have fewer coping resources available and less ability to mobilize help for themselves. The disabled are at risk of malnutrition, infectious disease in a shelter camp and lack of adequate health care. They are vulnerable to marginalization and isolation (Tanida, 1996). Lack of special support increases stress. Stress, in turn, may exacerbate their pre-existing mental and physical illness.

FAMILY CONTEXT

Lager Family

Caring for and obligation to others cause stress. In the classic experiment on two monkeys, the 'executive monkey' has to press a lever to prevent electric shock. The executive monkey had experienced stress, died on the 23rd day and was found having an ulcer (Brady, 1958). Having the responsibility to provide care and unable to do so intensified stress. In India, extended or joint families provide psychological security to their members in normal and critical periods (Kapadia, 1990). In larger families, adult members experiencing post-disaster stress are supposed to take care of other family members. In the Orissa supercyclone, members from larger fam-ilies having more than five members are found to experience more PTSD and anxiety than the members from smaller families having less than five members (Suar and Khuntia, 2004).

Marriage, Parenthood and Children

Marital stress is found to increase in post-disaster. Women who perceive themselves as having excellent spouse support are more vulnerable than the women having weaker ties. Husband's symptom severity predicts wife's symptoms strongly than the vice versa (Norris, 2005).

In India, the relationship between husband and wife is more enduring. With death of spouses, widows/widowers after supercyclone and tsunami are found to be more distressed than the married persons (Das, Suar and Hota, 2006; Kar et al., 2004). Their higher distress was because of permanent loss of life partner and sudden shouldering of unconventional economic-provider role for family and children.

In married families, mothers were at enhanced risk because of their concern over children's safety and security. Interpersonal conflict and lack of supportive climate in a family also increased children's trauma. In the Orissa supercyclone, parents were concerned for mental health of children (Kar et al., 2007). Children were directly and indirectly affected by experiences of death, destruction, terror, personal physical assault and by the absence or powerlessness of their parents. They were affected by the reactions of their parents and other trusted adults such as teachers and significant others in the community. Children's fears were intensified if parents and significant others in a community reacted with fear. Children have less ability to judge which fears are realistic or unrealistic. Their fear may also stem from their imagination. Most children respond sensibly and appropriately to a disaster if they experience the protection, support and stability of their parents and other trusted adults.

Persons with pre-disaster mental illness and substance abuse experience difficulty to recover from disaster trauma (Norris, 2005). Neurotic persons having emotional instability experience more trauma compared to stable and calm persons (Suar et al., 2002). A disaster further aggravates their pre-existing conditions.

Resource Context

Experiencing traumatic events, only about 25 per cent of people develop PTSD (Brady, 2001). What enables the remaining 75 per cent of trauma victims to psychologically recover despite their traumatic experiences? Though the trauma sufferers are more in developing countries following devastating disasters, the question essentially remains the same. Overcoming trauma depends on certain personality attributes and social support.

Mastery

Bandura (1986) suggests that individual reactions to severe stress are significantly related to self-appraisals of one's abilities to cope with the environmental demands. Coping self-efficacy is found to decrease survivors' PTSD in Oklahoma City bombing (Benight et al., 2000) and many severe natural disasters (Benight et al., 1999a; 1999b; 1999c).

Self-mastery refers to the personal feeling that one can control his/her destiny by dint of personal abilities, skills and talents. People who have a sense of self-mastery feel that they can control adverse situations and solve problems independently. Evidence suggests that a sense of self-mastery is associated with resilience in the face of stressful life circumstances (Hobfoll, 2001). In individualist cultures, individuals explain the success in terms of their own stable, internal attributes such as talent and ability. Individual mastery may be an important element of self-schema for persons from individualist cultures, but less effective in collectivist cultures (Triandis, 1996).

An alternative to individual mastery is communal mastery (Hobfoll, Schroder, Wells and Malek, 2002). It is a generalized sense that being a part of the closely-knit group generates ability for successful confrontation to stressors. Individuals can overcome life challenges and stresses because they are a part of closely-knit social network. In collectivist cultures, individuals will be resilient to stress depending on their social network and ties. Communal mastery is pivotal in coping with disaster stressors among persons from collectivist cultures (Hobfoll et al., 2002).

Attributional Style

Attributional style refers to a stable cognitive disposition for assigning causality for events that occur in one's life. Adoption of a maladaptive attributional style increases the risk for traumatic symptoms. Locus of control is a bipolar personality variable (internal and external) that depicts the attributional style of people (Rotter, 1966). People having internal locus of control attribute the success, failure and outcomes in life to themselves. On the contrary, those having external control attribute the happenings in life to external forces such as fate, luck or God. Studies in individualist cultures indicate that people with external attributions are more susceptible to trauma. External attribution and its cognitive processing induce helplessness in face of acute stress. In stress and coping research, external control or fatalism has been viewed as a risk factor for poor outcome (Wheaton, 1982) because it inhibits taking actions or seeking help when needed. The feeling of fatalism intensifies in post-disaster situations. The Orissa supercyclone-affected people, attributing control to external sources, experienced more traumas (Suar et al., 2002). They depended much on relief and help from external agencies rather than taking their own initiative for self-reliance. This acquired dependency on external agency for support following the supercyclone was referred to as 'weaning syndrome' (Mohanty, 2002). The analysis of secondary data revealed that after one year of supercyclone, the farming communities in coastal belt took more loans from agricultural credit cooperative societies and consumed more fertilizers in agricultural fields for more yield of crops (Suar and Kar, 2005). This suggested that the weaning syndrome dissipated after one year and gradually transferred to internal locus of control for reconstruction of life and livelihood.

Sense of Coherence

Sense of coherence (SOC) is a global orientation that expresses the extent to which one has a pervasive, enduring though dynamic feeling of confidence that: (a) the stimuli deriving from one's internal and external environments are structured, predictable and explicable; (b) the resources are available to one to meet the demands posed by these stimuli; and (c) these demands are challenges, worthy of investment and engagement (Antonovsky and Sagy, 1986). In other words, SOC is a coping mechanism characterized by the tendency to see life as predictable and manageable. It correlates positively with self-esteem, mastery, optimism and internal locus of control (Sack, Lamprecht and Forschungsaspekte, 1998). People with a strong SOC are less likely to perceive many stressful situations as threatening and anxiety provoking than their weak SOC counterparts. Accordingly, traffic accident victims having high SOC are found have more frustration tolerance, lower post-traumatic psychopathology, PTSD and anxious cognitions (Frommberger et al., 1999).

Social Support

Social support is a reciprocal or non-reciprocal interaction that may include the provision of emotional support, tangible support, informational support or some combination thereof. It provides survivors with actual assistance and embeds them into a network of social relationships that are perceived to be loving, caring and readily available at times of need. Social support comprises received support (actual receipt of support), perceived support (belief that help would be available when needed, cognitive appraisal of connectedness to others) and social embeddedness (quantity and type of relationships with other people).

Social embeddedness represents the structural component from which the other two functional components emerge. Disaster victims depend for social support on their formal network of families and informal networks of friends, neighbours, community, religious congregations, governmental and NGOs and external aid agencies. Supports available in the post-disaster are in the form of tangible goods such as food, cloth, shelter, medicine, money, tools/equipments and other consumables; information regarding the disaster, relief and rehabilitation; and emotional support, such as care and empathy. Social embeddedness decreases depression (Kaniasty and Norris, 1993; Norris et al., 1999) and received support decreases trauma (Carr, Lewin, Webster, Hazell, Kenardy and Carter, 1995).

Perceived support buffers trauma including depression (Kaniasty and Norris, 1993; Norris and Kaniasty, 1996), lower alcohol abuse and relapse (Lutgendorf et al., 1995). Continuance of support from non-kin members till the survivors return to normalcy can increase the perceived support or hope of getting support when needed and help buffering trauma.

The summary of risk and protective factors are presented in Table 20.3. We have learned that while certain populations are at risk of trauma, certain personality attributes buffer trauma and also the received and perceived social support. The risk factors suggest more care of certain populations who are more risk of trauma. More research is warranted on protective factors. Essentially, if the protective factors of communal mastery, internal attribution and SOC buffer post-disaster trauma, the post-disaster intervention strategies need to incorporate ways and means to revive and renew the mental strength of survivors for buffering trauma. Also, findings suggest for the delivery social support humanely to shield the survivors against trauma.

Table 20.3: Risk and Protective Factors of Trauma

Characteristics	Risk and Protective Factors
Level of exposure	Closeness to the epicentre of disaster
	Death of family member, injury to self/family members, threat to life, loss of property, (permanent or temporary) relocation
	More the stressors, the more the trauma
	Living in community that is highly disrupted and destroyed
Survivors' socio-demographic characteristics	Women, pregnant women, mothers having small children
	Older adults and children
	Low caste status
	Low socio-economic status
	Physically, mentally, and developmentally challenged
Family context	Larger families
	Husband's symptom severity predicts wife's symptoms strongly than the vice-versa
	Widow/widower, orphans
	Lack of supportive climate in family
	Pre-disaster mental illness, substance abuse, neurotic status aggravate trauma
Resource context	Communal mastery, internal control, sense of coherence, and social support buffer trauma.

Source: Author.

Why Trauma?

The four theories discussed here explain the varied causes of trauma. These are: (*a*) cognitive theory; (*b*) conservation of resources theory; (*c*) social support deterioration–deterrence model; and (*d*) impoverishment risk theory. Understanding these theories can help formulate strategies to arrest the causes of trauma.

Cognitive theory

The reactivation of emotional memories of the disaster manifests in trauma (Ehlers and Clark, 2000). The memory often includes an individual's reaction during a disaster (freezing, screaming, fearing, etc.). Perceiving the surrounding environment as dangerous elicits physiological (increased heart rate, faster respiration) and behavioural (flight response) reactions.

The reactivation of disaster memories expressing in trauma is also dealt in Indian psycho-philosophical literature and discussed earlier (Suar, 2004). Based on the happenings just before or during a disaster, some permanent emotional dispositions like fear, terror and grief, and transitory emotions like wonder, dejection, agitation, anger and mental derangement are excited. Such emotions in varied combinations manifest in traumas.

The emotional memory is retrieved getting cues from the environment. Disaster victims often fail to recall the emotional experiences. Such autobiographical memories entering consciousness, connect to specific and general information about a disaster, are poorly elaborated and inadequately linked to the context. Retrieval of associative memory is cue-driven and unintentional. A high-impact disaster makes an individual's threshold low for emotional arousal. Even a vague physical similarity of the stimulus in surroundings with the observed stimuli during a disaster becomes sufficient to trigger re-experiencing symptoms. Avoidance of reminder of trauma occurs when an individual changes from negative appraisal to how the event could have been avoided. It hinders the formation of organized memory.

Conservation of resources theory

The basic tenet of 'conservation of resources' (COR) theory (Hobfoll, 1988; 2001) is that individuals strive to obtain, retain, protect and foster those things that they value. These valued entities are termed as resources that include objects, conditions, personal characteristics and energy. Resources are valued in their own rights because those help in defining a person's identity and assist in acquiring and protecting other resources. Stress occurs when: (a) individuals' resources are threatened with loss; (b) individuals' resources are actually lost; or (c) individuals fail to gain sufficient resources following significant resource investment.

Acquiring and retaining resources promote mental health. The COR model proposes that individuals strive to minimize net loss of resources when confronted with stressors, and they strive to develop surplus resources in order to offset possibility of future resource loss. In catastrophic disasters, survivors may lose their homes (object resources) and with them a sense of safety and security. Survivors may lose their jobs and spouse (conditions resources) and with them a sense of status and belongingness. Survivors may lose their self-esteem and well-being (personal characteristics resources) and with them mental courage and conviction. Survivors may lose their money and knowledge (energy resources) and with them a desire to attain other resources. In a devastating disaster, either the resources are destroyed or become fragile. Those intensify trauma (Hobfoll, 2001; Hobfoll and Lilly, 1993).

In COR, resource loss is more important than resource gain. Given equal amounts of loss and gain, loss will have significantly greater impacts. While we tend to mourn our losses greatly and linger it for more time, we celebrate our gains mildly and briefly (Wells, Hobfoll and Lavin, 1999). People can invest resources in order to protect against resource loss. But, the poor possessing fewer and fragile resources are more vulnerable to experience resource loss in investing their resources to gain resources. They are vulnerable to both acute and chronic losses due to disasters, and also secondary resource losses (loss of optimism, hope) that can result in loss spirals. Contrarily, a resource-rich person may invest resources like money and social support after acute losses, preventing secondary losses and perhaps resulting in secondary gains, and thereby promoting a gain spiral.

Resource loss is also found to be a potential predictor of trauma (Ironson et al., 1997). Resource loss lowers coping self-efficacy, increases trauma (Benight et al., 1999a, 1999c) and overshadows the sense of coherence (Kaiser, Sattler, Bellack and Dersin, 1996). Disaster victims with fewer resources usually experience complete depletion of resources following a disaster, fail to find any resources to invest and experience more traumas. Even when there is some balance resources left with these people, such as hope, partially damaged house or good family relationships, when invested, these resources are likely to be lost trying to cope with the situational demands. Thus, the primary loss leads to secondary losses that finally culminate in loss spirals. People from low socio-economic status are found to have more resource loss because of their limited initial resources and also their failure to gain resources. They are less likely to muster post-disaster support and are more likely to be traumatized compared to their more resource-endowed counterparts.

Social support deterioration–deterrence model

The 'social support deterioration deterrence' (Kaniasty and Norris, 1993; 1995b; Norris and Kaniasty, 1996) model is based on evidences from Kentucky floods and hurricane Hugo. Most often, the help is provided to victims on the basis of their 'relative needs'. Victims more severely exposed to the stressors (injury to life, property loss) receive more help than the non-victims. But in some disasters, the rule of 'relative advantage' operates. Disaster victims who have greater economic resources are more educated or are members of ethnic majority groups marshal more support than their counterparts (Caldera et al., 2001; Kaniasty and Norris, 1995b). Victims having fewer resources, being less educated or members of ethnic minority groups receive less help than the equally affected victims having more resources, being more educated or members of ethnic majority. They experience a *pattern of neglect*. A few victims also experience a *pattern of concern* when they receive more help than the similarly affected victims. Older victims of Hurricane Hugo faced with threats to their lives and health received more help than the similarly affected victims from younger age groups.

The aftermath of a disaster disrupts the natural network with kin and non-kin members. The help and companionship of altruistic community initially rally and tend to dissipate with time. When survivor' initial received support deteriorates or needs are unmet, perceived social support and sense of social embeddedness decline. In other words, when received support becomes low relative to the needs, survivors' expectation of support deteriorates—support will not be available when needed. That increases trauma. When received support is adequate for the needs, disaster victims will maintain their expectations of available support that will buffer trauma.

In disasters, social support tends to dissipate with time. The poor and ethnic minority (Kaniasty and Norris, 1993; 1995b; Norris and Kaniasty, 1996) have less initial resources. They lose those resources in the disaster and are less likely to be linked to societal resource reserves and mobilize post-disaster resources. The inadequate received support with time decreases the perceived support. It increases trauma.

Impoverishment risk theory

Cernea's (2000) impoverishment risk model is developed studying the refugees of war and internal conflicts, and the displacees of big dams, factories and sanctuaries. The model explains resettlers' risks of landlessness, joblessness, homelessness, marginalization, food insecurity, increased morbidity and mortality, food insecurity, loss of access to common property and social disarticulation following forced displacement. The model is applicable to the risks in the aftermath of a disaster because displacement risks are similar to the problems of the disaster displacees, and resettlement is akin to post-disaster rehabilitation and reconstruction of communities.

It has been proposed that displacees experience trauma getting the warning to leave their ancestral place and property, losing their inherited land, vocation, relations, surroundings and finding them with strangers in the relocation site, and not regaining their earlier socio-economic status for inadequate planning. Along with socio-economic status, they lose their self-esteem and psychological infrastructure. Different losses causing the psychological distress are postulated (Good, 1996; Mahapatra, 1999) but not studied empirically.

In the cognitive theory, the reactivation of disaster memory expresses in trauma. The encoding of disaster memory depends on the number and magnitude of stressors. The running thread of COR theory and impoverishment risk model is the loss of resources. Furthermore, the COR model includes the failure to gain resources that intensifies trauma. While COR theory deals with loss of extrinsic and intrinsic resources, impoverishment risk model has only postulated about loss of extrinsic resources. The social support deterioration deterrence model mentions about the decrease of received support with time that deteriorates perceived support and increases trauma. Conclusively, these theories find three main drivers of trauma: (*a*) reactivation of disaster memories; (*b*) resource loss; and (*c*) inadequacy of received social support with time. Now there is ample evidence to support such contentions (Dass-Brailsford, 2007; Sattler et al., 2002). Hence, the counter strategy of building strength mentally and providing social support humanely to regain the lost resources can buffer trauma. Let us discuss how such interventions are made.

INTERVENTION PROGRAMME

In the aftermath of a disaster, it is important not to pathologize the reactions. Such symptoms are normal to highly abnormal situations. In India, the National Institute of Mental Health and Neuro Sciences (NIMHANS) has studied psychosocial support systematically since the Bangalore circus fire (1981) to Gujarat riots (2001). Organizations such as NIMHANS, Oxfam India, ActionAid India and CARE have developed community-based mental health programmes for affected communities of supercyclone in Orissa, earthquake and riot in Gujarat and tsunami in Tamil Nadu, Kerala, Pondicherry and Andaman and Nicobar islands. Here, we map the different stages of a disaster and specify mental health services for amelioration of trauma. Disaster management can be conceptualized as a cycle with four phases: impact, during, after and before disaster (Figure 20.1).

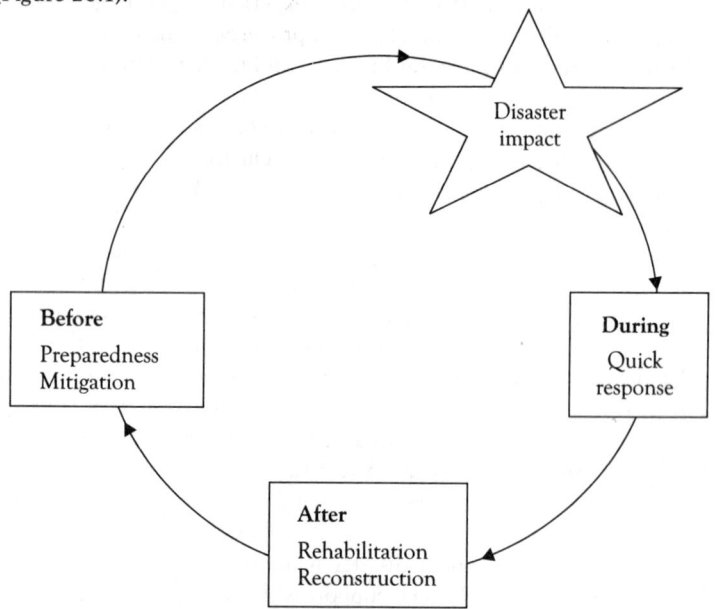

Figure 20.1: Disaster Management Cycle

Source: Author.

Impact Phase

Impact phase refers to the 'real time' of the disaster. The duration depends on the disaster. While ground shaking may occur only for few seconds during an earthquake, flooding may take place for a longer period. At this stage, individuals are at risk because of their inability to protect themselves. The common reactions of victims at this stage are confusion, anxiety, shock and panic. Confusion, anxiety and shock intensify, if: (a) the disaster threatens without warning, without information from trusted sources; (b) people have no previous experience of similar disasters; and (c) people have neither known nor learned the preparedness skills. Panic is shown if escape route is blocked, people are trapped and helpless. At this stage, mental health professionals have little to offer because the priorities are rescue and protection. After the Kobe earthquake (Japan) in 1955, survivors spurned the psychiatric clinics that had been set up (Shinfuku, 1999). For mental health services, it is the time for planning to set up mobile clinics, helplines and outreach programmes.

During Phase

During phase is the time in which lives and livelihoods are at risk. It lasts until the danger is over. This phase calls for disposal of dead bodies, clearing of debris and the provisions of relief. It includes setting up control room, issuing warning, action for evacuation, taking people to safe places, rendering food, drinking water and medicine, restoring communication, disbursement of assistance in cash or kind and coordination with local volunteers, state administration, NGOs and other agencies for quick response and relief.

A person's actions are geared to protection of oneself and others, especially children, family members and those who are weak and helpless. This behaviour is appropriate at the time but make people feel guilty that they are selfish. Some people are disorganized/stunned and may not respond appropriately to protect themselves and their families and such behaviour extends to post-disaster indicating their level of dissociation. Survivors experience the 'illusion of centrality', especially when they are isolated from others. They feel that the disaster is just happening to them and may not realize that the others have been affected (Raphael, 2000). Altruism is common and community volunteers and strangers place their life at risk to help others. With the disruption of information, misinterpretations, myths and rumours spread. Local sites for information about others, about appropriate actions, shelters, food, water and health care are of great value in providing assurance and guidance, and inform people to gather. Gathering together, sharing mutual concern and talking about what has happened are helpful to learn from one another. Such behaviour provides a natural outlet for 'debriefing' and preserves a sense of social embeddedness. It can so do for children through playing, drawing, etc. This is the time when many outsiders enter the disaster area. Survivors may gather, narrate their experiences, exaggerate their problems and often release their frustration and anger on outsiders.

Survivors begin to build a picture of what has happened. They want to reunite with kin members and community. Keeping family members in separate shelters are damaging, particularly to children and women. Survivors are further stressed and shocked by what they see and hear, and the realization of the death, damage and loss. People may appear confused, stunned or demonstrate high anxiety levels. This is the time when mental health problems surface.

Each family with its members suffer from psychological sequela. Intervention for children may be of limited effectiveness if the family is not treated as a whole. Providing solace to stressed parents can be the most effective ways to provide care and support to the children vis-à-vis family members. An approach to handle trauma of people is the psychological first aid (Raphael, 1986). It includes: (*a*) comfort and consolation; (*b*) protection from further threat and distress; (*c*) immediate physical care; (*d*) helping reunion with loved ones; (*e*) sharing experience (but not forced); (*f*) goal-oriented and purposeful behaviour; (*g*) linking survivors with source of support, (*h*) facilitating a sense of being in control; and (*i*) identifying those who need further help (triage). Essentially, it involves reassuring and providing food, clothes, shelter along with safety and security. If the survivor wishes to talk about their experience, emphasis is laid on listening and not on probing for psychological reactions. Attempts are made to link survivors with family and neighbours as it revives the natural support system. Trauma of survivors can be gradually buffered using techniques of active listening, natural ventilation, empathy, social support, relaxation, spiritual activities and externalization of interests. Helping individuals, families and communities to discover and use the resources and tools around them for livelihoods help in ventilation of trauma.

Individual-focused interventions are called for persons who are most distressed, who have weak psychological and social resources to begin with or suffered dire resource loss. Triage is for them who show acute cognitive, emotional and behavioural impairment. Because of their worst mental health, such sufferers are least likely to seek for external resource support. Outreach of mental health services to such persons and communities is essential.

Post-disaster Phase

Post-disaster phase aims to achieve rapid and durable recovery to counter the vulnerable conditions. This is a phase of rehabilitation and reconstruction. It often includes the activities undertaken immediately following the disaster that include debris clearance, immediate relief and needs' assessment. Rehabilitation includes provision of temporary public utilities and houses as interim measures. Reconstruction attempts to return communities to improved pre-disaster functioning. It comprises reconstruction of house/building, infrastructure, lifeline facilities and provisions of socio-economic support to promote livelihoods in long term.

Psychosocial care promotes the restoration of social cohesion, independence and dignity of individuals and groups and makes them more resilient (Loughry and Eyber, 2003). It is put in place once the search, rescue and the clean up have been completed and the rehabilitation of the community has begun. During this time, community comes together into an organization that did not exist in pre-disaster. They form groups such as self-help, advocacy and others. Emotional reactions may often express in the form of somatic complaints such as sleep disturbance, indigestion, fatigue, as well as social effects, such as relationship or work difficulties. To counter such reactions, counselling and mental health support should be available in readily accessible places of community. People who were socially and economically independent before the disaster may not come for assistance. Delivering physical assistance with psychological help in a supportive way can increase relevance. Survivors are more likely to accept help for 'problems in living' than for 'problems in mental health'.

Psychosocial care fosters social networks and communication, and information services. Maintaining social networks plays a vital role in the recovery from trauma. Psychosocial care fosters continued networking of friends, neighbours and respected members of the community so that stresses may be dealt with through social networks and support. Communication is vital after the disaster because it helps to dismiss myths, provides feedback to the affected community and promotes recognition of individual and community achievements. Psychosocial care is also about taking care of the symbolic needs of the community. Community rituals may evolve as symbolic and important steps in the recovery process. Memorial services, renewal projects, religious activities and involvement in livelihood activities constitute ways of externalizing trauma. The facilitative positive forces are: (*a*) recognizing and reinforcing people's strengths;

(b) providing clear and accurate information and education; (c) reinforcing supportive networks; (d) supporting and developing community strengths and processes; and (e) engaging in livelihood reconstruction using available resources and support (Colossi, 2000; Fonagi et al., 1994). Psychological care may range from consultation with disaster experts and community leaders to encouraging a supportive post-disaster environment, facilitating community networks, providing information, encouraging ceremonies and engaging in available livelihood activities to facilitate recovery. It might be helpful to educate the public about the reasons significant others may not always be able to provide them with the support they expect. In the Orissa supercyclone, collective prayer, play for children, construction of infrastructure, food-for-work and other activities decided and implemented by the participation of survivors helped in externalization of trauma.

In some instances, service-providers may encounter a person who is extremely agitated, seemingly unable to calm down, destructive and portrays suicidal actions. It is important for the helper to remain calm and to appear relaxed, confident and non-threatening. The interventions have to occur rapidly and the helper needs to take an active and directive role in helping the person. The initial goal of crises intervention is palliative and the ultimate goal is to refer such individuals to local service-providers for ongoing services.

After one year of the disaster, majority of the people recover from trauma. Those who do not recover, they require support and service on an ongoing basis. Complete reconstruction may take 6–8 years or more depending on the extent of devastation. In reconstruction phase, survivors make attempts to reach their earlier socio-economic status. Here, groups representing community stakeholders may identify their problem, seek consultation, find solutions, plan activities and implement them.

Pre-disaster

Pre-disaster is the period of time when a warning and/or alert is announced, mitigation and preparation activities are carried out. Mitigation activities are protective and preventive actions to lessen the hazardous consequences in the long run such as improved housing construction, reforestation in riverbanks, building disaster shelter, etc. Those cover structural engineering activities. Preparatory activities are stockpiling of food, water, cloth, medicine, etc., movement to safe places and training people at community level to decrease people's vulnerability to recurrent negative impacts.

Community members may be anxious when a disaster is imminent. Anxiety will be there if warning is absent or inadequate, preparedness skills are not learned and people have not experienced such a disaster in past. Preparedness of the communities before a disaster is necessary to lessen the adverse impact of that disaster.

Preparedness is a self-protective or precautionary behaviour. It emerges as a response to an impending danger to life and property. Preparedness enables individuals and communities to respond rapidly and effectively to disaster situations. For example, preparedness activities before a flood include some items to be kept ready such as torch lights, lantern filled with kerosene; ration, dry foods and baby foods with clean drinking water; ORS packets and first-aid box; animal feed; polythene bags for clothing and valuables; an umbrella and a bamboo stick for protection against snake; boats and rubber tubes for instant evacuation. Also, people need to act following the warning, know disaster shelter nearby, participate in mock drills, plant trees, keep sand bags in the riverbank and attend the meetings of community members, government authorities and civil societies for flood preparedness (see Table 20.4).

Natural disasters cannot be stopped. We need to educate people, create necessary resources and influence them to practise simulations at community level so that the adverse consequences of natural disasters can be arrested.

Table 20.4: Psychosocial Interventions at Various Phases of a Disaster

Phase	Reaction	Psychological Task	Intervention
Impact	Confusion, anxiety, shock, panic	Physical safety	Rescue and protection
During	Grief, anger, despair, blame, avoidance, flashbacks and nightmares or PTSD	Accommodation	Psychological first aid
Rehabilitation and reconstruction	PTSD, depression, family conflict, substance abuse, suicidal thought, inability to adjust, difficulties in livelihood	Assimilation and development	Psychosocial care, needs assessment, livelihood activities planning and implementation
			Supervision in individual and community activities, empowerment of communities
Pre-disaster	Anxiety	Preparedness	Disaster education, resources, simulation at community level

Source: Author.

REFERENCES

American Psychiatric Association. (1994). *Diagnostic and statistical manual for mental disorders* (4th ed.). Washington, DC: APA.

Antonovsky, H. and Sagy, S. (1986). The development of a sense of coherence and its impact on response to stress situations. *Journal of Social Psychology*, 126(2), 213-25.

Bandura, A. (1986). *Social foundations of thought and action*. New Jersey: Prentice-Hall.

Bem, S. L. (1974a). The measurement of psychological androgyny. *Journal of Consulting and Clinical Psychology*. 42(2), 155-62.

———. (1974b). *Bem sex-role inventory*. CA: Consulting Psychologists Press.

Benight, C. C., Ironson, G. and Durham, R. L. (1999a). Psychometric properties of a hurricane coping self-efficacy measure. *Journal of Traumatic Stress*, 12(2), 379-86.

Benight, C. C., Ironson, G., Klebe, K., Carver, C. S., Wynings, C., Burnett, K., Greenwood, D., Baum, A. and Schneiderman, N. (1999c). Conservation of resources and coping self-efficacy predicting distress following a natural disaster: A causal model analysis where the environment meets the mind. *Anxiety, Stress, and Coping*, 12(2), 107-26.

Benight, C. C., Swift, E., Sanger, J., Smith, A. and Zeppelin, D. (1999b). Coping self-efficacy as a mediator of distress following a natural disaster. *Journal of Applied Social Psychology*, 29(12), 2443-64.

Benight, C. C., Freyaldenhoven, R., Hughes, J., Ruiz, J. M., Zoschke, T. A. and Lovallo, W. (2000). Coping self-efficacy and psychological distress following the Oklahoma City Bombing: A longitudinal analysis. *Journal of Applied Social Psychology*, 30(7), 1331-44.

Bhatt, M. R. (2001). Gujarat: Lessons to be learnt. In N. Ravi (Ed.), *The Hindu survey of the environment 2001*(pp. 7-11). Chennai: Kasturi & Sons Ltd.

Brady, J. V. (1958). Ulcers in 'executive' monkeys. *Scientific American*, 199(3), 95-104.

Brady, K. T. (2001). Co-morbid post-traumatic stress disorder and substance use disorder. *Psychiatric Annals*, 31(5), 313-19.

Caldera, T., Palma, L., Penayo, U. and Kullgren, G. (2001). Psychological impact of the hurricane Mitch in Nicaragua in a one-year perspective. *Social Psychiatry and Psychiatric Epidemiology*, 36(3), 108-14.

Carr, V. J., Lewin, T. J., Webster, R. A., Hazell, P. L., Kenardy, J. A. and Carter, G. L (1995). Psychological sequelae of the 1989 Newcastle Earthquake: I. Community disaster experiences and psychological morbidity 6 months post-disaster. *Psychological Medicine*, 25(3), 539-56.

Center for Research on the Epidemiology of Disasters (CRED). (2005). *EM-DAT data base*. Universite Catholique de Louvain, Belgium: Author.

Cernea, M. M. (2000). Risks, safeguards, and reconstruction: A model for population displacement and resettlement. In M. M. Cernea and C. McDowell (Eds), *Risk and reconstruction: Experiences of resettlers and refuges* (pp. 11-55), Washington DC: World Bank.

Chen, H., Chung, H., Chen, T., Fang, L. and Chen, J. P. (2003). The emotional distress in a community after the terrorist attack on the World Trade Center. *Community Mental Health Journal*, 39(2), 157-65.

Colossi, M. M. (2000). *The community resilience manual*. Port Alberni, BC: Centre for Community Enterprise.

Denieli, Y. (Ed.). (1998). *International handbook of multigenerational legacies of trauma*. New York: Plenum Press.

Das, N., Suar, D. and Hota, L. B. (2006). *Social indicators affecting distress and physical health of tsunami survivors*. Paper presented at National Academy of Psychology Conference (India) at IIT Mumbai (Dec 14-16).

Dass-Brailsford, P. (2007). *A practical approach to trauma: Empowering interventions*. Los Angeles: Sage.

Ehlers, A. and Clark, D. M. (2000). A cognitive model of posttraumatic stress disorder. *Behavior Research and Therapy*, 38(3), 319-45.

Fonagi, P., Steele, M., Steele, H., Higgitt, A. and Target, M. (1994). The theory and practice of resilience. *Journal of Child Psychology and Psychiatry*, 35(2), 231-57.

Frommberger, U., Stieglitz, R-D, Straub, S., Nyberg, E., Schlickewel, W., Kuner, E. and Berger, M. (1999). The concept of 'sense of coherence' and the development of posttraumatic stress disorder in traffic accident victims. *Journal of Psychosomatic Research*, 46(4), 343-48.

Good, B. J. (1996). Mental health consequences of displacement and resettlement. *Economic and Political Weekly*, 31(24), 1504-08.

Hobfoll, S. E. (1988). *The ecology of stress*. New York: Hemisphere Publishing Corporation.

———. (2001). The influence of culture, community, and the nested-self in the stress process: Advancing conservation of resource theory. *Applied Psychology: An International Review*, 50(3), 337-421.

Hobfoll, S. E. and Lilly, R. S. (1993). Resource conservation as a strategy for community psychology. *Journal of Community Psychology*, 21(2), 128-48.

Hobfoll, S. E., Schroder, K. E. E., Wells, M. and Malek, M. (2002). Communal versus individualistic construction of sense of mastery in facing life challenges. *Journal of Social and Clinical Psychology*, 21(4), 362-99.

Hofstede, G. (1980). *Culture's consequences: International differences in work-related values*. Beverly Hills, CA: Sage Publications.

Holen, A. (1991). A longitudinal study of the occurrence and persistence of post-traumatic health problems in disaster survivors. *Stress Medicine*, 7(1), 11-17.

Howard, W. T., Loberza, F. R., Pfohl, B. M., Thorne, P. S., Magpantay, R. L. and Woolson, R. F. (1999). Initial results, reliability, and validity of a mental health survey of Mount Pinatubo disaster victims. *The Journal of Nervous and Mental Disease*, 187(11), 661-72.

Ironson, G., Wynings, C., Schneiderman, N., Baum, A., Rodriguez, M., Greenwood, D., Benight, C., Antoni, M., LaPerriere, A., Huang, H., Klimas, N. and Fletcher, M. A. (1997). Posttraumatic stress symptoms, intrusive thoughts, loss, and immune function after Hurricane Andrew. *Psychosomatic Medicine*, 59(2), 128–41.

Kaiser, C. F., Sattler, D. N., Bellack, D. R. and Dersin, J. (1996). A conservation of resources approach to a natural disaster: Sense of coherence and psychological distress. *Journal of Social Behavior and Personality*, 11(3), 459–76.

Kaniasty, K. and Norris, F. (1993). A test of the support deterioration model in the context of natural disaster. *Journal of Personality and Social Psychology*, 64(3), 395–408.

Kaniasty, K. and Norris, F. H. (1995a). In search of altruistic community: Patterns of social support mobilization following Hurricane Hugo. *American Journal of Community Psychology*, 23(4), 447–77.

———. (1995b). Mobilization and deterioration of social support following natural disasters. *Current Directions in Psychological Science*, 4(3), 94–98.

Kapadia, K. M. (1990). *Marriage and family in India* (3rd ed. twelfth impression). Calcutta: Oxford University Press.

Kar, N., Jagadisha, Sharma, P.S.V.N., Murali, M. and Mehrotra, S. (2004). Mental health consequences of the trauma of supercyclone 1999 in Orissa. *Indian Journal of Psychiatry*, 46(3), 228–37.

Kar, N., Mohapatra, P. K., Nayak, K. C., Pattanaik, P., Swain, S. P. and Kar, H. C. (2007). Post-traumatic stress disorder in children and adolescents one year after a super-cyclone in Orissa, India: Exploring cross-cultural validity and vulnerability factors. *BMC Psychiatry*, 7(8), 1–9.

Kessler, R. C., Sonnega, A., Bromet, E., Hughes, M. and Nelson, C. (1995). Posttraumatic stress disorder in the National Comorbidity Survey. *Archives of General Psychiatry*, 52(12), 1048–60.

Kuo, C. J., Tang, H. S., Tsay, C. J., Lin, S. K., Hu, W. H. and Chen, C. C. (2003). Prevalence of psychiatric disorders among bereaved survivors of a disastrous earthquake in Taiwan. *Psychiatric Services*, 54(2), 249–51.

Loughry, M. and Eyber, C. (2003). *Psychosocial concepts in humanitarian work with children*. Washington, DC: The National Academies Press.

Lutgendorf, S. K., Antoni, M. H., Ironson, G., Fletcher, M. A., Penedo, F., Baum, A., Schneiderman, N. and Klimas, N. (1995). Physical symptoms of chronic fatigue syndrome are exacerbated by the stress of Hurricane Andrew. *Psychosomatic Medicine*, 57(4), 310–23.

Mahapatra, L. K. (1999). *Resettlement, impoverishment and reconstruction in India*. New Delhi: Vikas Publishing.

McMillen, J. C., North, C. S. and Smith, E. M. (2000). What parts of PTSD are normal: Intrusion, avoidance or arousal? Data from the Northridge, California earthquake. *Journal of Traumatic Stress*, 13(1), 57–75.

Mehta, K., Vankar, G. and Patel, V. (2005). Validity of the construct of post-traumatic stress disorder in a low-income country: Interview study of women in Gujarat, India. *British Journal of Psychiatry*, 187(6), 585–86.

Mohanty, A. K. (2002). The weaning syndrome: Acquired dependence among super cyclone victims in Orissa. *Psychology and Developing Societies*, 14(2), 261–76.

Morgan, L., Scourfield, J., Williams, D., Jasper, A. and Lewis, G. (2003). The Aberfan disaster: 33-year follow up of survivors. *British Journal of Psychiatry*, 182(1), 532–36.

National Centre for Disaster Management (NDM). (2001). *Manual on natural disaster management in India*. Ministry of Agriculture, New Delhi: Author.

Norris, F. H. (2005). *Range, magnitude and duration of the effects of disasters on mental health: Review update 2005*. Dartmouth College, NCPTSD: RED.

Norris, F. H., Friedman, M. J., Watson, P. J., Byrne, C. M., Diaz, E. and Kaniasty, K. (2002). 60,000 Disaster victims speak: Part-I. An empirical review of the empirical literature, 1981-2001. *Psychiatry*, 65(3) 207–39.

Norris, F. H., Friedman, M. J. and Watson, P. J. (2002). 60,000 Disaster victims speak: Part II. Summary and implications of the disaster mental health research. *Psychiatry*, 65(3), 240–60.

Norris, F.H. and Kaniasty, K. (1996). Received and perceived social support in times of stress: A test of the social support deterioration deterrence model. *Journal of Personality and Social Psychology*, 71(3), 498–511.

Norris, F. H., Murphy, A. Kaniasty, K., Perilla, J. and Ortis, D. C. (2001). Postdisaster social support in the U.S. and Mexico: Conceptual and contextual considerations. *Hispanic Journal of Behavioral Sciences*, 23(4), 469–97.

Norris, F. H., Kaniasty, K., Conrad, M. L., Inman, G. L. and Murphy, A. D. (2002). Placing age differences in cultural context: A comparison of the effects of age on PTSD after disaster in the U.S., Mexico, and Poland. *Journal of Clinical Geropsychology*, 8(3), 153–73.

Norris, F. H., Perilla, J. L., Ibanez, G. E. and Murphy, A. D. (2001). Sex differences in symptoms of posttraumatic stress: Does culture play a role? *Journal of Traumatic Stress*, 14(1), 7–28.

Norris, F. H., Perilla, J. L., Riad, J. K., Kaniasty, K. and Lavizzo, E. A. (1999). Stability and change in stress, resources, and psychological distress following natural disaster: Findings from Hurricane Andrew. *Anxiety, Stress, and Coping*, 12(4), 363–96.

Ohta, Y., Araki, K., Kawasaki, N., Nakane, Y., Honda, S. and Mine, M. (2003). Psychological distress among evacuees of a volcanic eruption in Japan: A follow-up study. *Psychiatry and Clinical Neuroscience*, 57(1), 105–11.

Parasuraman, S. and Unnikrishnan, P. V. (2001). Disaster response in India: An overview. In S. Parasuraman and P. V. Unnikrishnan (Eds), *India disasters report: Towards a policy initiative* (pp. 3–24). New Delhi: Oxford University Press.

Phifer, J. and Norris, F. H. (1989). Psychological symptoms in older adults following disaster: Nature, timing, duration, and course. *Journal of Gerontology*, 44(3), 207–17.

Quarantelli, E. L. (2006). Emergencies, disasters, and catastrophes are different phenomena. Retrieved from http://www.udel.edu/DRC/preliminary/pp304.pdf on 20 October 2008.

Raphael, B. (1986). *When disaster strikes: How individuals and communities cope with catastrophe*. New York: Basic Books.

———. (2000). *Disaster mental health response handbook: An educational resource for mental health professionals involved in disaster management*. Sydney, Australia: NSW Health.

Rotter, J. B. (1966). Generalized expectancies for internal versus external control of reinforcement. *Psychological Monographs*, 80, (609 [Whole]).

Sack, M., Lamprecht, F. and Forschungsaspekte, Z. (1998). Sense of coherence. In W. B. U. Schuffel, R. K. V. Johnen, F. Lamprecht and U. Schnyder (Eds), *Handbuch der Salutogenese* (pp. 325–36). Wiesbaden: Ullstein.

Salcioglu, E., Basoglu, M. and Livanou, M. (2003). Long-term psychological outcome for non-treatment-seeking earthquake survivors in Turkey. *Journal of Nervous and Mental Disease*, 191(3), 154–60.

Sattler, D. N., Preston, A., Kaiser, C. F., Olivera, V. E., Valdez, J. and Schlueter, S. (2002). Hurricane Georges: A cross-national study examining preparedness, resource loss, and psychological distress in the U. S. Virgin Islands, Puerto Rico, Dominican Republic, and the United States. *Journal of Traumatic Stress*, 15(5), 339–50.

Sharan, P., Chaudhary, G., Kavathekar, S. A. and Saxena, S. (1996). Preliminary report of psychiatric disorders in survivors of a severe earthquake. *American Journal of Psychiatry*, 153(4), 556–58.

Shinfuku, N. (1999). To be a victim and a survivor of the Great Hanshin Awaji Earthquake. *Journal of Psychosomatic Research*, 46(6), 541–48

Srinivas, M. N. (1996). *Village, caste, gender and method: Essays in Indian social anthropology* (1st ed. second impression). New Delhi: Oxford University Press.

Suar, D. (2004). Disaster and emotion. *Psychological Studies*, 49(2 and 3), 177–84.

———. (2007). *Concept paper on disaster management*. New Delhi: Report submitted to DIPR.

Suar, D. and Kar, S. (2005). Social and behavioural consequences of Orissa supercyclone. *Journal of Health Management*, 7(2), 263–75.

Suar, D. and Khuntia, R. (2004). Caste, education, family and stress disorders in Orissa supercyclone. *Psychology and Developing Societies*, 16(1), 77–91.

Suar, D., Das, N., Hota, L. B. and Prasad, H. C. S. (2008). Do age and gender influence psychological distress? Evidence from two disasters. *Psychological Studies*, 53(2 &3), 226–32.

Suar, D., Mandal, M. K. and Khuntia, R. (2002). Supercyclone in Orissa: An assessment of psychological status of survivors. *Journal of Traumatic Stress*, 15(4), 313–19.

Suar, D., Mishra, S. and Khuntia, R. (2007). Placing age difference in the context of Orissa supercyclone: Who experiences psychological distress? *Asian Journal of Social Psychology*, 10(2), 117–22.

Tanida, N. (1996). What happened to elderly people in the great Hanshin Earthquake. *BMJ*, 313(2), 1133-35.
Ticehurst, S., Webster, R. A., Carr, V. J. and Lewin, T. J. (1996). The psychological impact of an earthquake on the elderly. *International Journal of Geriatric Psychiatry*, 11(11), 943-51.
Tolin, D. F. and Foa, E. B. (2002). Gender and PTSD: A cognitive model. In R. Kimerling, P. Ouimette and J. Wolfe (Eds), *Gender and PTSD* (pp. 76-97). New York: Guilford Press.
Triandis, H. C. (1996). The psychological measurement of cultural syndromes. *American Psychologist*, 51(4), 407-15.
Wells, J. D., Hobfoll, S. E. and Lavin, J. (1999). When it rains, it pours: The greater impact of resource loss compared to gain on psychological distress. *Personality and Social Psychology Bulletin*, 25(9), 1172-82.
Wheaton, B. (1982). A comparison of the moderating effects of personal coping resources on the impact of exposure to stress in two groups. *Journal of Community Psychology*, 10(3), 293-311.
Yang, Y. K., Yeh, T. L., Chen, C. C., Lee, C. K., Lee, I. H., Lee, L. C. and Jeffries, K. J. (2003). Psychiatric morbidity and posttraumatic symptoms among earthquake victims in primary care clinics. *General Hospital Psychiatry*, 25(4), 253-61.

About the Editors and Contributors

Editors

Ajit K. Dalal is Professor of Psychology at the University of Allahabad, India. He has obtained his doctoral degree from the Indian Institute of Technology, Kanpur, India, and has published widely in the areas of causal attribution, school education and health psychology. He received the Fulbright Senior Fellow at the University of California, Los Angeles, USA. He also received UGC Career Award and ICSSR Senior Fellowship. He was a visiting faculty at the Queen's University, Canada; National Institute of Health and Family Welfare, New Delhi, India and Indian Institute of Management, Ahmedabad, India. He has published about 70 research articles and book chapters, in addition to eight books, including *Attribution Theory and Research*, *New Directions in Indian Psychology (Vol.1)* (with G. Misra), *Social Dimensions of Health* (with S. Ray) and *Handbook of Indian Psychology* (with K.R. Rao and A. Paranjpe). He has conducted several evaluation studies of NGOs working with communities in the disability sector. Presently, he is the editor of *Psychology and Developing Societies*.

Girishwar Misra is Professor of Psychology at University of Delhi, India. During an academic career spanning over four decades, he has taught at Deen Dayal Upadhyay Gorakhpur University, University of Allahabad and Barkatullah University, Bhopal, all based in India. He has been a Senior Fulbright Fellow at Swarthmore College, Philadelphia, and University of Michigan, USA; visiting professor at the Ruhr University of Bochum, Germany, and an ESRC Fellow at Sussex University, UK. His teaching and research interests include social psychology, human development, cultural processes and psychological knowledge. He has published widely on deprivation, self-processes, emotions and well-being. He has been Convener and President of the National Academy of Psychology, India, and National Fellow of the Indian Council of Social Science Research (ICSSR), India. He has authored and edited *Psychological Consequences of Prolonged Deprivation* (with L.B. Tripathi), *Deprivation: Its Social*

Roots and Psychological Consequences (with D. Sinha and R.C. Tripathi), *Perspectives on Indigenous Psychology* (with A.K. Mohanty), *Psychological Perspectives on Health and Stress, Psychology of Poverty and Social Disadvantage* (with A.K. Mohanty), *Applied Social Psychology in India, New Directions in Indian Psychology, Vol. 1: Social Psychology* (with A.K. Dalal), *Towards a Culturally Relevant Psychology* (with J. Prakash), *Rethinking Intelligence* (with A.K. Srivastava), *Psychology and Societal Development: Paradigmatic and Social Concerns, Psychology in India: Advances in Research* and *Handbook of Psychology in India*. He is editor of *Psychological Studies*.

Contributors

Jyoti Anand is a practising counsellor and a freelance researcher. She has a PhD from Awadhesh Pratap Singh University, Rewa, Madhya Pradesh, India and has done work in the area of healing and suffering. She has published her work in the areas of spiritual and emotional healing. She has authored a book, *Healing Narratives of Women: A Psychological Perspective*.

Shalini Bharat is Professor at the Tata Institute of Social Sciences, Mumbai, India. Having a PhD in psychology from the University of Allahabad, she is engaged in applied and interdisciplinary research on diverse aspects of the family. Some of her recent work focuses on adoptive families; women, work and family and familial and social dimensions of HIV/AIDS. Her publications include *Family Measurement in India, Child Adoption: Trends and Emerging Issues, and Research on Families with Problems in India*. She was a member of the Editorial Board of the *Indian Psychological Abstracts and Reviews*.

Sudhir Kakar, a practising psychoanalyst based in Goa, India, was trained at Sigmund Freud Institute in Frankfurt, Germany. He has taught at several universities in India, USA and Europe. His many honours include the Boyer Prize for Psychological Anthropology of the American Anthropological Association; the Bhabha, Nehru, and ICSSR National fellowships as well as fellowships at the Institutes for Advanced Study in Princeton (USA) and Berlin (Germany). Some of his important publications are: *The Inner World, Shamans, Mystics and Doctors, The Colors of Violence, Culture and Psyche, The portraits of Indians, The Analyst and the Mystic, The Indians* and *Mad and Divine*.

About the Editors and Contributors

R.L. Kapur was Emeritus Professor at the National Institute of Advanced Studies, Shimla, India, and was a Fellow at the Royal College of Psychiatrists, London, UK; the Indian Academy of Sciences, Bangalore, India; and the National Academy of Medical Sciences, New Delhi, India. Subsequently, he had worked as Professor of Psychiatry at the Kasturba Medical College, Manipal, India, and was Professor of Community Psychiatry and the Head of the Department of Psychiatry at the National Institute of Mental Health and Neuro Sciences (NIMHANS), Bangalore, India. He has been a consultant to World Health Organization. He was awarded the Hari Om Ashram Medical Council of India Award, D.L.N. Murthy Rao Oration Award and Eminent Psychiatrist Award. He was on the Editorial Board of *Transcultural Psychiatric Research Review* of the McGill University, Montreal, Canada, and *Culture, Medicine and Psychiatry* published from the Harvard University, USA. His books include: *The Twice Born* (co-author), *The Great Universe of Kota* (co-author), *Cross-cultural Psychiatry*, *Psychological Basis of Creativity* and *Contributions of Indian Philosophical Traditions to the Study of Psychology*.

Lina Kashyap, Professor and Chairperson of the Centre for Disability Studies and Action, School of Social Work, Tata Institute of Social Sciences, Mumbai, India. She has published in the areas of social work with children, families and persons with disability—policies, programmes and interventions and ethical issues. She has conducted several training programmes for family counsellors in the field of persons with disabilities. She was awarded the 2005–06 Rotary Foundation Ambassadorial Grant for Visiting Professor.

A. Kiranmayi received her PhD in Psychology in 1999. She has worked in Ali Yavar Jung National Institute for the Hearing Handicapped (AYJNIHH), Secunderabad, India, as psychologist, as a HR in a software company, and has taught soft skills for M.S. Students in St. Ann's College for Women, Hyderabad, India. Since 2004 she has started independent practice, focusing on personal counselling and supporting and guiding parents of children with autism and other special needs.

David J. Lam was associated with the Department of Psychology, University of Hong-Kong, Hong-Kong. Recently, he has shifted to Honolulu, Hawaii, where he has established a clinical and consultancy service. His research interests include stress and clinical psychology.

Radha Krishna Naidu has a PhD from the University of Allahabad, India, where he is currently Professor of Psychology. Prior to this, he was at Pandit Ravishankar Shukla University, Raipur, India. He served as the convener of National Academy of Psychology (India), 1991–1993, and was a Fulbright Scholar at the Institute of Social Research, University of Michigan, USA in 1981. He was initially interested in the study of stress and coping, but later shifted his focus to indigenous concepts, and initiated survey investigations of detachment, an indigenous transpersonal concept, as a moderator of the stress–strain relationship.

M. N. Palsane has retired as Professor of Psychology at the University of Pune, India. He has worked extensively in the areas of stress and coping, traditional Indian perspectives, Yoga as psychotherapy and environmental psychology. He has been convener of the UGC programme on the production of video lectures in psychology. He has edited a volume on applied psychology in Marathi. He is Fellow at the National Academy of Psychology, India.

Namita Pande is Professor of Psychology at University of Allahabad, India. Her areas of research interest are mediators of stress and well being, self processes and indigenous psychology. She has published in the areas of detachment, disability attitudes and visual imagery. She is the co-author of *Mind Matters*, a volume related to rehabilitation of the disabled people.

Alok Pandey, MD Psychiatry, is pursuing spiritual therapy at Sri Aurobindo Ashrama, Pondicherry, India. He has written extensively in the areas of spiritual health, self and consciousness and integral Yoga psychology of Shri Aurobindo. Presently he is the editor of the journal *Namah: New Approaches to Medicine and Health*. He has authored a book, *Death, Dying and Beyond*.

Satwant Pasricha is a Professor of Clinical Psychology at the NIMHANS, Bangalore, India. For the past over three decades, she has been engaged in the scientific investigation of cases of the reincarnation type, near-death experiences and other paranormal experiences that contribute to the evidence for survival of personality (or mind) beyond bodily death. She has published extensively in the national and international, peer-reviewed journals of psychology, psychiatry, parapsychology and scientific exploration. She has authored books such as *Claims of Reincarnation: An empirical study of cases in India* (1990, 2006; also published in Japanese) and *Can* the Mind Survive Beyond Death? In pursuit of scientific evidence (2 Volumes; 2008). She is a recipient of several prestigious national and international awards and honours.

Namita Ranganathan is Senior Reader in the Department of Education, University of Delhi, India. She has specialized in Educational Psychology and teaches courses and guides research in child and adolescent development, personality, guidance, counselling and mental health. She also works on the psychology of gender. She is involved in action research with schools aimed at building up a mental health perspective in schools, particularly with teachers. She is also engaged in research in collaboration with the development sector in relation to girls' education, empowerment and mobility.

Sagar Sharma is former Professor and Chairman, Department of Psychology at Himachal Pradesh University, Shimla, India. After retirement, he has been associated with Punjab University, Chandigarh, India, as UGC Emeritus Fellow. He has been Fellow at East-West Center, Hawaii, and Visiting Professor at University of South Florida, Tampa, USA; State University at Buffalo, New York, USA; and University of Bergen, Norway. He was a UGC National Lecturer and participated in the Indo-Hungarian and Indo-Portuguese cultural exchange programmes. His contributions have been in the areas of stress, anxiety and health-psychology. He is a Fellow of the National Academy of Psychology, India.

Amar Kumar Singh was Professor and Head, Department of Psychology, Ranchi University, Ranchi, India. He was the Honourary Editor of *Social Change*. Dr Singh was formerly a Fellow at Harvard University, USA. His main research interests included modernization and social change, national integration and secularism, health and population education.

Arvind Sinha has a PhD in organizational behaviour area. He has published as many as 40 articles and about as many conference papers. He has mainly worked in the area of organizational behaviour and social psychology. He has served on several academic and administrative positions as well. Currently, he is Professor of Psychology at the Department of Humanities and Social Sciences, Indian Institute of Technology, Kanpur, India.

Durganand Sinha was the founding Head and Professor of Psychology, Department of Psychology at the University of Allahabad, India. He has been the President of the International Association for Cross-cultural Psychology as well as its Fellow. He has published extensively on psychological dimensions of poverty and deprivation, cross-cultural psychology and indigenization in psychology. His publications include *Indian Villages in Transition: A Motivational Analysis, Motivation and Rural Development: The Mughal Syndrome, Psychology in a Third World Country: The Indian Experience, Social Values and Development: Asian Perspectives* and *Effective Organisations and Social Values*.

R. Srinivasa Murthy was Professor and Head of the Department of Psychiatry, NIMHANS, Bangalore. He was MD in psychiatry from Postgraduate Institute of Medical Education and Research (PGI), Chandigarh, India. He has published extensively in national and international journals (over 200 publications). He functioned as Editor-in-Chief of the *World Health Report 2001* which focused on mental health. He assisted in the development of national programmes of mental health in many developing countries (Bhutan, Iran, Kuwait, Myanmar, Nepal, Pakistan, Sri Lanka and Yemen). His field of interest was community mental health.

Ashok K. Srivastava, PhD, is Professor in Educational Psychology at National Council of Educational Research and Training (NCERT), New Delhi. After earning a PhD in Psychology from Utkal University, Bhubaneswar, India, he taught at North Eastern Hill University, Shillong, India. During his academic career spanning over two decades, he has been associated with designing courses and training teaching educators. His research interests include development of values, creativity and intelligence. He has authored or edited *Conflicts and their Resolutions, Readings on Child and Adolescent Psychology* and *Child Development: The Indian Perspective* and *Rethinking Intelligence*.

Sweta Srivastava is PhD from the Indian Institute of Technology Kanpur, India. Currently, she is a faculty in organizational behaviour area at Indian Institute of Foreign Trade (IIFT), New Delhi. Her areas of interest include stress and well-being in organizations.

Damodar Suar, PhD, is a Professor at the Indian Institute of Technology, Kharagpur, India. He is Associate Editor of *Psychological Studies*. He has done research on social issues, and also has run many research/consultancy projects and training programmes. His areas of interest include leadership, laterality, human values, stress and environmental behaviour. Apart from journal articles, he has authored and and edited *Psychological Aspects of Polarisation Phenomenon and Management through Interpersonal Relationships* (co-editor), *Psychology Matters: Development, Health and Organization* (co-editor), and *Time in Indian Culture: Diverse Perspectives* (co-editor).

V. Vijayalakshmi, PhD, is Faculty-Counsellor in Indian Business School (IBS), Hyderabad. Her areas of interest are health psychology, counselling, child psychology and psychometric testing. She has written articles related to soft skills and counselling. She has conducted 'Faculty Development Programmes' at IBS and 'Management Development Programmes' for government organizations. She has conducted workshops on stress management and prepared handbooks and brochures on counselling. She was a recipient of the Durganand Sinha Research Award presented at the 12th Annual Conference of the National Academy of Psychology, 2000.

U. Vindhya is currently Professor of Psychology, Tata Institute of Social Sciences, Mumbai. Earlier she was with Andhra University, Visakhapatnam, India, and the Centre for Economic and Social Studies, Hyderabad, India. Her research concerns are located in the interface of psychology and feminism and include mental health of women, domestic violence, the psychological dynamics of women's political activism and the linkages between reproductive health and psychological well-being. She has edited *Psychology in India: Intersecting Crossroads* (2003) and co-edited *Handbook of International Feminisms: Perspectives on Psychology, Women, Culture and Rights* (2011). She has published widely in national and international journals. She was the recipient of the South Asian Visiting Scholarship at University of Oxford, UK, and the Fulbright Visiting Lecturership.

Index

abnormal behaviour, 59
accessibility, 206
Acquired immune deficiency syndrome (AIDS), 355-56, 409
    association with moral denigration and lifestyles, 411
    metaphoric use of language, 411
    scenario in India, 412-13
    social dimensions of, 412
    study in Mumbai
        findings of, 415-24
        methodology of, 414-15
        observations of, 424-25
        research setting and socio-cultural context, 413-14
    Thailand, in, 411
ActionAid India, 456
adjustment, 97
adolescence
    as age of challenge and potential, 141-42
    disaster trauma, response after, 437
adulthood, 207
adversity. *See* Suffering
affordability, 206
Akbar Allahabadi, 358
alchemical transformation, of self, 224. *See also* Healing
Allahabad University, 304
Alma Ata Declaration, 34, 57
American Social Indicator. *See* Happiness
Analects, 87
anasakti
    action, 289

    behavioural referents of, 290-91
    Bhagavadgita, in, 289
    computation of, 295-96
    features of, 286
    meaning of, 286
    measurement of, 291-92
    and mental health, 292-94
    multiple regression analysis, 298
    perception of distress and strain, 299-301
    predictor of strain, 301-2
    spiritual lore, in, 298
ancient Vedic texts, 2
anger proneness. *See* Trait anger (T-anger)
anger suppression, 391-92
anti-professional feelings, 61
anti-psychiatry movement, 61
anxiety, xi
Apsara syndrome, 2
Arya Samaj, 215
Asanas, 252
ashtanga, 252
Atharvaveda, 2
average distress rating (ADR), 295
    multiple regression analysis, 298
average person, 329
Ayurveda, xi
    emphasis on *samatva*, xii
    indigenous model of health and well-being, 15-19

belief(s)
    rebirth and *karma* principle, in (*see* Suffering, mediators of)
    types of, 312

Bhagavadgita, 18, 84, 104, 258
   anasakti (*see* Anasakti)
   task excellence (*see* Task excellence)
bhakti yoga, 92
bhäva, 233
Bhopal gas tragedy, 430
Bhore Committee Report (1946), 3, 34
Bihar, Madhya Pradesh, Rajasthan and Uttar Pradesh (BIMARU), 35
Biomedical model of health care, 9-10
birth, 81
blindness, 181. See also Disability, categories of
blood pressure (BP), 389
body immune system
   stress and (*see* Stress and body immune system)
brahmcharya, 136
breast development, of urban adolescent girls, 145-46
Buddhism, 54
   method of meditation, 267

Carakasamhita, 84, 95
cardiovascular disorders (CVD), 389
CARE, 456
causal belief, reported by patients, 309-10
Centre for Research on the Epidemiology of Disasters (CRED), 431
Charaka Samhita, 15
Chernobyl nuclear explosion, 430
chronic diseases, 135
   coping with, 28-30
   illness beliefs and psychological adjustment, 312-13
   interview with hospital patients, 308
   symptoms of, 305
   treatment decisions and affective reactions, 310-11

cognitive adaptation theory, 90
Cognitive theory, 452
Community Health Workers (CHWs), 34
competence
   aspects of, 105
   West, in, 105
Conservation of resources (COR) theory, 452-54
coping
   Asian perspectives of, 77
   modern concepts of, 80-81
   urban adolescent girls, of, 150-51
   Western literature, in, 91
coronary heart disease (CHD), xi
Corticotrophine-releasing Factor (CRF), 64
counsellor-client relationship, in Indian thought, 276-78
criminal, 59
culture and health, 40

Dalai Lama, 111, 234
deafness, 181. See also Disability, categories of
depression, 160
desires, 84
detachment. See Suffering, mediators of
devotional surrender, 213
Dharana, 253
Dharma. See Suffering, mediators of
Dhyana, 253
diabetes, xi
Disability Adjusted Life Years (DALY), 155
disability(ies)
   categories of, 181
   meaning of, 180
disabled person
   implications for
      social policy, 192-95
      social work practice, 192-95
      teaching, 192-95

research on family members
coping strategies, of family members, 190-91
effect on family, of disabled individual presence, 183-87
influencing factors within family, 187-90
professional intervention, for helping families to cope, 191-92
disaster management cycle, 456
disaster(s)
India, in
potential victim, 430-35
intervention programme
impact phase (see Impact phase)
during phase, 457-58
post-disaster phase, 459-60
pre-disaster phase, 460-61
origin of, 429
psychosocial interventions, at various phases of, 462
disaster trauma, 435-36
categories of
members of community, 436
mentally disturbed persons, 436
primary victims, 436
researchers and clinicians, 436
secondary victims, 436
tertiary victims, 436
children responses, after trauma, 437
family context
lager family, 447
marriage life, stress on, 447-48
multiple symptoms of, 436
normal traumatic reactions to, 439
resource context, 448-51
risk and protective factor, 441
severity of exposure, 441
socio-demographic characteristics
age, 443-44
caste status, 445

gender, 442-43
physically, mentally and developmentally challenged, 446-47
socioeconomic status, 445-46
theories of
cognitive theory (see Cognitive theory)
conservation of resources (COR) theory (see Conservation of resources [COR] theory)
impoverishment risk theory (see Impoverishment risk theory)
social support deterioration-deterrence model (see Social support deterioration-deterrence model)
dukha, 53. See also Suffering
dysthymia, 160

education
and happiness, 125
emotional pain, 207. See also Healing
experience of, 236-38
isolation from contemporary events, 232
meaning of, 232
as natural consequence of living, 232
emotional vital signs (EVS), 390
equalitarianism, 363
equanimity, 124-25
extraversion, 114. See also Happy people

faith, 279
family-centred programmes, for disabled persons, 193
forgiveness, 233

Gandharva syndrome, 2
gender differences, patterns of, 160
general adaptation syndrome, 13

Index • 479

Gita, 70
  integral thought of, 267-69
good health, 99
grihastha, 136
groups, sources of change in, 335-36
growth. See Health, domains of
Growth Chart, Oral Re-hydration, Breast Feeding, Immunization, Food Supplement and Family Planning (GOBI-FF), 384
Guru(s)
  ambience of affective acceptance, 225
  dangers of self-fragmentation, awareness about, 225
  dominant image, in Hindu tradition, 212
  as healer, 211
  healing techniques of, 227
  importance of healing, 215
  Jnaneshvara views on, 214
  Satyanand views on, 221
  Upanishadic (see Upanishadic guru)

handicap, 180-81
happiness, 333, 335-36. See also Subjective well-being (SWB)
  Bhutan government, 109
  complementarity in, 123-24
  construal of, 117-19
  and education (see Education and happiness)
  enhancement of, 118
  experience of, 110
  importance of, 109
  Indian view of, 120-22
  meaning of, 111-13
  measurement of, 338
  quality of equanimity, importance of, 124
  relational nature of, 122-23
  research in West, 113-14
  stable trait, 119-20
  as state of mind, 110
  wealth and (see Wealth and happiness)
happy, 114
  comparison between unhappy people and, 119
happy people, characteristics of, 114
healer
  Guru as (see Guru, as healer)
healing
  alchemical transformation, 224
  forgiveness (see Forgiveness)
  India, in, 36, 205
    Kohut theory (see Kohut theory)
    supportive-suggestive processes, 206
  narratives
    analysis and interpretation, 236
    closing of emotions, 241-42
    emotional pain experience, 236-38
    method of, 235-36
    reclamation of self, in depression, 238-41
    release of emotions, 244-46
    sublimation of emotional self, 242-44
  psychoanalytic view of, 220
  at social and spiritual planes, 205
health, 1
  Ayurveda (see Ayurveda)
  definition of, 100
  domains of, 21
  Indian perspective on, 49
  pathway for attaining, all life goals, 49
  promotion of, 31-33
  psychological factors shaping
    cognitive and attitudinal factors in recovery, 23-24
    health beliefs and affective reactions, 24-26

health impairing behaviours
    and lifestyle changes, 26-28
individual dispositions and
    temperament, 22-23
schematic model, 19-20
and well-being, 8
WHO definition of, 7, 57
health beliefs shares, research focusing on, 30
health education, for mothers, 355
Health for All by 2000, 33, 37
health modernity, 357
    education, 382-84
        content of, 384
    importance of, 365-67
    omission of, 365
    political modernity, determination by, 367
    profile of, 372
    survey of, 373
Health modernity scale (HMS), 370-71
health psychology
    beginnings of, 2-4
    changing scenario if, 5-6
    social support system (see Social support system)
health scenario, in India, 33-35
health status, in India, 373-82
HIV infection, 412
Homeostasis, 101-2
human activity, aim of, 109
human immunodeficiency virus (HIV), 12
humanity, 88
human lifespan, stages of, 136
hypertension (HT), 355
    patients diagnosis with, 392
    unemployment or lowered occupational status, impact of, 389
hypertensive patients, 391-93
    vs. normotensive controls, 395-97

impact phase
    meaning of, 456
    victims reactions, 457
impairment, 180
Impoverishment risk theory, 455
impulse control. See Suffering, mediators of
Indian Council for Social Science Research (ICSSR), xiii, 33
Indian Council of Medical Research (ICMR), 34, 382-83
individualism, xi
individual lives, study of, 136
industrialization, 359
infant mortality differentials, in India, 381
inner differentiation, 206
inner-directedness, xii
inner purification, 209
    ideal of, 264-66
inner technology. See *Tantra* tradition
intense self-object experience, 224
intervention programme, primary goal of, 181
intimacy, 225-26
involuntary mental mechanisms, 12
Islamic tradition, sufferings in, 81

jnana yoga, 92

kapha. See *Tridoshas*
karma yoga, 92
Kohutian psychology, 218
Kohut theory, 207

leprosy, 410
level of living, components of, 106
liberation, 246
life crises, 332
life events stress scale (LESS), 393
life satisfaction, meaning of, 331-32
live, ways of, 223

Mahatma Gandhi, 111, 123, 359-60
maintenance. *See* Health, domains of
maladjustment, 97
manomayakosha, 299
mantra, 37
materialism, xi
mayavadin, 260
meditation, techniques of, 267
menstruation, 145-46
mental disorders, women, in, 155
mental handicap, 181. *See also* Disability, categories of
  attention from family members, 182
mental health, 57, 59-65
  Alma Ata Declaration (*see* Alma Ata Declaration)
  anasakti and (*see anasakti* and mental health)
  Indian view of, 68-71
  prevention and promotion of, 65-66
  primary health care (*see* Primary health care)
  programme development, 71-73
  scope of, 58-59
mental-hygiene movement, 60
mental illness(es), 3, 59-65, 73
  women and, 158-63
metaphysical beliefs
  cultural differences in, 307
  traditional Indian society, in, 307
modernity
  characteristics of, 364-65
  commitment of, 354
  correlates of, 359-60
  definition of, 365
  dimensions and themes of, 368-69
  foundations of, 354
  health (*see* Health modernity)
  and Indian society, 361-62
  reigning ideology of, xi
  relation to time, 357

sankritization and, 362-63
scientific rationalism, acceptance of, 358
social science scholarship, in, 354
social science usages of, 360-61
Westernization and, 362-63
Westernization of styles and manners, 357
Modernization, meaning of, 363
moha, 2
Mother Teresa, 30
multi-disciplinary team approach, 180

National AIDS Control Organisation (NACO), 413
National Health Policy, 33-34
National Institute of Mental Health and Neuro Sciences (NIMHANS), 319, 456
National Institute of Mental Health (NIMH), 159-60
National Institute of Visual Handicap, 182
National Mental Health Programme (NMHP), 161, 163
natural disasters, 430-31, 434
Near-death experiences (NDEs), 286-87
  systematic survey in Channapatna
    material and methods, 319-21
    result of, 321-25
Nidan parivarjana, 51
Niyamas, 252
normalization principle, 180

obesity, xi
obsessive-compulsive disorder, 160
optimism, 114
orthopaedic handicap, 181. *See also* Disability, categories of
out-of-the-body-experience (OBE), 325
Oxfam India, 456

panchakosha, 298
Patanjali. *See also* Yoga
  meaning of, 249
phobias, 160
pitta. See Tridoshas
positive health, Indian tradition emphasis on, xi
positive mental health, 329
positive psychology, 329
post-disaster trauma, research on difficulties, 429-30
Post-traumatic stress disorder (PTSD), 356, 437-38
Prakriti, 250-51
Pratyahara, 252
Prauayama, 252
primary health care, importance of, 58
primary health centres (PHC), 9
psychiatrist, advantage in developing countries, 73
psychic consciousness, 272
psychoanalysis, 219
psychological adjustment(s), 97
  homeostatic phenomena, 102
psychological disorders, 137
psychological recovery, linkages between physical and, 313
psychological state, influence on person health, 2
psychological stress, 3-4
psychological suffering, negative vedantin solution to, 260-64
Psychological well-being (PWB), 331-32
Psychologists, role of, 4
psycho-social well-being, 95
psychotherapy
  categories of, 259-60
  goal of, 210, 278
  Indian thought, of
    grand synthesis, 271-74
    harmony of body and mind, 266-67

  inner purification, ideal of, 264-66
puberty, 137, 141
  urban adolescent girls, experience of, 144-45

quality of life, 106

Ramakrishna Mission, 215
recovery belief, reported by patients, 309-10
rehabilitation, meaning of, 181
research, emerging issues for
  culture and health, 40
  efficacy of psychological interventions, 37
  healing practices, 36-37
  health status, enhancement of, 37-38
  mapping of meaning of health and illness, 38-39
  rethinking well-being, 39
  stress research, 36
resilience, 331
  definition of, 332
  measurement of, 338-39
restoration. *See* Health, domains of

sacred, 206
Sai Baba, 225-26
Samadhi, 253
Samkhya, 250
Samsamana, 51
Samsodhan, 50
sanyas, 136
satisfaction, 55
  enhancement of, 118
  meaning of, 111-13
second birth, 218
secularisation, 363
self-actualization, 107
self-aggrandizement, xii
self-esteem, 114, 336
  individual assessments of, 334

meaning of, 333-34 (*see also* Happy people)
susceptible to, situational influences, 334
self-generated pain, 83
self-transcendence, xiii
self-transformation process, 208
Sense of coherence (SOC), 450
sense of personal mastery, 114. See also Happy people
sexual aberrations, 230
sexuality, 137
urban adolescent girls, of, 150-51
Sexually Transmitted Disease (STD), 412
Siddha, 33
silent killer, 389
simple stress score (SSS), 295
Social support deterioration-deterrence model, 454
Social support system
health psychology, in, 30
mechanisms of, 31
spiritual healing, 207
spirituality, xii
Western behavioural science, in, 5
spiritual life, 68
Sri Aurobindo, 209, 271-73, 281
state of mind
yoga and (*see* Yoga and state of mind)
State-Trait anger expression inventory (STAXI), 393
State-Trait anxiety inventory (STAI), 394
strain scores
computation of, 295-96
difference between means of stress and, 297
stress, xi, 285. See also Anasakti
Asian perspectives of, 77
and body immune system, 11-13
computation of, 295-96

contextual differences in study of, 78-80
and health paradigm, 11
modern concepts of, 80-81
research on, 36
stress-free life, 53
stressful life events, 13-15
subjective mental states, yoga effects on, 256-58
subjective well-being (SWB), 8, 33
components of, 331
meaning of, 111-13
suffering, 53
Asian thought, in, 81-83
causes of, 83-87
consequences of, 87-88
mediators of, 88-93
sukhaswarup, 101
surrender
to master, 222
of self, 222
svadharma, 258
Swami Satyanand Saraswathi, 221
swastha, 50

Taittiriya Upnishad, 8
tamas, 8
tantra tradition, 205
path of, 269-71
Taoism, 92
task excellence, 290
technological disaster, 431
terrestrial divine perfection, 274-76
T-group learning method, 331, 334-35
Three Mile Island accident, 430
total detachment, action, in, 87
tradition. See Modernity
Trait anger (T-anger), 390
Trance onset, 63
physiologic signs of, 64
transcendence. See Suffering, mediators of

transformational object, 224
Tridoshas, 50. See also Ayurveda
Type A Personality, 3

Unani-Tibb, 33
unhappiness, complementarity in, 123-24
unhappy people, 119
UNICEF, 366, 384
University Grants Commission, 194
Upanishadic era, 212
Upanishadic guru, 212
urban adolescent girls
    analysis of experience
        bodily changes and allied feelings, 147-48
        breast development and menstruation, 145-46
        experience of puberty, 144-45
        home, school and peer-related experiences, 148-50
        sexuality and coping, 150-51
urbanization, 3959

vanprastha, 136
vata. See Tridoshas

wealth and happiness, 115-17
Weighted stress score (WSS), 295
    multiple regression analysis, 298
welfare, 96
well-being, 1, 331-32
    all economic growth contribution to, 116
    Ayurveda (*see* Ayurveda)
    economic growth, impact of, 117
    health and (*see* Health and well-being)
    meaning of, 96
    neutral economic growth, 117
    promotion of, 31-33

psychological factors shaping
    cognitive and attitudinal factors in recovery, 23-24
    health beliefs and affective reactions, 24-26
    health impairing behaviours and lifestyle changes, 26-28
    individual dispositions and temperament, 22-23
    psychological growth, of individual, 99
    schematic model, 19-20
West
    happiness research in (*see* Happiness, research in West)
Western behavioural science, 5
Western psychiatrists, focus of, 219
woman disease. See Acquired Immune Deficiency Syndrome (AIDS)
women
    mental disorders in (*see* Mental disorders, in women)
    and mental illness (*see* Mental illness, women and)
World Health Organization (WHO), 65, 304
    definiton of health (*see* Health, WHO definition of)
    Health for All by 29000, 33

Yajurveda, 2
Yamas, 252
Yoga, xi. *See also* Samkhya
    definition of, 208
    emphasis on *samatva*, xii
    and state of mind, 208
        of cosmic and psychological reality, 250-53
        subjective mental states, effect of, 256-58